POCKETBOOK OF

Differential Diagnosis

T0195476

Differential Diagnosis

Thomas A. Slater MRes, MBBS, MRCP, AFHEA
Speciality Registrar in Cardiology
Leeds, West Yorkshire, UK

Mohammed Abdul Waduud BSc, MBChB,
MSc, MRCS, PgCert (Health Res), AFHEA, RCPathME
Clinical Research Training Fellow and Speciality Registrar in Vascular
Surgery
Leeds, West Yorkshire, UK

Nadeem Ahmed BSc, MSc, MBChB, MRCGP, MPH,
RCPathME, PGCHE, FHEA
General Practitioner
Birmingham, West Midlands, UK

FIFTH EDITION

ELSEVIER

International ISBN: 9780702077784

Library of Congress Control Number: 2021933289

Content Strategist: Jeremy Bowes
Content Development Specialist: Andrae Akeh
Project Manager: Beula Christopher
Design: Margaret Reid
Illustration Manager: Anitha Rajarathnam
Marketing Manager: Deborah Watkins

Printed in Scotland

Last digit is the print number: 9 8 7 6 5 4 3 2

Working together
to grow libraries in
developing countries

www.elsevier.com • www.bookaid.org

We are grateful to the publishers, Elsevier, for the opportunity to produce the fifth edition of the *Pocketbook of Differential Diagnosis*. This edition sees a change in authorship from our previous authors ATR, EL and AJKO to a new team as they hand down the reins. The text has been updated with modern medical terminology, new differential diagnoses and updated end-of-chapter hazard comments in line with current research and general guidance. The colour coding continues in this edition, as this has worked very well previously but now with the added depth of highlighting particular diagnoses that are life threatening and need serious consideration by a hazard symbol. We have also taken into account suggested additions and corrections in this new edition and updated the frequency of some conditions. We have also continued with the theme of history, examination and investigations, as we want the reader to be able to quickly navigate between these common presenting complaints rather than the management. Moreover, management varies between countries and even between clinicians. Finally, we encourage feedback from readers for ideas they would like to see in future editions.

Medicine has moved at a considerable pace from traditional lectures, self-directed problem-based learning, to small group work and seminars, and having a book which offers a quick didactic approach offers merits. This is the book to use in the wards, in clinics and even in primary care settings. We would like to broaden the scope of this book, which has relevance to advanced nurse practitioners, paramedics, physician associates and beyond.

NB – At the time of writing this book the world was in the grip of the COVID-19 pandemic, which resulted in high fatalities across the globe. We dedicate this book to the health care teams and services across the world.

Andrew T. Raffety, Sheffield
Eric Lim, London
Andrew J. K. Ostor, Cambridge
Thomas A. Slater, Leeds
Mohammed A. Waduud, Leeds
Nadeem Ahmed, Birmingham
2020

We are grateful to Elsevier and in particular to Jeremey Bowes (Content Strategist) as well as Andrae Akeh (Content Development Specialist) for their support with this project. We wish to thank all those who have contributed to the successive editions of this book. We would especially like to thank the previous lead author, Mr Andrew Raftery, for his guidance and wish him very well in retirement. We would also like to thank our junior staff and medical students who have suggested corrections, amendments and improvements to the book. We do our best to mitigate errors but maintain responsibility to deliver information in an accurate format.

TS, MAW and NA would also like to thank their families, including their parents and partners, for their patience and encouragement throughout the production of this fifth edition.

FIGURE ACKNOWLEDGEMENTS

Firstly, we are also indebted to our consultant radiologist colleagues at the Sheffield Teaching. Additionally, the following images are reproduced, with kind permission, from other Elsevier titles:

Burkitt, Quick, Reed and Deakin: *Essential Surgery – Problems, Diagnosis and Management*, Fourth Edition
Figures 3, 8, 19, 20, 24, 28, 37, 43, 48, 52, 54, 58, 63

Cross: *Underwood's Pathology – A Clinical Approach*, Sixth Edition
Figure 51

Forbes and Jackson: *Color Atlas and Text of Clinical Medicine*, Third Edition
Figures 18, 21, 22, 27, 31, 41, 44, 49A and B, 60, 64A and B, 65

Adam and Dixon: *Grainger and Allison's Diagnostic Radiology*, Fifth Edition
Figure 29

Henry and Thompson: *Clinical Surgery*, Third Edition
Figure 17

Lim, Loke and Thompson: *Medicine and Surgery – An Integrated Textbook*
Figures 6, 7, 9, 10, 12, 14, 23, 25, 26, 30, 32, 36, 42, 45, 47, 56, 61, 62

Raftery, Delbridge and Wagstaff: *Churchill's Pocketbook of Surgery*, Fourth Edition
Figures 1, 13, 15, 33, 35, 38, 39, 40, 48

Swartz: *Textbook of Physical Diagnosis: History and Examination*, Sixth Edition
Figure 16

This book has been written in three sections: Clinical Presentations, Biochemical Presentations and Haematological Presentations.

In the Clinical Presentations section (Section A), we have attempted to indicate the relative frequency of the conditions causing the various symptoms and signs by colour coding them in green, orange and red, according to whether they are considered common, occasional or rare, respectively.

●	A common cause of the symptom or sign
●	Might occasionally give rise to the symptom or sign
●	Will only rarely cause the symptom or sign

This has been no easy task (and indeed in the Biochemical Presentations and Haematological Presentations sections, we found it so difficult that we abandoned it), but we hope that it will indicate to readers whether they are dealing with a common, occasional or rare disorder. It is appreciated that some conditions may be common in the UK and rare in other parts of the world (and vice versa). Where this is the case, the appropriate colour coding is indicated in brackets, e.g. *Campylobacter* is a common cause of diarrhoea in the UK and therefore coded green but rare in tropical Africa and therefore coded red and in brackets. We have tried to indicate the importance of the condition, not only in causing a particular symptom or sign but also in its overall incidence; e.g. diverticular disease is a common condition and is a common cause of pain in the left iliac fossa and is therefore coded green but it is only an occasional cause of large bowel obstruction and in this context and therefore coded orange.

We have also now added hazard symbols next to certain diagnoses to highlight the need for caution and rapid action for investigation and management. It is hoped that this will add an extra depth to the colour coding of differential diagnosis, as a rare condition could indeed be life threatening and should not be ignored.

Finally, at the end of each chapter, the reader will find a box containing either what we consider to be updated and important learning points or indicating symptoms and signs suggestive of significant pathology that require urgent action. A focus has also been placed on excluding malignancy.

5HIAA	5-hydroxyindoleacetic acid
ßHCG	beta-human chorionic gonadotropin
AC	air conduction
ACE	angiotensin converting enzyme
ACTH	adrenocorticotropic hormone
ADH	antidiuretic hormone
AFP	alpha fetoprotein
AGB	arterial blood gas
AIDS	acquired immune deficiency syndrome
ANA	antinuclear antibody
ANCA	antineutrophil cytoplasmic antibodies
AOM	acute otitis media
AP	anteroposterior
APTT	activated partial thromboplastin time
ARF	acute renal failure
ARMD	age related macular degeneration
ATA/TTG	anti-tissue transglutaminase
AVNRT	atrioventricular nodal reentry tachycardia
AVRT	atrioventricular reentry tachycardia
AXR	abdominal X-ray
BC	bone conduction
BCC	basal cell carcinoma
BPPV	benign paroxysmal positional vertigo
C&S	culture and sensitivities
CCF	congestive cardiac failure
CCP	cyclic citrullinated protein
CMV	cytomegalovirus
CNS	central nervous system
COPD	chronic obstructive pulmonary disease
CREST	calcinosis/Raynauds/esophageal dysmotility/sclerodactyly/telangiectasia
CRF	chronic renal failure
CRP	c-reactive protein
CSF	cerebrospinal fluid
CT	computed tomography
CVA	cerebrovascular accident
CXR	chest X-ray
DaT scan	dopamine transporter scan
DDH	developmental dysplasia of the hip
DHEA	dehydroepiandrosterone
DIC	disseminated intravascular coagulation
DIP	distal interphalangeal
DMARDS	disease-modifying antirheumatic drugs
DMSA	dimercaptosuccinic acid
DVT	deep vein thrombosis
EBV	Epstein-Barr virus
ECG	electrocardiogram
EEG	electroencephalogram

EMG	electromyography
ENT	ears/nose/throat
ERCP	endoscopic retrograde cholangiopancreatography
ESR	erythrocyte sedimentation rate
FBC	full blood count
FNAC	fine needle aspiration cytology
FSH	follicle stimulating hormone
G6PD	glucose-6-phosphate dehydrogenase
GBM	glomerular basement membrane
GCS	glasgow coma score
GIST	gastrointestinal stromal tumour
GPA	granulomatosis with polyangiitis
GUM	genito-urinary medicine
Hb	haemoglobin
HbA1c	glycated haemoglobin
HIV	human immunodeficiency virus
HSV	herpes simplex virus
IGF-1	insulin-like growth factor 1
ITP	idiopathic thrombocytopenic purpura
IVC	inferior vena cava
IVP	intravenous pyelogram
IVU	intravenous urogram
JVP	jugular venous pressure
KUB	kidneys/ureters/bladder
LDH	lactate dehydrogenase
LFTs	liver function tests
LH	luteinising hormone
LSD	lysergic acid diethylamide
MAG 3	mercaptoacetyltriglycine
MCHC	mean corpuscular hemoglobin concentration
MCP	metacarpophalangeal
MCV	mean corpuscular volume
MEN	multiple endocrine neoplasia
MRA	magnetic resonance angiography
MRCP	magnetic resonance cholangiopancreatography
MRI	magnetic resonance imaging
MSU	mid-stream urine
MTP	metatarsophalangeal
NAAT	nucleic acid amplification test
NSAID	non-steroidal anti-inflammatory drug
OGD	oesophageal gastro-duodenoscopy
pCO2	partial pressure of carbon dioxide
PCR	polymerase chain reaction
PCV	packed cell volume
PIP	proximal interphalangeal
pO2	partial pressure of oxygen
PPPD	persistent postural-perceptual dizziness
PR	per rectum
PSA	prostate serum antigen
PT	prothrombin

PTC	percutaneous transhepatic cholangiography
PTH	parathyroid hormone
PV	per vaginum
RAST	radioallergosorbent test
RDW	red cell distribution width
RhF	rheumatoid factor
SAAG	serum-ascites albumin gradient
SCC	squamous cell carcinoma
SIADH	syndrome of inappropriate antidiuretic hormone secretion
SLE	systemic lupus erythematosus
SNRI	serotonin and norepinephrine reuptake inhibitors
STD	sexually transmitted disease
TB	tuberculosis
TFTs	thyroid function tests
TIA	transient ischaemic attack
TIBC	total iron binding capacity
TMJ	temporomandibular joint
TSH	thyroid stimulating hormone
TT	thrombin time
U&Es	urea and electrolytes
US	ultrasound
UTI	urinary tract infection
VBG	venous blood gas
VDRL	venereal disease research laboratory
VQ	ventilation-perfusion
WCC	white cell count

SECTION A

CLINICAL PRESENTATIONS

SECTION B

BIOCHEMICAL PRESENTATIONS

SECTION C

HAEMATOLOGICAL PRESENTATIONS

SECTION A

CLINICAL PRESENTATIONS

ABDOMINAL PAIN

Abdominal pain is an extremely common presenting symptom. The pain may be acute (sudden onset) or chronic (lasting for more than a few days or presenting intermittently). It is important to be able to distinguish causes of abdominal pain which need urgent surgery (e.g. ruptured aortic aneurysm, perforated bowel, or acute mesenteric ischaemia) from those that do not (e.g. biliary colic, ureteric colic, acute pancreatitis). The causes of abdominal pain may be described based on anatomical location or the region affected on clinical examination. The list below contains some of the more common causes but is not intended to be comprehensive.

Figure 1 Diverticular disease. A barium enema showing numerous diverticulae in the sigmoid colon (see arrow).

CAUSES

GASTROINTESTINAL

GUT

Gastroduodenal
- Gastritis
- Gastric/peptic ulcer
- Oesophageal/gastric malignancy
- Gastric/duodenal perforation
- Gastric volvulus ⚠

Intestinal
- Constipation
- Appendicitis
- Obstruction ▲
- Diverticulitis (Fig. 1)
- Gastroenteritis
- TB ● *(common in parts of the world where TB is endemic)*
- Strangulated hernia ▲
- Inflammatory bowel disease
- Intussusception ▲
- Volvulus ▲
- Mesenteric adenitis
- Merkel's diverticular

HEPATOBILIARY
- Cholecystitis
- Biliary colic
- Cholangitis ▲
- Hepatitis

PANCREATIC
- Pancreatitis ▲
- Malignancy
- Pancreatic pseudocyst

SPLENIC
- Infarction
- Spontaneous rupture ▲

URINARY TRACT
- Acute retention of urine
- Urinary tract infection/acute pyelonephritis
- Ureteric colic
- Cystitis
- Hydronephrosis
- Tumour
- Pyonephrosis ▲
- Polycystic kidney

GYNAECOLOGICAL
- Ectopic pregnancy ▲
- Torsion of ovarian cyst ▲
- Ovarian cyst
- Severe dysmenorrhoea

SECTION A

- Mittelschmerz
- Endometriosis
- Uterine fibroid
- Salpingitis

VASCULAR

- Abdominal aortic aneurysm ▲
- Mesenteric embolus ▲
- Ischaemic colitis ▲
- Acute aortic dissection (i.e. type B) ▲
- Mesenteric angina (claudication)
- Mesenteric venous thrombosis ▲

ABDOMINAL WALL

- Cellulitis
- Strangulated hernia ▲
- Rectus sheath haematoma

REFERRED PAIN

- Myocardial infarction ▲
- Lobar pneumonia
- Testicular torsion ▲
- Pleurisy
- Pericarditis ▲
- Herpes zoster
- Thoracic spine disease, e.g. disc, tumour

'MEDICAL' CAUSES

- Diabetic ketoacidosis ▲
- Hypercalcaemia
- Uraemia
- Sickle cell disease
- Addison's disease
- Acute intermittent porphyria
- Henoch–Schönlein purpura
- Tabes dorsalis

HISTORY

Age

Certain conditions are more likely to occur in certain age groups,
e.g. mesenteric adenitis in children, diverticular disease in the elderly.

Past history

- Previous surgery, e.g. adhesions may cause intestinal obstruction.
- Recent trauma, e.g. delayed rupture of spleen.
- Menstrual history, e.g. ectopic pregnancy.

Pain

- Site
  Right upper quadrant- consider biliary, gallbladder, hepatic causes.
  Epigastric- consider gastric, pancreatic, or referred cardiac pain.
  Left upper quadrant- consider splenic causes. Left/Right lumber/
  flank- consider bowel, renal, ureteric causes. Umbilical- consider
  mesenteric or an abdominal aortic aneurysm. Right iliac fossa-
  consider appendicitis, ovarian, ilio-caecal causes. Left iliac fossa-
  consider diverticulitis, ovarian. Suprapubic- consider urinary tract
  infections or cystitis.

- Onset/Timing
  Pathologies may develop suddenly or over a period of time. This
  should guide the urgency of your investigations to exclude life-
  threatening causes.

- Character
  Pain described as colicky or constant with acute exacerbations may
  signify constipation, bowel obstruction, gastroenteritis, ureteric
  calculi, biliary/gallbladder pathology etc. Constant pain may be an
  indication of peritonitis.

- Radiation
  Pain associated with ureteric calculi typically radiates from loin to
  groin. Pain associated with appendicitis typically migrates from the
  umbilicus to the right iliac fossa.

- Associated symptoms
  Absolute constipation, abdominal distention, and faecalant
  vomiting is suggestive a bowel obstruction. Hard stools, rectal
  bleedings and localised left sided peritonism may be indicate
  diverticulitis. Haematemesis/ coffee ground vomit may indicate
  gastro-intestinal ulceration.

- Exacerbating factors
  Pain on or after food ingestion may indicate gastric reflux or ulcer
  disease. Productive cough with upper abdominal pain may be
  suggest referred pain or muscle strain. Exacerbation by movements
  or palpation may be indicative of muscular strain.

- Severity
  Assess severity out of 10 and administer analgesia. Constant severe
  pain despite analgesia may be indicative of further assessment.

Fever

- Any rigors, sweats and temperatures may suggest infection.

EXAMINATION

General

Is the patient lying comfortably? Is the patient lying still but in pain, e.g. peritonitis? Is the patient writhing in agony, e.g. ureteric colic? Is the patient flushed, suggesting pyrexia?

Pulse, temperature, respiration

Pulse and temperature are raised in inflammatory conditions. They may also be raised with impending infarction of bowel. An increased respiratory rate might suggest chest infection referring pain to the abdomen.

Cervical lymphadenopathy

Associated with mesenteric adenitis or even cancer.

Chest

Assess for respiratory signs implicating referred pain from lobar pneumonia.

Abdomen

- Inspection. Does the abdomen move on respiration? Look for scars, distension, visible peristalsis (usually due to chronic obstruction in patient with very thin abdominal wall). Check the hernial orifices. Are there any obvious masses, e.g. visible, pulsatile mass to suggest aortic aneurysm?
- Palpation. The patient should be relaxed, lying flat, with arms by side. Be gentle, and start as far from the painful site as possible. Check for guarding and rigidity. Check for masses, e.g. appendix mass, pulsatile expansile mass to suggest aortic aneurysm. Carefully examine the hernial orifices. Examine the testes to exclude torsion.
- Percussion, e.g. tympanitic note with distension with intestinal obstruction; dullness over bladder due to acute retention.
- Auscultation. Take your time (30–60 s); e.g. silent abdomen of peritonitis; high-pitched tinkling bowel sounds of intestinal obstruction.

Rectal examination

Always carry out a rectal examination.

Vaginal examination

There may be discharge or tenderness associated with pelvic inflammatory disease. Examine the uterus and adnexa, e.g. pregnancy, fibroids, ectopic pregnancy.

GENERAL INVESTIGATIONS

- **FBC, ESR, CRP**
  Hb ↓ peptic ulcer disease, malignancy. WCC and CRP ↑ infective/
  inflammatory disease, e.g. appendicitis, diverticulitis.
  ESR ↑ Crohn's disease, TB.

- **U&Es**
  Electrolyte disturbances in vomiting and diarrhoea.
  Pseudo-obstruction.

- **LFTs**
  LFTs may be deranged in cholangitis and hepatitis.

- **Serum amylase**
  Usually raised (x3 baseline) in acute pancreatitis.

- **Venous blood gas**
  Metabolic acidosis in infective, ischaemic aetiologies and diabetic
  ketoacidosis.

- **MSU**
  Leucocytes and nitrates in UTIs. Blood, leucocytes and nitrates in
  pyelonephritis. Blood in ureteric colic.

- **βHCG**
  Pregnancy. Ectopic pregnancy.

- **Erect CXR**
  Gas under diaphragm (perforated viscus). Lower lobar pneumonia
  (referred pain).

- **AXR**
  Obstruction – dilated loops of bowel. Site of obstruction. Local
  ileus (sentinel loop) – pancreatitis, acute appendicitis. Toxic
  dilatation – dilated, featureless, oedematous colon in ulcerative
  colitis or Crohn's disease. Renal calculi. Calcified aortic aneurysm.
  Air in biliary tree (gallstone ileus). Gallstones (10% radio-opaque).

- **US**
  Localised abscesses, e.g. appendix abscess, paracolic abscess
  in diverticular disease. Free fluid – peritonitis, ascites. Aortic
  aneurysm. Ectopic pregnancy. Ovarian cyst. Gallstones. Empyema,
  mucocele of gall bladder. Kidney – cysts, tumour.

SPECIFIC INVESTIGATIONS

- **Blood glucose**
  Raised in diabetic ketoacidosis.

- **Serum calcium**
  Hypercalcaemia.

- **VDRL**
  Syphilis (tabes dorsalis).

- **Sickling test**
  Sickle cell disease.

- **Urinary porphobilinogens**
  Acute intermittent porphyria.

- **ECG**
  Myocardial infarction (referred pain).

- **CT (i.e. abdomen, angiography)**
  Abscess. Aortic aneurysm. Pancreatitis. Tumour. Mesenteric
  ischaemia. Mesenteric thrombosis.

- **OGD colonoscopy**
  Peptic ulcer. Malignancy.

- **IVU**
  Stones. Obstruction.

- **Barium enema**
  Carcinoma. Volvulus. Intussusception.

- **Small bowel enema (i.e. gastrograffin follow through)**
  Small bowel Crohn's disease. Lymphoma of small bowel. Carcinoma
  of small bowel.

- **MRCP/ERCP**
  Biliary tract disease.

- **Don't forget to examine the hernial orifices.**
- **Perform specific examinations in order to narrow your
  differential diagnosis.**

ABDOMINAL SWELLINGS

Abdominal swellings are a common surgical problem. Abdominal swellings may be divided into generalised and localised swellings. Generalised swellings are classically described as the 'five Fs', namely fat, faeces, flatus, fluid or fetus. For the purpose of description of localised swellings, the abdomen can be divided into nine areas, i.e. right upper quadrant, left upper quadrant, epigastrium, umbilical, right lumbar, left lumbar, right iliac fossa, left iliac fossa and suprapubic area. Many of the swellings that occur in the different abdominal regions have similar aetiological causes and therefore have been described according to the organ affected. Hepatomegaly, splenomegaly and renal masses are dealt with under the relevant heading in other sections of the book.

Figure 2 Autosomal dominant polycystic kidney disease. Both kidneys are greatly enlarged by numerous cysts of various sizes.

CAUSES

ABDOMINAL WALL

- Lipoma
- Hernia (i.e. paraumbilical, umbilical, spigelian hernia)
- Metastatic deposits (i.e. Sister Joseph Mary nodule)
- Other (i.e. urachal cyst)

LIVER

- See hepatomegaly, p. 215.

GALL BLADDER

- Secondary to carcinoma of the head of the pancreas
- Mucocele
- Empyema
- Carcinoma

STOMACH

- Carcinoma
- Gastric distension (acute dilatation, pyloric stenosis)
- Acute gastric volvulus

PANCREAS

- Carcinoma
- Pseudocyst

KIDNEY

- Hydronephrosis
- Solitary cyst
- Carcinoma
- Polycystic kidney (Fig. 2)
- Pyonephrosis/perinephric abscess
- Tuberculosis (TB)
- Wilms' tumour (nephroblastoma)

SPLEEN

See splenomegaly, p. 393.

COLON

- Appendix abscess
- Carcinoma (i.e. caecal mass)
- Faeces
- Diverticular mass
- Volvulus (i.e. caecal, sigmoid)
- Intussusception

SMALL BOWEL

- Crohn's disease
- Carcinoma
- Mesenteric cysts
- Lymphoma
- Ileo-caecal TB

BLADDER

- Acute retention
- Chronic retention
- Carcinoma

OVARY/UTERUS/FALLOPIAN TUBE

- Ovarian cyst
- Ovarian neoplasm
- Pregnancy
- Ectopic pregnancy
- Tubo-ovarian abscess
- Uterine fibroid
- Uterine carcinoma

RETROPERITONEUM

- Arterial aneurysm (i.e. aortic, iliac)
- Lymphadenopathy (lymphoma, secondaries from testicular carcinoma)
- Neoplasm of the iliac bone, e.g. osteogenic sarcoma, Ewing's tumour

OMENTUM

- Omental secondaries, e.g. stomach and ovary

HISTORY

Abdominal wall

The patient may indicate a soft, subcutaneous swelling, which may be a lipoma or a hernia containing extraperitoneal fat. The latter always occurs in the midline through a defect in the linea alba. The patient may have had a lump for a long time. The development of a soft mass that is slow growing, suggestive of a lipoma.

A hernia may present with incarceration or with a tender painful swelling occasionally with erythematous overlying skin, suggesting strangulation. An umbilical hernia presents in infancy as an umbilical swelling which is reducible, and will usually have been noted at birth. Paraumbilical hernias usually occur in obese adults, often female. A spigelian hernia occurs just lateral to the rectus muscle, halfway between the umbilicus and symphysis pubis.

Occasionally a patient may indicate a firm bony lump in the upper epigastrium, which is in fact a normal xiphisternum. This may have become apparent due to either a deliberate attempt to lose weight or sudden weight loss as a result of underlying disease.

Metastatic deposits may present as single or multiple fixed lumps in the skin or subcutaneous tissue, e.g. from breast or bronchus. Sister Joseph's nodule presents as a hard lump at the umbilicus. It is due to secondary deposits of carcinoma of the stomach, colon, ovary or breast.

Umbilical discharge may suggest a urachal cyst or abscess.

Liver

See hepatomegaly, p. 215.

Gall bladder

Known history of gallstones. History of flatulent dyspepsia. Jaundice. Dark urine. Pale stools. Pruritus. Recent weight loss may suggest carcinoma of the head of the pancreas or carcinoma of the gall bladder.

Stomach

Vomiting may suggest pyloric stenosis, acute dilatation of the stomach and carcinoma.

Vomiting food ingested several days previously suggests pyloric stenosis. A baby may present with projectile vomiting. The infant thrives for the first 3–4 weeks of life, and then develops projectile vomiting after feeds. The first-born male child in a family is most commonly affected. There may be a history of a familial tendency, especially on the maternal side.

Lethargy, loss of appetite and weight loss are seen in carcinoma of the stomach.

Pancreas

There may be a history of acute pancreatitis, which would suggest the development of a pseudocyst. Weight loss, backache and jaundice will suggest carcinoma of the pancreas. Recent onset of diabetes may occur with carcinoma of the pancreas.

Kidney

See kidney swellings, p. 276.

Spleen

See splenomegaly, p. 393.

Colon

Colicky abdominal pain, constipation and faecal blood loss may suggest colonic carcinoma or diverticular disease. Identify any known history of diverticular disease. A change in bowel habit and unintentional weight loss are suggestive of carcinoma. The patient may have also noticed a development of a mass.

Lassitude, weakness, lethargy, suggesting anaemia from chronic blood loss.

There may be a history of gross constipation to suggest faecal loading.

Caecal volvulus will present with central abdominal colicky pain and abdominal distension. Sigmoid volvulus will present with lower abdominal colicky pain and a tense, palpable mass in the left abdomen, which is tympanitic on percussion.

History of attacks of crying, abdominal pain, blood and mucus in the stool ('redcurrant jelly' stool) will suggest intussusception in infants.

A short history of central abdominal, colicky pain followed by a sharply localised pain in the right iliac fossa will suggest the diagnosis of acute appendicitis. After 48 hours, if there is not generalised peritonitis, an appendix mass will have formed, and an abscess may subsequently form in the right iliac fossa.

Large bowel Crohn's disease will present with a sausage-like, palpable mass, which may be tender and is associated with diarrhoea.

Small bowel

The patient may present with central abdominal colicky pain, vomiting and diarrhoea, suggestive of Crohn's disease or more rarely a carcinoma of the small bowel.

Ileo-caecal TB causes abdominal pain, diarrhoea which is associated with malaise and weight loss.

Bladder

Sudden onset of suprapubic pain with inability to pass urine suggests acute retention. There will usually be a history of difficulty in starting and a poor stream. A history of dribbling may suggest chronic outflow obstruction. Haematuria, frequency or dysuria may suggest bladder carcinoma.

Ovary/uterus/fallopian tube

The patient herself may feel a lump in the abdomen (ovarian cyst, fibroid) or notice generalised abdominal swelling, which may be associated with a massive ovarian cyst or ascites associated with ovarian cancer. Ectopic pregnancy will present with a missed period and abdominal pain, bleeding per vaginal (PV), and collapse with hypovolaemic shock if it ruptures. Salpingo-oophoritis will present with lower abdominal pain and tenderness and associated fever and often a purulent vaginal discharge. Menorrhagia, lower abdominal pain and dyspareunia may suggest fibroids. Missed periods and early morning vomiting will suggest pregnancy. Menorrhagia and dyspareunia will suggest fibroids. Intermenstrual bleeding suggests carcinoma.

Retroperitoneum

A history of backache may suggest an aortic aneurysm or the patient may complain of a pulsatile epigastric swelling. Backache may also be a presenting symptom of retroperitoneal lymphadenopathy. The patient may present having noticed a pulsatile swelling in the iliac fossa, suggesting an iliac aneurysm.

Pelvic lymphadenopathy may be suspected by history of removal of a malignant lesion from the lower limb, especially malignant melanoma. There may be an existing lesion present on the limb. A dull, boring pain may be suggestive of an iliac bone lesion. A palpable bony lesion suggests an osteogenic sarcoma or Ewing's tumour of bone.

Omentum

Patient may have a history of cancer.

EXAMINATION

Abdominal wall

A soft, lobulated mass suggests a lipoma. It will be mobile over the tensed abdominal musculature. A fatty, occasionally tender, nonmobile swelling in the midline will suggest an epigastric hernia. The majority of epigastric hernias are composed of extraperitoneal fat, although there may be a sac with bowel contents. A cough impulse will be palpable. The swelling may be reducible. Hard, irregular, fixed lumps in the abdominal wall suggest metastatic deposits, especially if there is a history of carcinoma of the breast or bronchus. Sister Joseph's nodule presents as a hard lump or lumps at the umbilicus. Check for carcinoma of the stomach, colon, ovary or breast.

In infants, there may be an obvious large umbilical defect. The swelling is usually wide-necked and reducible. In adults, there may be a reducible paraumbilical hernia. Occasionally, it is soft, containing extraperitoneal fat. Frequently, there is a sac containing omentum. Incarceration may occur. A tender red swelling suggests strangulation. A Richter's-type hernia may occur at this site.

Liver

See p. 215.

Gall bladder

A mucocele is either nontender or only mildly tender. It is large and smooth and moves with respiration, projecting from under the ninth costal cartilage at the lateral border of rectus abdominis. Empyema presents with an acutely tender gall bladder, which is difficult to define due to pain and tenderness. The patient may be jaundiced due to Mirizzi syndrome (external pressure from a stone impacted in Hartmann's pouch on the adjacent bile duct).

Carcinoma of the gall bladder may present as a hard, irregular mass in the right hypochondrium, but normally presents as obstructive jaundice due to secondary deposits in the nodes at the porta hepatis causing external compression of the hepatic ducts. A smooth enlarged gall bladder in the presence of jaundice may be due to carcinoma of the head of the pancreas (Courvoisier's law: 'in the presence of obstructive jaundice, if the gall bladder is palpable, the cause is unlikely to be due to gallstones').

Stomach

Gastric distension may present with a vague fullness and a succussion splash. Carcinoma will present with a hard, craggy, immobile mass. Pancreatic tumours may be impalpable or present as a fixed mass, which does not move with respiration. Pancreatic pseudocysts are often large and smooth and may be tender.

Pancreas

Painless jaundice may indicate pancreatic cancer. A mass may be palpable at the epigastria, suggesting pancreatic cancer, cyst or pseudocyst.

Kidney

See kidney swellings, p. 276.

Spleen

With massive splenomegaly, the spleen may be palpable extending into the right lower quadrant.

Colon

Faeces are usually soft and putty-like and can be indented. However, they may also be felt as a mass of rocks in the colon, suggesting constipation. Carcinoma is usually a firm to hard irregular mass, which may be mobile or fixed. A diverticular mass is usually tender and ill-defined, unless there is a large paracolic abscess. With caecal volvulus, there is a tympanitic mass, which may be tender with impending infarction. With intussusception, there will be a smooth, mobile, tender, sausage-shaped mass in the right hypochondrium. The mass may move as the intussusception progresses.

Small bowel

Small bowel masses are usually very mobile, may be sausage shaped and may be tender. If there is a mass palpable in the right iliac fossa, the site of pathology is likely to be in the terminal ileum.

Bladder

In acute retention, there will be a smooth, tender swelling extending towards (but not above) the umbilicus. It is dull to percussion, and it is impossible to get below it. Digital rectal examination will usually reveal benign prostatic hypertrophy or occasionally a hard, irregular prostate associated with carcinoma. With carcinoma of the bladder, a hard, irregular craggy mass may be felt arising out of the pelvis.

Ovary/fallopian tube/uterus

Examination may reveal a greatly distended abdomen, which may be due to a huge ovarian cyst or ascites associated with an ovarian neoplasm. Huge ovarian cysts are often smooth and loculated. It is impossible to get below them as they arise out of the pelvis. Signs of ascites include shifting dullness and a fluid thrill.

With ectopic pregnancy, there may be a palpable mass in either iliac fossa. This may be associated with shock if rupture of the ectopic pregnancy has occurred. Shoulder-tip pain may occur from irritation of the undersurface of the diaphragm with blood. With tubo-ovarian abscess, there may be a palpable mass arising out of the pelvis, or merely lower abdominal tenderness. Vaginal examination will reveal tenderness in the pouch of Douglas. Uterine fibroids may be extremely large and palpable as nodules on the underlying uterus.

A smooth, regular swelling arising out of the pelvis suggests a pregnant uterus. Later, as the uterus enlarges, fetal heart sounds may be heard. Fibroids are usually smooth and firm and may become very large. Uterine carcinoma is hard and craggy. Bimanual examination may confirm the diagnosis.

Retroperitoneum

An aneurysm presents as a pulsatile expansile mass. Check the distal circulation (emboli, associated peripheral ischaemia). Retroperitoneal lymph node metastases from testicular cancer may present as a large retroperitoneal mass. Check the testes for swellings. Check all other sites for lymphadenopathy (especially the left supraclavicular node). Lymphadenopathy may also result from lymphoma. Check for lymphadenopathy elsewhere and for splenomegaly. A hard, craggy, mobile mass, especially in the presence of ascites, suggests omental secondaries (ovary, stomach – check for Virchow's node, i.e. left supraclavicular node).

Omentum

There may be palpable mass on deep palpation.

GENERAL INVESTIGATIONS

- **FBC, CRP, ESR**
  Hb ↓, e.g. carcinoma of the colon, haematuria with renal lesions.
  Hb ↑, e.g. hypernephroma (polycythaemia associated with hypernephroma).
  WCC and CRP ↑ appendicitis, diverticulitis, renal infections.
  ESR ↑, malignancy, Crohn's disease, ileo-caecal TB.

- **U&Es**
  Vomiting and diarrhoea resulting in electrolyte losses and dehydration. Ureteric obstruction with renal lesions, leading to uraemia. Renal lesions.

- **LFTs**
  Alkaline phosphatase ↑ with primary liver lesions or liver secondaries.

- **Serum amylase**
  Acute pancreatitis.

- **MSU**
  Renal lesions – red blood cells, pus cells, malignant cells.
  Organisms. C&S.

- **USS**
  Liver lesions. Gallstones. Mucocele. Empyema. Bile duct dilatation. Splenomegaly. Pancreatic pseudocyst. Renal lesions. Paracolic abscess. Ovarian lesions. Uterine lesions. Tubo-ovarian abscesses. Pregnancy. Ectopic pregnancy. Aortic/iliac artery aneurysms. Lymphadenopathy. Appendix mass. Crohn's mass. Fibroids. Bladder tumour. Urachal cyst.

- **AXR**
  Obstruction. Dilated loops of bowel. Ovarian teratoma (teeth, etc.).
  Erosion of iliac bone – bone tumours. Gallstones (10% are radio-opaque). Caecal volvulus. Constipation. Calcification in renal lesions.

SPECIFIC INVESTIGATIONS

- **βHCG**
  Raised in pregnancy.
- **Finger prick blood glucose**
  Glucose may be abnormal in pancreatic carcinoma or pancreatitis.
- **PSA**
  Carcinoma of the prostate.
- **CT: abdomen and pelvis**
  Liver lesions. Gall bladder lesions. Renal lesions. Carcinoma of the pancreas. Pancreatic pseudocyst. Liver secondaries. Splenomegaly. Ovarian lesions. Uterine lesions. Bladder lesions. Urachal cyst. Ectopic pregnancy. Aortic/iliac artery aneurysm. Lymphadenopathy. Appendix mass. Bone tumours. Omental deposits. Guided biopsy/FNAC.
- **Barium enema**
  Carcinoma. Diverticular disease. Intussusception.
- **Small bowel enema**
  Crohn's disease. Carcinoma. Lymphoma.
- **Colonoscopy**
  Carcinoma. Diverticular disease. Biopsy.
- **Gastroscopy**
  Carcinoma. Pyloric stenosis. Biopsy.
- **Laparoscopy**
  Carcinoma. Omental secondaries. Carcinomatosis peritonei. Biopsy.
- **Cystoscopy**
  Bladder tumour. Biopsy.
- **Bone scan**
  Bone tumour.
- **Mantoux test**
  Ileo-caecal TB.

- Abdominal mass in conjunction with weight loss is suggestive of malignancy and requires urgent investigation.
- An abdominal mass in association with pyrexia, tachycardia and localised tenderness suggests an infective cause.
- Always check the βHCG in women of childbearing age.

ANORECTAL PAIN

Anorectal pain is a common presenting complaint. The majority of patients have an obvious cause, e.g. fissure-in-ano, perianal abscess or thrombosed haemorrhoids.

Figure 3 Thrombosed haemorrhoids. Note the oedematous, congested purplish mass seen at the anal margin.

CAUSES

ACUTE

- Fissure-in-ano
- Perianal haematoma
- Thrombosed haemorrhoids (Fig. 3)
- Anorectal abscess (i.e. perinal, interspincteric, ischiorectal)
- Trauma
- Anorectal gonorrhoea
- Herpes

CHRONIC

- Fistula-in-ano
- Anorectal malignancy
- Chronic perianal sepsis, e.g. Crohn's disease, TB ⚠

- Proctalgia fugax
- Solitary rectal ulcer
- Cauda equina lesions

HISTORY

Constipation with pain on defecation and blood (usually on the paper) will suggest fissure-in-ano. A sudden onset of pain with a tender lump in the perianal region will suggest perianal haematoma. A past history of prolapsing piles, with failure to reduce them, associated with pain and tenderness suggests thrombosed haemorrhoids. Gradual onset of pain and tenderness with swelling is suggestive of abscess formation. A careful history must be taken of trauma. A history of anal sexual exposure will suggest gonorrhoea or herpes. With gonorrhoea, there may be irritation, itching, discharge and pain. With herpes, there will be pain and irritation. Proctalgia fugax is diagnosed on the history of perineal pain, which is spasmodic, the spasms lasting up to 30 min. The pain often feels deep inside the rectum. The cause is unknown but may be related to paroxysmal contraction of levator ani. Anorectal malignancies will be suggested in alteration of bowel habit and bleeding on defecation. Pain will only be apparent if the tumour involves the anal canal below the dentate line, where sensation is of the somatic type. Solitary rectal ulcer may present with pain but more usually presents with bleeding PR, passage of mucus and difficulty with defecation. Chronic perianal sepsis may be the presenting symptom of Crohn's disease or TB. These diseases may already be manifest at other sites of the body. Rarely, lesions of the cauda equina may cause anal pain.

EXAMINATION

- Rectal examination
  - Inspection may reveal a fissure-in-ano, perianal haematoma, thrombosed piles or a tumour growing out of the anal canal. A digital examination should be carried unless the diagnosis is obvious.
  - A tense, red, tender area may be present, representing a perianal abscess.
  - A fullness in the buttock with redness may indicate a large ischiorectal abscess.
  - The presence of vesicles in the anal area will suggest herpes.
- Other examinations
  - If a cauda equina lesion is suspected, a full neurological examination should be carried out.
  - No abnormality is usually found with proctalgia fugax.

SECTION A

GENERAL INVESTIGATIONS

- **FBC, ESR, CRP, U&Es**
  WCC & CRP ↑ infections, e.g. abscess. ESR ↑ Crohn's disease, TB and malignancy. U&Es to assess for renal function for intravenous antibiotics. Diabetes may pre-dispose to infections.

- **Proctoscopy**
  Haemorrhoids. Anorectal malignancy. Anorectal gonorrhoea. Swab ↑ Gram-negative intracellular diplococci.
  With gonococcal proctitis, proctoscopy may reveal pus and blood in the rectal ampulla with oedematous and friable mucosa.

- **Sigmoidoscopy**
  Anorectal malignancy.
  Solitary rectal ulcer is usually diagnosed on sigmoidoscopy when redness and oedema of the mucosa is seen, usually, but not always, in association with frank ulceration.

SPECIFIC INVESTIGATIONS

- **Endo-anal ultrasound**
  This may demonstrate intersphincteric abscesses or fistulae-in-ano.

- **MRI**
  This will delineate complex fistula problems or may indicate a cauda equina lesion.

- **Barium enema**
  This may help identify fistula tracts.

- **Antigen detection tests**
  Herpes.

- **PCR**
  For fast diagnosis of herpes.

- **Recurrent perianal abscesses may be the first presentation of diabetes.**

- **Recurrent perianal problems, especially fissures in unusual places, may be a presentation of Crohn's disease.**

- **Do not treat perianal abscesses with antibiotics. Perianal abscesses should be incised and drained. Failure to do so may result in development of a fistula-in-ano.**

ARM PAIN

This section deals with pain in the upper limb unrelated to joint pains, and focuses on causes related to either neurological or vascular lesions. Musculoskeletal causes of arm pain are covered in the chapter on Joint Disorders (p. 247).

Figure 4 A trans-axial image showing a right-sided acute disc bulge at C6–C7 level, which is compressing the C7 nerve root in the exit foramen (arrow). The patient will experience pain in the right arm radiating into the middle finger (dermatomal distribution of C7) and weakness of extension of the elbow (weak triceps-myotomal distribution of C7). There will be a reduced or absent triceps reflex.

CAUSES

CERVICAL LESIONS

- Disc lesion (Fig. 4)
- Cervical spondylosis
- Syringomyelia
- Infection, e.g. osteitis, TB ⚠
- Tumours ⚠
  - Spinal cord
  - Meninges
  - Nerves
  - Vertebral bodies

BRACHIAL PLEXUS

- Cervical rib
- Malignant infiltration, e.g. Pancoast's tumour
- Thoracic inlet syndrome

VASCULAR LESIONS

- Myocardial ischaemia (left arm) ⚠
- Embolism ⚠
- Arterial/venous thrombosis ⚠
- Subclavian artery stenosis
- Steal syndrome
  - I.e. coronary-subclavian steal syndrome, arterio-venous fistula
- Upper limb lymphadema

OTHERS

- Repetitive strain injury
- Carpal tunnel syndrome
- Peripheral neuropathy
- Bone tumours
- Compartment syndrome ⚠
  - Acute, e.g. crush injuries
  - Chronic, e.g. exertional

HISTORY

Symptoms of cervical lesions causing cervical cord compression include: pain and stiffness in the neck; pain radiating down the arm.

Cervical spondylosis represents 'wear and tear' of the cervical spine. It is common over the age of 60 years. Acute disc lesions usually occur in the younger patient. A careful history is needed to exclude trauma.

Brachial plexus lesions refer pain down the arm and may result from localised lesions, e.g. a cervical rib causing extrinsic compression will affect T1 and cause wasting of the small muscles of the hands and paraesthesia in the dermatomal distribution, i.e. the inner aspect of the upper arm.

Subclavian artery stenosis will result in 'claudication' in the arm, i.e. pain brought on by exercise, relieved by rest, due to inadequate blood flow. A history of cardiac problems, e.g. atrial fibrillation or arterial disease, will suggest embolism or thrombosis. A sudden onset of a painful, swollen, cyanotic limb will suggest axillary vein thrombosis. Pain radiating into the left arm brought on by exercise and related to central chest pain and pain radiating into the neck suggests myocardial ischaemia. Pain associated with occupation, e.g. writing, word-processing (keyboard occupations), suggests repetitive strain injury. A history of diabetes mellitus, renal failure, liver failure, alcohol abuse, vitamin B_{12} deficiency, drugs, e.g. phenytoin or vincristine, suggests peripheral neuropathy.

Pain, paraesthesia in the thumb, index and middle finger, which is worse in bed at night and relieved by hanging the arm out of bed, would suggest carpal tunnel syndrome. The latter may be associated with pregnancy, rheumatoid arthritis, myxoedema, anterior dislocation of the lunate, gout, acromegaly, amyloidosis and arteriovenous fistula at the wrist created for haemodialysis.

Localised bone pain may be due to primary or secondary tumours. The latter are most common and may result from a primary in the breast, bronchus, thyroid, prostate or kidney. Pathological fractures may occur. With compartment syndrome, there may be a history of crush injury, vascular injury or vascular surgery. Chronic compartment syndrome may result from unusual exertion, e.g. weightlifting. Occupation will suggest repetitive strain injury.

EXAMINATION

- Neurological examination
  A full neurological examination should be carried out, looking for cervical lesions, brachial plexus lesions or carpal tunnel syndrome. There may be limitation in movements of the cervical spine. Horner's syndrome (ptosis, miosis, enophthalmos and anhidrosis) suggests Pancoast's tumour.

- Vascular examination
  The limbs should be examined for swelling, e.g. axillary vein thrombosis, when there will be cyanosis and dilated veins. Examine for signs of ischaemia and feel for pulses. The classical signs of an ischaemic limb, i.e. pain, pallor, pulselessness, paraesthesia, 'perishing cold' and paralysis, may be present.

- Musculoskeletal examination
  With bone tumours, there will be localised swelling and tenderness. With compartment syndrome, there will be a swollen tender compartment in the forearm, paraesthesia and paralysis. Pulses may be normal initially; later, they are reduced or absent.

GENERAL INVESTIGATIONS

- FBC, ESR, CRP, D-dimer, U&Es, LFTs
  WCC ↑ infection, e.g. osteomyelitis or cervical spine TB.
  ESR & CRP ↑ infection and malignancy. D-dimer will indicate likelihood of thrombosis.

- Cervical spine X-ray
  Cervical spondylosis, bony metastases, cervical spine fractures.

- CXR
  Malignancy resulting in bone secondary. Pancoast's tumour (apical lung tumour spreading to involve brachial plexus). Cervical rib (13 ribs).

- ECG
  Cardiac ischaemia.
- Cardiac enzymes
  Cardiac ischaemia.

SPECIFIC INVESTIGATIONS

- CT
  Cervical stenosis, bony injury, tumours.
- MRI
  Cervical disc lesions, tumours.
- Nerve conduction studies
  Brachial plexus lesions, peripheral neuropathy, carpal tunnel syndrome.
- Duplex Doppler
  Arterial or venous lesions.
- MR angiography
  Arterial lesions. Venous lesions, e.g. axillary vein thrombosis.

- Angina may present only with pain in the left arm. Take a careful history.

- Paraesthesia and weakness in association with arm pain suggests nerve compression.

ARM SWELLINGS

Swelling may be localised or generalised. Localised swellings may be related to joints or fractures. Localised swellings around joints are covered in the section on Joint Disorders (p. 247). This section includes only those conditions that may cause generalised swelling of the arm.

CAUSES

- Trauma
- Infection, e.g. cellulitis, lymphangitis, phlebitis
- Acquired lymphoedema
- Venous thoracic outlet syndrome
- Venous thrombosis
- Congenital lymphoedema
  - Congenital
  - Acquired, e.g. carcinoma, infection, lymph node removal, iatrogenic, radiotherapy
  - Infection, e.g. filariasis
  - Lymph node removal
  - Radiotherapy
- Compartment syndrome

HISTORY

A history of trauma will be obvious in many cases, although pathological fractures may occur with little trauma. Congenital lymphoedema of the arm is rare; however, secondary lymphoedema is not, and a history of carcinoma of the breast, operations on the axilla or radiotherapy to the axilla should be sought. There may be a history of a puncture wound or flea bite, suggesting cellulitis or lymphangitis. Streptococcal cellulitis is common following puncture wounds in patients who already have lymphoedema of a limb. Axillary vein thrombosis may come on after excessive or unusual exercise and has been nicknamed 'effort thrombosis'. An example is a patient who has been painting a ceiling who is not used to doing that sort of thing. It may occur in patients with cervical ribs or thoracic inlet obstruction. Thrombosis may also occur following insertion of a central line.

EXAMINATION

There may be localised swelling and tenderness together with crepitus associated with a fracture. There may be generalised non-pitting oedema suggestive of lymphoedema. Examination of the axilla may reveal a mass of lymph nodes, a scar suggestive of previous surgery or the skin changes of previous radiotherapy. Examination of the breast may reveal the site of a primary tumour that has resulted in secondary axillary lymphadenopathy. With axillary vein thrombosis, there will be swelling, cyanosis and prominent dilated veins on the arm. With cellulitis, there may be redness and heat in the arm, and in lymphangitis, there may be red, inflamed streaks along the line of lymphatic vessels. With reflex sympathetic dystrophy, the limb becomes painful, swollen and stiff, with a reddened, smooth, shiny appearance to the skin.

GENERAL INVESTIGATIONS

- **FBC, ESR, CRP, U&Es**
  Hb ↓ tumour. WCC & CRP ↑ infection. ESR ↑ tumour or infection. Platelet count may indicate platelet consumption. U&Es may highlight dehydration, increasing the risk of thrombosis.

- **CXR**
  Cervical rib (associated with thoracic outlet syndrome).

- **Arm X-ray**
  Identify any underlying fractures causing the swelling. Possible foreign body associated with cellulitis.

- **US +/− duplex**
  Imaging with provocation (i.e. Roos test) will help identify thoracic outlet syndrome. Axillary vein thrombosis. Axillary mass.

SPECIFIC INVESTIGATIONS

- **Swab**
  C&S of any lesion that may have resulted in cellulitis, phlebitis or lymphangitis.

- **MR**
  Identify any mechanical obstruction to the thoracic outlet

- **Venography**
  Axillary vein thrombosis.

- **Always take a careful and detailed history. Trauma may have been minimal and forgotten, e.g. an insect bite.**
- **Always examine the breast and axillary nodes.**

ASCITES

Ascites is the accumulation of excess free fluid in the peritoneal cavity (Fig. 5).

Figure 5 CT scan of ascites. *There is free fluid throughout the peritoneal cavity (arrows).*

CAUSES

HEPATIC

- Cirrhosis
- Hepatic tumours

MALIGNANT DISEASE

- Peritoneal metastases
- Abdominal/pelvic tumour (primary or secondary)
- Pseudomyxoma peritonei
- Primary mesothelioma

CARDIAC

- Cardiac failure
- Constrictive pericarditis
- Tricuspid incompetence

RENAL
- Nephrotic syndrome

PERITONITIS
- TB ⚠
- Spontaneous bacterial ⚠

VENOUS OBSTRUCTION
- Budd–Chiari syndrome
- Veno-occlusive disease
- Hepatic portal vein obstruction
- Inferior vena cava obstruction

GASTROINTESTINAL
- Pancreatitis ⚠
- Malabsorption
- Bile ascites

HISTORY

Symptoms

Patients with ascites can present with abdominal discomfort, increasing abdominal girth, weight gain and ankle or sacral swelling.

Onset

The development of ascites is usually gradual, but sudden onset can result from acute decompensation of liver cirrhosis, malignancy, portal or splenic vein thrombosis and Budd–Chiari syndrome.

Past medical history

Any history of malignancy in the abdomen or pelvis is relevant; however, abdominal metastasis can also result in ascites, especially from breast, ovarian, prostatic, testicular and haematological malignancies. Cirrhosis of the liver may result from alcohol-related liver disease, nonalcoholic fatty liver disease previous hepatitis, Wilson's disease, primary and secondary biliary cirrhosis and haemochromatosis. A previous history of TB should raise suspicion of secondary disease.

Associated symptoms

Shortness of breath can result from splinting of the diaphragm due to tense ascites itself, or as part of the syndrome of congestive cardiac failure when it is the underlying cause.

EXAMINATION

Classical findings are shifting dullness and a fluid thrill. As liver disease and cancers account for 90% of the cases presenting with ascites, a detailed examination of all systems is required. The next commonest causes are cardiac failure and nephrotic syndrome.

Inspection

Evidence of liver disease would be suggested by the presence of jaundice, spider naevi, loss of body hair, gynaecomastia, palmar erythema and caput medusae. The jugular venous pressure (JVP) is elevated in the presence of cardiac failure, and a prominent v wave is seen with tricuspid regurgitation. Further elevation of the JVP on inspiration (Kussmaul's sign) may be observed with right heart failure or constrictive pericarditis.

Palpation

Careful abdominal examination should be performed to look for possible abdominal or pelvic tumours. Hepatomegaly and splenomegaly can occur with portal hypertension and hepatic and haematological malignancies. Displacement of the apex beat with cardiomegaly may result from cardiac failure. Pedal oedema occurs with cirrhosis, cardiac failure, malabsorption, obstruction of lymphatic flow due to intra-abdominal or pelvic tumours and nephrotic syndrome.

Auscultation

A third heart sound, systolic murmurs (functional tricuspid and mitral regurgitation) and crepitations (pulmonary oedema) may be audible with cardiac failure. Heart sounds are muffled with pericardial effusions. A pericardial friction rub is occasionally audible in pericarditis.

Percussion

Dullness of the lung bases occurs with pulmonary oedema and pleural effusions (which may occur secondary to ascites).

Internal examination

A rectal examination may reveal ulceration or a fixed mass suggestive of a carcinoma. In women, an adnexal mass PV may be the first indication of a pelvic tumour.

GENERAL INVESTIGATIONS

History and examination findings may reveal the underlying cause. General investigations can be used to confirm or indicate the possible aetiology.

- **Urine dipstick**
  Will be strongly positive for protein in nephrotic syndrome. If so, a 24-hour urine collection for protein should be undertaken: more than 3.5 g/24 h is indicative of nephrotic syndrome.

- **FBC**
  A raised white count may indicate an infective aetiology, but a differential white count is more specific.

- **U&Es**
  Elevated urea and creatinine implies severe renal impairment, and may occur as a component of hepatorenal syndrome, which is renal impairment secondary to liver failure.

- **LFTs**
  May be deranged in the presence of liver disease. The serum albumin will be able to indicate hypoalbuminaemia, but the underlying cause must still be sought.

- **CXR**
  Findings suggestive of cardiac failure are cardiomegaly, upper venous diversion of blood, the presence of Kerley B lines, pulmonary oedema and pleural effusions. Occasionally, the presence of carcinoma may be suggested by a lesion in the lung fields.

- **US abdomen/pelvis**
  In addition to confirming the presence of ascites, US will detect any intra-abdominal masses that are not palpable on clinical examination, and visualise fatty deposits in the liver in the presence of cirrhosis. Dilated collateral veins may be seen in conditions that result in obstruction of the venous outflow of the liver, including cirrhosis and Budd–Chiari syndrome.

- **Abdominal paracentesis**
  Aspiration of the ascitic fluid is very useful to help determine the underlying cause. A sample should be sent to microbiology, clinical chemistry and pathology.

Ascitic fluid

Appearance

Chylous   The milky white appearance of chylous ascites is due to obstruction of the lymphatic ducts.

Bile-stained   Is suggestive of bile peritonitis.

Haemorrhagic   Can occur in malignancy, trauma and TB.

Straw-coloured   The usual appearance with most other causes.

Biochemistry

Protein   Used to classify ascites based on the serum-ascites albumin gradient (SAAG). SAAG is calculated by serum albumin – ascitic fluid albumin. $>11g/L$ = high SAAG = transudate (cardiac causes, cirrhosis): $<11g/L$ = low SAAG = exudate (infective causes, malignancy, bile leak).

Amylase Usually elevated in pancreatic ascites.

Glucose Low in bacterial infections.

Triglyceride Elevated in chylous ascites; may indicate obstruction of drainage of the thoracic duct.

Bilirubin Elevated in bile ascites.

Microbiology

Gram and Ziehl–Neelsen staining with cultures may be positive with a bacterial aetiology.

Cytology

WCC Neutrophilia is suggestive of a bacterial peritonitis, while tuberculous peritonitis usually results in a lymphocytosis. Malignant cells may be identified, and a primary source may possibly be located.

SPECIFIC INVESTIGATIONS

- ■ Echocardiography
  Cardiac failure will manifest as a dilated and poorly contracting ventricle with a reduced ejection fraction. A pericardial effusion is visible as an echo-free space between the left ventricle and the pericardium. Tricuspid regurgitation can be visualised with colour-flow Doppler imaging.

- ■ Liver biopsy
  Will be able to confirm and may be able to ascertain the underlying cause of liver cirrhosis.

- ■ Renal biopsy
  Reveals the underlying cause of nephrotic syndrome.

- • Ascites can result from abnormalities in a number of different systems, and a detailed examination of all systems is required to avoid missing potentially treatable conditions, such as cardiac failure and TB.

AXILLARY SWELLINGS

The great majority of axillary swellings are enlarged lymph nodes. Axillary nodes can be enlarged due to secondary deposits from carcinoma of the breast. Most axillary swellings are easily diagnosed from clinical examination alone.

CAUSES

SUPERFICIAL

- Acute abscess
- Sebaceous cyst
- Lipoma
- Viral or bacterial infections
- Hidradenitis suppurativa

DEEP

- Lymphadenopathy (e.g. lymphoma, leukaemia, lupus)
- Benign or malignant breast lump (arising in the axillary tail) ⚠
- Lipoma
- Chronic abscess (e.g. TB)
- Axillary artery aneurysm ⚠

HISTORY

Superficial

Acute abscess

This presents as a tender erythematous swelling in the skin. There may be a purulent discharge. Common in diabetics.

Sebaceous cyst

A sebaceous cyst will present as a firm swelling in the skin, often with a punctum. It may be tender if it becomes inflamed along with discharge.

Lipoma

These present as a soft, lobulated swelling in the subcutaneous tissues and are often not tender.

Hidradenitis suppurativa

The patient presents with multiple tender swellings in the superficial tissue of the axilla, with the infection occurring in the apocrine sweat glands. A purulent discharge usually occurs. There may be a history of diabetes.

Deep

Lymphadenopathy

The patient may have noticed a lump in the axilla, which may be tender or nontender. Consider infection or malignancy in the region of drainage of the nodes, i.e. the arm, the chest wall and the abdominal wall as far down as, and including, the umbilicus, the skin of the back (as far down as the iliac crest) and the breast. Has the patient noticed any lumps elsewhere? Check for malaise, pyrexia, night sweats, cough and weight loss. There may be a history of bruising or epistaxis to suggest a haematological condition. Is there any evidence of scratches on the arm to suggest cat scratch disease, caused by Bartonella henselae, causing regional lymph node swelling?

Breast lumps

Occasionally a lump in the medial wall of the axilla may be a swelling from the axillary tail of the breast (e.g. fibroadenoma or carcinoma).

Lipoma

The patient may notice a firm swelling which appears intermittently, slipping out from under cover of the muscles.

Chronic abscess

Check for a history of TB. There may also be a history of night sweats.

Axillary artery aneurysm

This is rare and potentially life threatening. The patient may notice a pulsatile swelling under the arm. When the swelling becomes large, the patient may notice the arm moving away from the side of the body with each heart beat. Occasionally, there may be symptoms in the hand due to distal embolisation.

EXAMINATION

Superficial

Acute abscess

There may be a tender, red, fluctuant swelling with a purulent discharge.

Sebaceous cyst

A small, well-defined swelling in the skin. A punctum may be visible. If it is infected, the surrounding skin will be red and the lesion tender. Discharge may be present.

Lipoma

There will be a soft, lobulated swelling in the subcutaneous tissue.

Hidradenitis suppurativa

Multiple tender swellings with surrounding erythema and discharge of pus are present.

Deep

Lymphadenopathy

Single discrete node, e.g. lymphoma. Numerous hard nodes or matting of nodes (carcinoma). Tender fluctuant nodes (abscess). Check for infection or tumour in the area of drainage of the lymphatics. Examine the breast. Check all other sites of nodes, e.g. cervical, inguinal; check for hepatosplenomegaly.

Breast lumps

A lump on the medial wall of the axilla may be a lump in the axillary tail of the breast.

Lipoma

Deep lipomas are usually intermuscular and may be felt only in certain positions. They may slip in and out between the pectoral muscles. They may be firmer and not have the lobulated feel of a more superficial lipoma.

Chronic abscess

A fluctuant swelling presents in the axilla. With TB, there may be little or no signs of inflammation.

Axillary artery aneurysm

A pulsatile mass will be palpable within the axilla. Check the distal circulation. If an axillary artery aneurysm is large, when the patient stands with the arms by the sides, the arm moves away from the side of the body as the lump pulsates.

GENERAL INVESTIGATIONS

- **FBC, ESR**
  Hb ↓ malignant disease. WCC ↑ infection or leukaemia.
  ESR ↑ infection and malignancy. Platelets ↓ leukaemia.

- **Swab**
  Microscopy culture and sensitivity of any discharge.

SPECIAL INVESTIGATIONS

- **CXR**
  TB.

- **USS**
  Identify lymphadenopathy, lipoma or aneurysm.

- **Mantoux test**
  TB.

- **FNAC**
  Differentiate benign versus malignant.

- **Mammography**
  Characterise lumps. Part of breast cancer work-up and often used as a screening tool.
- **Arteriography**
  Assess distal circulation with axillary artery aneurysm and may also include Doppler assessment to assess blood flow.

- Cautiously examine lumps which are painless, increasing in size or not resolving.

- Consider examination of the breast in patients presenting with axillary swellings – in both male and female patients (and remember a chaperone).

- Consider systemic examination for lymphadenomathy (i.e. inguinal/hepatosplenomegaly).

BACKACHE

Backache is one of the most common complaints seen in general practice and orthopaedic clinics. Most causes are either traumatic or degenerative, but other causes are numerous and may occur as a result of pathology in almost any system of the body.

Figure 6 Bamboo spine. *Lateral radiograph of the lumbosacral spine in a patient with ankylosing spondylitis showing syndesmophytes with bamboo appearance. (Courtesy of Drs A Iagnocco and G Valesini and the EULAR Image Database.)*

CAUSES

CONGENITAL

- Kyphoscoliosis
- Spina bifida
- Spondylolisthesis

ACQUIRED

TRAUMATIC
- Vertebral fractures
- Ligamentous injury
- Joint strain
- Muscle tears

INFECTIVE ⚠
- Osteomyelitis – acute and chronic
- TB ● *(common in parts of the world where TB is endemic)*
- Discitis

INFLAMMATORY
- Ankylosing spondylitis (Fig. 6)
- Rheumatology disorders

NEOPLASTIC
- Metastases – multiple myeloma
- Primary sarcomas

DEGENERATIVE
- Osteoarthritis
- Intervertebral disc lesions

METABOLIC
- Osteoporosis (associated vertebral fractures)
- Osteomalacia

ENDOCRINE
- Cushing's disease (osteoporosis)

IDIOPATHIC
- Paget's disease
- Scheuermann's disease

PSYCHOGENIC
- Psychosomatic backache

VISCERAL
- Penetrating peptic ulcer
- Carcinoma of the pancreas
- Carcinoma of the rectum

VASCULAR ⚠
- Aortic aneurysm
- Acute aortic dissection

RENAL

- ● Renal calculus ⚠
- ● Carcinoma of the kidney
- ● Inflammatory disease

GYNAECOLOGICAL

- ● Pelvic inflammatory disease
- ● Endometriosis
- ● Uterine tumours

HISTORY

Congenital

The diagnosis is usually apparent from the history, although with spondylolisthesis, the symptoms, i.e. low lumbar backache, worse on standing, may not present until late childhood or early adult life.

Acquired

General

The speed of onset is important. Sudden onset back pain may be due to trauma or disc lesions, whereas gradual onset of pain may be due to conditions such as degenerative disease. Mechanical lesions impinging on the cord can result in neurological symptoms such as bladder dysfunction (urinary retention). Symptoms worse on movement and relieved by rest suggest a mechanical cause, whereas pain that is severe and unrelenting can occur with malignant causes. In addition, there may be symptoms (other than musculoskeletal) related to the underlying cause such as abdominal pain, dysuria or menorrhagia.

Traumatic

There will usually be a clear history of trauma. Care must be taken in moving the patient. Neurological sequelae may be obvious.

Infective

There may be a history of TB; the patient may have had night sweats or cough. Osteomyelitis of the spine may also occur in diabetes and the immunocompromised. With spinal TB, the patient is usually young and complains of malaise, fever, pain, tenderness and limitation of movement of the spine. Discitis usually presents with mild backache accompanied by leg pain.

Inflammatory

Ankylosing spondylitis usually affects young adult males. The sacroiliac joints are affected initially, then the whole spine. The patient usually presents with lumbar stiffness, especially when rising in the morning. Iritis and plantar fasciitis may also occur. Rheumatology disorders may present with symptoms in other joints.

Neoplastic

The patient is usually unwell with severe unrelenting pain, often localised to a particular area of the spine. There may be a past history of a primary tumour (e.g. bronchus, breast, thyroid, prostate or kidney) or the primary may not be apparent. The pain may have been of sudden onset with a pathological fracture, resulting in a collapsed vertebra. Rarely paraplegia may be a presenting symptom. Myeloma may present with backache.

Degenerative

Osteoarthritis usually presents in the older patient, with pain made worse on movement and relieved by rest. With intervertebral disc lesions, there is usually sudden onset of pain radiating down the back of the leg (sciatica). The pain is worse on movement, coughing and straining. Neurological symptoms may be present, e.g. weakness of a limb or bladder symptoms.

Metabolic

Osteoporosis is commonest in postmenopausal women. Osteoporosis itself does not cause pain, but pathological fractures of the vertebra may occur, causing pain. Bone pain and pathological fractures occur. Osteomalacia may occur in adults with a history of gastrectomy, steatorrhoea, renal failure or anticonvulsant therapy.

Endocrine

There may be a history of Cushing's disease or long-term steroid therapy.

Idiopathic

Paget's disease of bone may cause backache. This usually occurs over the age of 40 years. The patient may have noted other changes, e.g. enlargement of the face or bowing of the leg. Scheuermann's disease is osteochondritis of the spine. It causes backache in adolescence. The patient may present because the parents have noticed round shoulders.

Psychogenic

This is very common. Check for anxiety and depression.

Visceral

With penetrating peptic ulcer, the patient complains of epigastric pain radiating straight through to the back. The pain may be relieved by food and antacids. With carcinoma of the pancreas, the patient will describe a boring pain in the back, which is unrelenting. There will be a history of anorexia and weight loss. The patient may be jaundiced. With carcinoma of the rectum, invasion of the sacrum and the sacral plexus may occur, causing low back pain with sciatica.

Vascular

Aortic aneurysm may cause back pain by eroding into the vertebral bodies. Alternatively, it may cause severe back pain due to rupture.

The patient may have noticed a pulsation in the abdomen. Acute aortic dissection usually gives a severe tearing back pain associated with chest pain. The patient is usually shocked.

Renal

There is usually a dull, boring ache with carcinoma of the kidney. The patient may also complain of haematuria. With ureteric colic, the pain radiates from loin to groin and is severe, the patient being unable to get into a comfortable position. Inflammatory disease of the kidney presents with upper lumbar back pain. The patient may be feverish with rigors, and complain of frequency and dysuria.

Gynaecological

The pain is usually low back pain associated with pelvic discomfort. The patient may also complain of dysmenorrhoea, menorrhagia or post-menopausal bleeding.

EXAMINATION

General

Acute cord compression will cause bilateral leg pain with lower motor neurone signs at the level of the compression, and upper motor neurone signs below. Check for sphincter disturbance. Acute cauda equina compression causes root pain in the legs, saddle anaesthesia and disturbances of bladder and bowel function. In any patient with acute backache, the above signs should be sought and, if found, the appropriate urgent referral made to a neurosurgeon or spinal surgeon.

Congenital

Kyphoscoliosis and spina bifida are usually obvious on examination. With spondylolisthesis, a 'step' may be palpable in the line of the spinous processes, with a skin crease below. It usually involves L5 slipping on S1, or, less commonly, L4 slipping on L5. Occasionally, there are neurological signs in the limbs.

Acquired

Traumatic

This will usually be obvious. Careful positioning of the patient and full neurological examination should be carried out. Always check for associated injuries.

Infective

With acute osteomyelitis, there is pyrexia, malaise and local tenderness and spasm. With chronic osteomyelitis, e.g. due to TB, there will be wasting of the paraspinal muscles, spasm and restricted movements. There may be a localised kyphosis or 'gibbus' due to vertebral collapse. A psoas abscess may be present in the groin. Paraplegia may occur. With discitis, there will be reduced movement of the spine.

Inflammatory

The patient with ankylosing spondylitis will present with a stiff spine. There will be flexion of the hips and spine. In the advanced case, the patient cannot raise the head to see in front. Check for iritis and plantar fasciitis. Rheumatological disease will also present with problems in other joints.

Neoplastic

With myeloma, in addition to backache, there may be pain in the ribs, long bones and skull. Bone tenderness will be present with secondary deposits. Palpate along the spine for tenderness. Check the chest, thyroid, breast, kidney and prostate for malignancy. Check for any neurological signs.

Degenerative

There will be limitation of movement of the spine with osteoarthritis. With acute disc lesion, there will be limitation of spine movement, lordosis and neurological symptoms of the lower limbs. Carry out a full neurological examination.

Metabolic

There may be evidence of recent vertebral collapse. Loss of height and curvature of the spine may eventually occur. With osteomalacia, apart from bone pain, there may be proximal myopathy, resulting in a waddling gait.

Endocrine

There may be signs of Cushing's disease or prolonged steroid therapy, e.g. cushingoid facies, buffalo hump, proximal myopathy, abdominal striae, etc.

Idiopathic

In Paget's disease, check for changes in the skull and long bones (bowing of the tibia). Compressive symptoms due to skull enlargement may result in blindness, deafness or cranial nerve entrapment. There may be signs of high-output cardiac failure due to vascularity of bone. In Scheuermann's disease, there will be a smooth, thoracic kyphosis and, below this, a compensatory lumbar lordosis. The chest is flat.

Psychogenic

This is often difficult to assess. Signs may vary from examination to examination. There may be exaggeration of symptoms during the examination. It is best to watch from a distance as the patient leaves the consulting room.

Visceral

Check for epigastric tenderness or mass. Jaundice may be present in pancreatic cancer, and the gall bladder may be palpable (Courvoisier's law). Carry out a digital rectal examination to check for rectal carcinoma.

Vascular

A pulsatile abdominal mass may be palpable. The patient may be shocked. With acute aortic dissection, there may be shock with disparity of pulses in the extremities.

Renal

Check for renal masses or loin tenderness.

Gynaecological

Check for pelvic masses. Carry out bimanual examination.

GENERAL INVESTIGATIONS

- **FBC, ESR**
  Hb ↓ malignancy, peptic ulceration. WCC ↑ infection, e.g. osteomyelitis. ESR ↑ malignancy, e.g. myeloma or secondary deposits. TB. Ankylosing spondylitis.

- **CRP**
  ↑ infection, inflammation.

- **U&Es**
  May be abnormal in renal disease.

- **LFTs**
  Bilirubin and alkaline phosphatase will be raised in biliary tract obstruction related to carcinoma of the head of the pancreas. Alkaline phosphatase may also be raised in Paget's disease, osteomalacia and secondary deposits in bone. This is bony alkaline phosphatase and isoenzymes should be checked.

- **CXR**
  Primary tumour, e.g. bronchial carcinoma. Secondary tumours.

- **Spine X-ray**
  Trauma – fractures. Osteoarthritis – narrowed disc spaces and osteophytes. Prolapsed intervertebral disc – mild scoliosis, loss of lumbar lordosis, loss of disc space, Schmorl's node. Scheuermann's disease – wedging of vertebra and irregularity of vertebral end plates. Chronic osteomyelitis – erosion of joint surfaces, destruction of bone and intervertebral discs, soft-tissue shadows, e.g. psoas abscess. Myeloma – punched-out lesions. Secondary deposits – osteolytic or osteosclerotic (prostate). Osteoporosis – thinned bones, vertebral collapse. Ankylosing spondylitis – 'bamboo' spine; irregularity, sclerosis and fusion of sacroiliac joints. Paget's disease of bone – 'sclerotic' white vertebrae.

- **US**
  Aortic aneurysm. Renal lesions. Uterine lesions.

SPECIFIC INVESTIGATIONS

- **PSA**
  Prostatic carcinoma.
- **Serum calcium**
  Raised in malignancy, myeloma and bony metastases.
- **Urinary Bence Jones protein**
  May be raised in myeloma.
- **Plasma protein electrophoresis**
  Monoclonal gammopathy in myeloma.
- **CT**
  Pancreatic lesions. Aortic lesions. Pelvic lesions.
- **Technetium scan**
  Hot spots with bony secondaries. Occasional hot spots with inflammatory disease.
- **MRI**
  Location of disc lesion.

- In men over 55 years of age with low back pain, consider metastatic prostatic cancer. Perform a digital rectal examination.

- Acute cauda equina compression may cause bilateral sciatica, saddle anaesthesia and disturbances of bladder and bowel function. In any patient with acute backache, the above signs should be sought and, if found, urgent referral made to a neurosurgeon.

- Always remember renal and pancreatic disease and aortic aneurysm as a cause of backache.

BREAST LUMPS

A lump in the breast is a common clinical presentation. In every case of a breast lump, in both males and females, carcinoma must be excluded.

Figure 7 Left-sided breast cancer. Note the skin tethering and the nipple retraction.

CAUSES

DISCRETE LUMPS

MALIGNANT
- Carcinoma (Fig. 7) ▲
- Phyllodes tumour (some behave in benign fashion)

BENIGN
- Fibroadenoma
- Cyst (in cystic mastitis)
- Duct ectasia
- Sebaceous cyst
- Galactocele
- Fat necrosis
- Lipoma
- Tuberculous abscess ● (*common in parts of the world where TB is endemic*)

GENERALISED SWELLING

- Pregnancy
- Lactation
- Puberty
- Mastitis

SWELLINGS BEHIND THE BREAST

- Retromammary abscess from chest disease ⚠
- Tietze's disease
- Rib deformities
- Chondroma of the costal cartilages

HISTORY

A diagnosis of carcinoma is suggested by a strong family history, nulliparous state, early menarche, late menopause and history of cystic hyperplasia. The patient may have found a breast lump (carcinoma is painless in 85% of cases) or may have noticed nipple retraction, skin dimpling, axillary swelling. Jaundice may have occurred due to liver secondaries or porta hepatis node involvement. Bone pain may be due to secondary deposits and pathological fractures. Breathlessness may be due to lung secondaries or a pleural effusion. Personality change, fits, headaches suggest cerebral metastases. A patient who presents in pregnancy or lactation may have mastitis, abscess or galactocele. A history of trauma suggests fat necrosis. A patient in the fifth decade with retroareolar pain, nipple retraction and a thick, creamy nipple discharge suggests duct ectasia. The patient presenting between the ages of 15 and 25 years with a nontender swelling suggests fibroadenoma. A patient with a history of painful breasts may have one of the conditions described under breast pain (p. 48). Enquiries should be made of a past history of TB, as rarely a tuberculous abscess may form within the breast or erode through the chest wall from the lung.

EXAMINATION

Carcinoma

Hard irregular swelling. May be fixed to the skin or fixed deeply. Skin dimpling. Nipple retraction. *Peau d'orange*. Paget's disease of the nipple. Axillary lymphadenopathy. Supraclavicular lymphadenopathy. Hepatomegaly. Pathological fractures – spine, ribs, long bones.

Phyllodes Tumour

Mobile mass may become very large.

Fibroadenoma

Smooth, rounded, mobile mass. Breast 'mouse' (so-called because it darts about under the examining fingers).

Cyst

Smooth, mobile swelling. May be tender. May be associated with generalised lumpiness of the breast.

Galactocele

Smooth, mobile swelling occurring in the lactating breast.

Fat necrosis

Hard, irregular swelling. May be overlying bruising of the skin or teeth marks! Occasionally, the lesion is fixed to the skin and is difficult to distinguish from carcinoma.

Lipoma

Soft, lobulated swelling. Rare on the breast. 'Pseudolipoma' is a bunching of fat between retracted suspensory ligaments of the breast and is associated with an underlying carcinoma.

Duct ectasia

Tender retroareolar area. Retroareolar erythema. Nipple retraction. Thick, creamy nipple discharge.

Sebaceous cyst

Mobile swelling fixed to the skin. May be a punctum. May be infected, with discharge and surrounding redness.

Generalised swellings

Generalised swelling of the breast may occur in pregnancy, lactation and puberty. It may also occur with mastitis, when the breast is enlarged, red, tender and hot.

Swellings behind the breast

These are rare. Tietze's disease is the most common. There will be prominence and tenderness over the second, third and fourth costal cartilages. With retromammary abscess, chest signs may be obvious on percussion and also on auscultation of the chest.

GENERAL INVESTIGATIONS

- **FBC, ESR & CRP**
  Hb ↓ widespread malignancy. ↑ WCC & CRP breast abscess.
  ESR ↑ malignancy and TB.
- **LFTs**
  Alkaline phosphatase ↑ with liver secondaries and bone secondaries (isoenzymes).
- **Serum calcium**
  ↑ in bone secondaries.

SPECIFIC INVESTIGATIONS

- **Mammography**
  Infiltrating radio-opaque mass or microcalcification indicates malignancy. Dilated retroareolar ducts and skin indentation suggests duct ectasia. Coarse calcification may occur with long-standing fibroadenomas.

- **US**
  US of breast is better than mammography in young women. US of liver for metastases. US-guided FNA/core biopsy/Mammotome®.

- **FNAC +/− core biopsy**
  Benign versus malignant. Cystic versus solid. A biopsy may be considered when malignancy is suspected and FNAC inconclusive.

- **Open excision biopsy**
  E.g. fibroadenoma, fat necrosis.

- **CXR**
  Secondary deposits in lung and rib. Underlying chest disease, e.g. TB or empyema.

- **CT**
  Abdomen, chest, brain. Metastases.

- **Bone scan**
  Metastases.

- **BRCA1, BRCA2**
  Gene mutations in breast cancer.

- Skin dimpling and nipple retraction indicate carcinoma until proved otherwise.

- Breast lumps after the menopause are most likely to be due to carcinoma.

BREAST PAIN

Pain in the breast is a common symptom in general surgical practice. Most cases are benign and due to cyclical mastalgia, but occasionally pain may be the presenting symptom of carcinoma.

Figure 8 A large abscess of the left breast. Note the redness and swelling.

CAUSES

- Cyclical mastalgia (fibroadenosis, cystic mastitis)
- Noncyclical mastalgia
- Duct ectasia
- Breast abscess (Fig. 8) ▲
- Pregnancy
- Lactation
- Carcinoma (15% of lumps are painful) ▲
- Fat necrosis
- Mastitis
- Tietze's disease
- Mondor's disease ▲
- Rib secondaries
- Herpes zoster

HISTORY

Cyclical mastalgia causes soreness, frequently in the upper and outer quadrants of the breast in the week preceding a period. The pain usually disappears after the period, and there is freedom from soreness or pain for 2 weeks, when it recommences. Symptoms are common in the 20–45-year age group. Noncyclical mastalgia may occur and is more common in the fourth and fifth decades. Duct ectasia occurs in the fifth decade. The pain is usually behind the nipple and associated with subareolar erythema and a thick, creamy nipple discharge. Fat necrosis will be suggested by a history of trauma, which occasionally the patient will be embarrassed to admit (often the partner's teeth!). Breast abscess or mastitis will be obvious. It usually occurs during pregnancy or lactation, but it may occur in a retroareolar position in a patient with duct ectasia. Breast fullness and soreness is a symptom of early pregnancy. Patients may indicate breast pain where the condition is not actively in the breast but behind it. Tietze's disease (costochondritis of the costal cartilages) will present with pain related to the breast. Mondor's disease (superficial thrombophlebitis of the subcutaneous veins of the chest wall) also presents with pain in the breast. It may be associated with an underlying carcinoma. Rib secondaries may also present with pain behind the breast. Herpes zoster may present with pain radiating round into the breast and precedes the development of a vesicular eruption by 2–3 days.

EXAMINATION

A hard, irregular lump is suggestive of carcinoma (this is discussed in the section on Breast lumps). Tenderness and lumpiness, occasionally with a smooth, mobile swelling (cyst), is suggestive of cyclical mastalgia. The tenderness and lumpiness is most often palpated in the upper and outer quadrants of the breast. In the early stages of fat necrosis, there may be bruising over the breast, and the lump is tender. In the later stages, it becomes hard and irregular and may be tethered to the skin. Breast abscess will present with redness, swelling, heat and pain in the breast during pregnancy or, more commonly, lactation. The swelling will be fluctuant and usually there is associated fever. Duct ectasia presents with subareolar erythema, tenderness and occasionally a subareolar lump. Nipple retraction may be present in longstanding cases, and there may be a thick, creamy discharge that can be expressed from the nipple. Pregnancy will present with fullness of the breast and increased circumareolar pigmentation. In Tietze's disease, there will be tenderness, and occasionally swelling over the second, third and fourth costal cartilages. In Mondor's disease, the veins of the chest wall are felt as red, tender cords, often extending onto the anterior axillary fold. The breast should be carefully checked for an underlying mass, as the condition may be associated with carcinoma of the breast. Herpes zoster will usually present with a characteristic vesicular eruption a few days after the pain.

GENERAL INVESTIGATIONS

- **FBC, ESR, CRP**
  WCC & CRP ↑ in inflammatory pathologies (i.e. mastitis and breast abscess). ESR ↑ widespread carcinoma.

- **LFTs**
  Alkaline phosphatase may be raised with liver or bony secondaries.

- **Serum calcium**
  May be raised with bone secondaries.

- **βHCG**
  Positive in pregnancy.

- **Swab**
  C&S if there is any discharge from an abscess or from the nipple.

- **CXR**
  Secondaries in lung or ribs. Pleural effusion in carcinoma.

SPECIFIC INVESTIGATIONS

- **Mammography**
  Carcinoma. Duct ectasia.

- **US**
  US of breast is better than mammography in young women.

- **FNAC +/− core biopsy**
  Benign versus malignant. Cystic versus solid. Biopsy may be considered if a malignant pathology is suspected and FNAC inconclusive.

- **Bone scan**
  Rib secondaries. Myeloma.

- Always examine the breasts in a patient with breast pain, even if the history strongly suggests cyclical mastalgia.

- Pain is a relatively uncommon presenting symptom of breast cancer.

- In women of childbearing age, always consider the likelihood of pregnancy as a cause of breast pain.

CHEST PAIN

Chest pain is a common presenting symptom of disorders that can range from trivial to life-threatening.

Figure 9 Anterior ST segment elevation myocardial infarction (STEMI).

CAUSES

CARDIOVASCULAR

- Angina
- Myocardial infarction ⚠
- Pericarditis/myocarditis
- Acute aortic dissection ⚠

GASTROINTESTINAL

- Gastro-oesophageal reflux disease
- Peptic ulcer disease
- Oesophageal spasm

PULMONARY

- Pneumonia
- Pneumothorax ⚠
- Pulmonary embolism ⚠

MUSCULOSKELETAL

- Chest wall trauma
- Herpes zoster
- Costochondritis
- Secondary tumours of the rib

MISCELLANEOUS

- Fibromyalgia
- Depression

HISTORY

Character

The character of angina is tight and crushing, while the pain from aortic dissection has a tearing quality. Pericarditis typically causes pain of a sharp, stabbing nature. Oesophageal reflux may be described as a burning pain, and peptic acid-related pain tends to be deep and gnawing.

Location

The pain from angina and oesophageal reflux may be located retrosternally, and they both can radiate to the jaw or down into the left arm. The pain from pericarditis may be centrally located and radiate to the shoulders (trapezius ridge pain). Pain from aortic dissection often radiates into the back and occasionally into the abdomen (depending on the extent of the dissection). Pulmonary pain can be located anywhere in the thorax.

Precipitating factors

Stable angina may be precipitated by effort, a defining characteristic. Other known precipitants of angina are emotion, food and cold weather. Anginal symptoms occurring at rest may represent unstable or crescendo angina and should be treated in the same manner as a myocardial infarction. Oesophageal reflux is often related to meals and precipitated by changes in posture, such as bending or lying flat. Pain originating from pericarditis and pulmonary origin is often pleuritic, i.e. worse on inspiration; however, musculoskeletal pain can also be worse on breathing due to movement of the thorax. Musculoskeletal pain is usually tender, helping to differentiate it from other causes.

Relieving factors

Both oesophageal spasm and angina may be relieved by nitrates, which relax smooth muscle. Antacids will relieve the pain of oesophageal reflux but not angina. The pain associated with pericarditis may be relieved by sitting forwards and anti-inflammatory analgesics.

Trauma

A history of a blunt or stretching injury immediately suggests the underlying aetiology of chest wall tenderness, and it is important to diagnose rib fractures that can result from more severe trauma. Pathological rib fractures that result from minor injuries may be due to bony metastasis or osteoporosis.

Miscellaneous

Fibromyalgia may present with symptoms of chest pain very similar in nature to angina. Occasionally, chest pain is a somatic manifestation of patients with depression or anxiety. In both cases, it is essential to exclude all organic causes before accepting either as the underlying cause. Moreover, a serious aetiology may co-exist.

EXAMINATION

Temperature

Pyrexia can occur with pneumonia, myocardial infarction, pericarditis and herpes zoster infection.

Pulse

Heart rate on its own is not discriminating, as pain invariably leads to tachycardia. However, palpating both upper and lower limb pulses may be useful. Occasionally, peripheral pulses are absent in patients with aortic dissection.

JVP

The JVP is elevated with congestive cardiac failure and acute right ventricular failure, an occasional complication of inferior myocardial infarction and pulmonary embolism (when more than 60% of the pulmonary vascular supply is occluded).

Palpation of the chest

Chest wall tenderness would imply a musculoskeletal cause. The presence of unilateral tenderness confined to a single or adjacent group of dermatomes would suggest either central (vertebral or spinal origin) or peripheral nerve pathology (herpes zoster infection). The trachea deviates away from the side of a tension pneumothorax, and chest expansion is decreased on the same side for pneumonia and pneumothorax. Dullness to percussion will be noted in an area of consolidation with pneumonia and hyperresonance with pneumothorax (a difficult sign to interpret).

Auscultation of the chest

The unilateral absence of breath sounds is consistent with a pneumothorax; more localised loss occurs over an effusion. Bronchial breath sounds are audible over a segment of consolidation and sometimes above the level of an effusion. Localised areas of crepitations are audible with lobar pneumonia, whereas widespread crepitations suggest multilobar involvement or pulmonary oedema secondary to left ventricular failure (from myocardial infarction).

A friction rub may be auscultated with both pericardial and pleuritic disease, but only a pericardial rub will be present when the patient holds their breath.

Lower limbs

Hemiparesis can occur with aortic dissection, and a hot, swollen, tender calf or thigh may give a clue to an underlying deep vein thrombosis. Measurements of the mid-thigh or mid-calf circumference may demonstrate a larger circumference on the side of a DVT.

GENERAL INVESTIGATIONS

- FBC
  An elevated white cell count will be expected with pneumonia and, to a lesser extent, in a myocardial infarction.

- Serum cardiac markers
  Following a myocardial infarction, cardiac troponin rises within six hours and remains elevated for up to 2 weeks.

- ECG (Fig. 9)
  Angina or a myocardial infarct will result in ECG changes following the anatomical pattern of coronary vascular insufficiency. Involvement of the left main coronary artery would result in ECG changes of ischaemia or infarction in the anterior (V3–4) and left lateral (V4–6) leads. Involvement of the left anterior descending artery will be reflected in the anterior leads, and right coronary artery occlusion will produce changes in the inferior leads (II, III, aVF). Changes suggestive of ischaemia or NSTEMI are ST segment depression and T wave inversion. Elevated serum cardiac markers distinguish NSTEMI from angina. ST segment elevation infarcts (STEMI), by definition, produce ST segment elevation in the corresponding leads. Pulmonary emboli can result in nonspecific ECG changes, such as tachycardia, right axis deviation, right ventricular strain and atrial fibrillation. Occasionally, one may find the S1Q3T3 pattern (S wave in lead I, Q wave and an inverted T wave in lead III), indicative of right heart strain.

- CXR
  The line of the pleura with absence of lung markings distal to it is the usual finding for a pneumothorax. Areas of consolidation on a chest film may be confined to a lobe or widespread in bronchopneumonia. The classic wedge-shaped shadow (base is distal) of a pulmonary embolus is rare, and occurs only if pulmonary infarction resulted. Dissection of the aorta may widen its width, causing a bulge to appear at the right mediastinal border. Rib fractures or secondary deposits in ribs may be visible.

SPECIFIC INVESTIGATIONS

- Coronary angiography
  Usually indicated in the case of myocardial infarction or unstable angina. It allows visualisation of the coronary arteries and occlusions or significant stenosis may be treated with angioplasty and stenting.

- Functional cardiac imaging
  Usually used in the context of stable angina to assess for significant inducible ischaemia by examining cardiac function when myocardial demand is increased, either through exercise or drug therapy. Imaging modalities include stress echocardiography, nuclear myocardial perfusion imaging or stress perfusion cardiac MRI.

- **CT Pulmonary angiography**
  Pulmonary emboli will be delineated. It is possible to visualise the site and extent of the embolism, as well as any signs of right heart strain.
- **CT aortography**
  Confirm and assess the extent and site of the dissection of the aorta.
- **Upper GI tract endoscopy**
  Oesophagitis.
- **Oesophageal manometry**
  Abnormal oesophageal pressures.

- It is important to perform a prompt history, examination and initial investigations in patients who present with chest pain, as a number of conditions require urgent management.
- If tension pneumothorax is suspected as a cause of chest pain, do not wait for a chest film. Decompress the pneumothorax immediately with a large-bore cannula inserted into the 2nd intercostal space in the midclavicular line.

CLUBBING

Clubbing is the selective bulbous enlargement of the distal segments of fingers or toes due to proliferation of connective tissues (Fig. 10).

Figure 10 Clubbing. Note the exaggerated longitudinal curvature and the loss of angle between the nail and the nailbed.

CAUSES

RESPIRATORY

- Bronchial carcinoma
- Chronic suppurative lung disease
  - Bronchiectasis
  - Lung abscess
  - Empyema
  - Cystic fibrosis
- Interstitial lung disease (fibrosing alveolitis, pulmonary fibrosis)

CARDIOVASCULAR

- Infective endocarditis ● *(common in developing countries)*
- Congenital cyanotic heart disease

GASTROINTESTINAL

- Cirrhosis
- Ulcerative colitis
- Crohn's disease
- Coeliac disease

OTHER

- Graves' disease (hyperthyroidism)
- Familial

Clubbing is said to be present when there is loss of the normal angle between the base of the nail and the nailfold. In the presence of clubbing, when the fingernails from each hand are placed together, the gap is lost, and this is known as Schamroth's sign. Other features are increased curvature of the nailbed (in all directions), sponginess or fluctuation and expansion of the end of the digit to resemble a drumstick.

HISTORY

A systematic approach to the history is required to determine the cause of clubbing. Respiratory, cardiovascular and gastrointestinal system enquiries should be made in an attempt to determine the underlying cause. A detailed discussion on the diagnosis of congenital cyanotic heart disease (tetralogy of Fallot, transposition of great arteries, total anomalous pulmonary venous drainage) is beyond the scope of this text.

Duration

The duration of clubbing may give an indication of the underlying aetiology. Clubbing present since infancy would suggest a familial trait or congenital cyanotic heart disease. Alternatively, it may be a secondary manifestation of hereditary disorders, such as coeliac disease and cystic fibrosis.

Respiratory symptoms

A history of cough, haemoptysis, dyspnoea and weight loss in a chronic smoker should alert the clinician to the diagnosis of bronchial carcinoma. Symptoms of metastasis (bone pain, jaundice) and paraneoplastic involvement (neuropathy, thirst and polyuria from hypercalcaemia) should also be ascertained. With bronchial carcinoma, clubbing may be part of a generalised arthritic manifestation of hypertrophic pulmonary osteoarthropathy.

Cough productive of copious amounts of purulent sputum is usually the main complaint with bronchiectasis. With a chronic lung abscess or empyema, the symptoms are often less specific and may be preceded by a history of pneumonia or aspiration secondary to neurological disorders, dysphagia or alcoholism. Patients may present with a persistent low-grade pyrexia, malaise, weight loss and productive cough. Shortness of breath and a nonproductive cough characterise interstitial lung disease.

Gastrointestinal symptoms

Malaise, diarrhoea, abdominal pain and weight loss are experienced by most patients with inflammatory bowel disease and coeliac disease. The presence of aphthous ulceration, fistulae and perianal sepsis are suggestive of Crohn's disease. Predominantly rectal involvement with tenesmus, mucus and rectal bleeding is more characteristic of ulcerative colitis; however, differentiation based on history alone can be very difficult. Symptoms of coeliac disease tend to be very variable and nonspecific, with nonbloody diarrhoea with steatorrhoea.

Heavy alcohol consumption or previous infection with hepatitis B will predispose to cirrhosis of the liver. Patients may complain of jaundice, abdominal distension due to ascites (p. 27), upper gastrointestinal haemorrhage due to varices or bruising from impaired clotting (p. 513). Severely affected individuals may present with encephalopathy or even coma (p. 61).

Family history

A family history of clubbing or cystic fibrosis will suggest a hereditary cause. Approximately 15% of patients with coeliac disease will have an affected first-degree relative.

EXAMINATION

Inspection

The presence of wasting may be accounted for by cachexia of malignancy or chronic lung or gastrointestinal disease. The mucous membranes should be inspected for central cyanosis, which may be a feature of, or sequel to, congenital cyanotic heart disease. Cyanosis may also be noticeable with any of the previous causes of severe lung disease. Aphthous ulceration occurs with Crohn's and coeliac disease. A goitre, exophthalmos, ophthalmoplegia and a resting tremor are features of Graves' disease.

With infective endocarditis, splinter haemorrhages, Osler's nodes (raised tender lesions on the pulps of the fingers) and Janeway lesions (flat nontender macules on the palms and soles) may also be present.

Temperature

Pyrexia is notable in several important causes of clubbing, namely suppurative lung disease, infective endocarditis and active inflammatory bowel disease.

Examination of the chest

Auscultation of the precordium may reveal new or changing murmurs with infective endocarditis. Widespread coarse crepitations of the lungs occur with retained secretions of bronchiectasis. Fine quality end-inspiratory crepitations are suggestive of interstitial lung disease. More localised coarse crepitations and dullness to percussion may be found with a lung abscess. Findings suggestive of pleural effusion (unilateral decreased expansion, dullness to percussion and absent breath sounds) may be due to malignancy. However, when this is associated with pyrexia in an ill patient, it should lead to the consideration of a thoracic empyema.

Abdominal examination

On abdominal examination, signs of chronic liver disease (p. 29) may be present; however, there may be few specific features to suggest inflammatory bowel disease. When this diagnosis is suspected, a sigmoidoscopy should always be performed. Occasionally, right iliac fossa tenderness or a mass may be found in Crohn's disease. The presence of splenomegaly may indicate portal hypertension with liver disease, or enlargement accompanying infective endocarditis.

GENERAL INVESTIGATIONS

- FBC
  Hb ↓ carcinomatosis, inflammatory bowel disease, infective endocarditis.
  WCC ↑ lung abscess, empyema, inflammatory bowel disease.
- ESR/CRP
  Malignancy, inflammatory bowel disease, infective endocarditis.
- LFTs
  Liver disease.
- CXR
  Should be performed if respiratory symptoms are present.
  Bronchial carcinoma may manifest as a hilar or peripheral opacity, cavitating mass, collapse of a segment of lung due to luminal obstruction, pleural effusion, elevated hemidiaphragm due to phrenic nerve palsy or destruction of an adjacent rib due to invasion. Lung abscesses present as a spherical shadow with a central lucency or air-fluid level. Bronchiectatic lungs have visibly dilated bronchi and multiple areas of consolidation. With fibrosing alveolitis, hazy shadowing of the lung bases produces a honeycomb appearance.

SPECIFIC INVESTIGATIONS

In view of the diverse nature of causes of clubbing, further investigations should be guided by the history and findings on clinical examination.

- **Urinalysis**
  Blood from microemboli in infective endocarditis.
- **Blood cultures (three sets in total: two sites at the same time, and then one taken 12 hours later)**
  Infective endocarditis.
- **Echocardiography**
  Useful in the diagnosis of infective endocarditis, especially in the presence of large vegetations.
- **Sigmoidoscopy**
  Inflammatory bowel disease – characteristic findings include erythematous mucosa, areas of haemorrhage, contact bleeding and ulceration.
- **Rectal and colonic biopsy**
  Ulcerative colitis and Crohn's disease.
- **Colonoscopy**
  Inflammatory bowel disease.
- **Barium enema**
  Inflammatory bowel disease.
- **Small bowel enema**
  Crohn's disease.
- **Anti-tissue transglutaminase (ATA)**
  Coeliac disease.
- **Jejunal biopsy**
  Coeliac disease. May reveal subtotal villous atrophy reversible with a gluten-free diet.
- **CT thorax**
  Should be performed if bronchial carcinoma or thoracic empyema is suspected. Also useful to confirm the diagnosis of bronchiectasis and idiopathic pulmonary fibrosis.

- Malignancy must be excluded when clubbing develops. Localising features such as respiratory or gastrointestinal disease associated with weight loss and raised inflammatory markers are ominous signs. Investigation is tailored to the presentation.

COMA

Coma can be defined as a state of prolonged unconsciousness from which a person cannot be roused, or numerically categorised as a GCS score of <8.

Figure 11 CT of the head. There is a left-sided extradural haematoma (arrow). The haematoma is confined, giving rise to its characteristic biconvex shape, with a well-defined margin.

CAUSES ⚠ (ALL CAUSES OF COMA REQUIRE EMERGENCY ASSESSMENT)

TRAUMA

- Head injury (diffuse axonal injury)
- Extradural haemorrhage (Fig. 11)
- Subdural haemorrhage

METABOLIC

- Diabetic ketoacidosis
- Hypoglycaemia
- Hypothermia

- Hyperglycaemia
- Hyponatraemia
- Hypernatraemia

ORGAN FAILURE

- Cardiac/circulatory failure
- Respiratory failure
- Liver failure (encephalopathy)
- Renal failure (uraemic coma)
- Hypothyroidism

VASCULAR

- Ischaemic stroke
- Subarachnoid haemorrhage

INFECTIVE

- Meningitis
- Encephalitis
- Cerebral malaria in the developed world ● *(common in endemic areas)*

TOXIN/DRUG-INDUCED

- Alcohol
- Overdose (opiates, tricyclics, benzodiazepines)
- Carbon monoxide poisoning

CEREBRAL

- Epilepsy
- Brain tumour
- Brain abscess

HISTORY

The history for the comatose patient is usually obtained collaterally from relatives, friends, witnesses or ambulance crew. Other sources of information are previous hospital notes, records kept by general practitioners and tablets or prescriptions that have been found at the patient's premises.

Presentation

The circumstances regarding discovery of the patient is usually the first piece of information to be reported. Trauma patients may have been transported from sites of road traffic accidents, fire or have been found assaulted on the street. When teenagers are brought in unconscious from a night club, it is important to exclude alcohol intoxication, epilepsy, hypoglycaemia and the effects of illicit drugs (e.g. malignant hyperthermia with 'ecstasy'). Attempted suicides may have an accompanying note or drug bottles may have been recovered from the scene. Carbon monoxide poisoning occurs with suicide attempts in enclosed areas with running engines or may be a complication in victims involved with fires. Patients who have been brought in from cold environments may also have hypothermia in addition to the primary event.

Onset

When witnessed, information regarding the speed of onset of coma may help in determining a cause. Sudden onset of unconsciousness is characteristic of a seizure or a vascular event.

Trauma

Head injuries are a common cause of coma, but not all causes are due to blunt trauma to the cranium. Diffuse axonal injury results from severe shearing forces on the brain, a sequel to rapid acceleration and deceleration forces. Blunt head injuries may cause extradural haemorrhages as a result of skull fractures with laceration of meningeal arteries. There is usually a history of an injury with transient loss of consciousness, a lucid interval in which the patient feels and appears well, followed by drowsiness, headache, vomiting, progressive hemiplegia and eventually coma. Subdural haemorrhages are a consequence of severe trauma, with cortical lacerations or less severe trauma, with laceration of bridging veins. Chronic subdural haemorrhages may result even in the absence of trauma; elderly patients with cortical atrophy are predisposed to this type of injury.

In addition to head injury, coma may also complicate any other condition severe enough to result in circulatory or respiratory insufficiency.

Headache

The onset of severe headache prior to coma may be caused by trauma, subarachnoid haemorrhage (classically, patients complain of a sudden onset of blinding headache, the worst ever experienced) or meningitis (headache associated with photophobia and neck stiffness). Progressive headache, worse in the mornings and associated with vomiting, may be due to raised intracranial pressure from a cerebral tumour.

Predisposing factors

The history of possible predisposing factors is useful when assessing the comatose patient. The presence of diabetes should lead to the consideration of ketoacidosis and hypoglycaemia (oral hypoglycaemic or insulin dosage errors). Patients with known hepatic or renal failure may deteriorate to coma as a result of encephalopathy or uraemia, respectively. Coma may also complicate severe hypothyroidism. Previous suicide attempts or a history of depression should lead to the consideration of drug overdose. Epileptic patients may be in status epilepticus or in a post-ictal recovery state. Pre-existing cardiac or respiratory disease may result in coma as a terminal event.

EXAMINATION

Temperature

Body temperature should be recorded, and a series of normal body temperatures will exclude hypothermia and hyperpyrexia as a consequence of heat stroke or illicit drug use.

General examination

A thorough inspection should be performed. This will necessitate removal of clothing, log rolling (to examine the back) and a detailed examination of the scalp for bleeding, haematomas and fractures. The presence of bilateral periorbital haematomas or cerebrospinal fluid rhinorrhoea may indicate an anterior fossa fracture of the skull. Bruising over the mastoid (Battle's sign) or cerebrospinal fluid otorrhoea may be due to a middle cranial fossa fracture. Patients with carbon monoxide poisoning may appear bright red. Patients with myxoedema are characteristically obese, with coarse features, dry skin and brittle hair. The arms should be carefully scrutinised for lacerations and needle puncture sites suggestive of drug abuse and thus the possibility of opiate overdose. A petechial rash may be visible with meningococcal meningitis.

The organ systems should be examined in turn; suspect encephalopathy if signs suggestive of liver disease are present (p. 29) or uraemia with chronic renal failure. The pulse should be examined for arrhythmias, which may precipitate cardiac failure. The JVP may also be elevated. Other causes of JVP distension include tension pneumothorax and cardiac tamponade, both of which may embarrass the circulation and precipitate unconsciousness.

Auscultation of the chest may reveal bilateral crepitations with pulmonary oedema from left ventricular failure, bronchopneumonia, chronic bronchitis or aspiration.

Neurological examination

The neurological examination should begin with the GCS score. Patients who are not involved in trauma should be assessed for neck stiffness, which may result from meningitis or subarachnoid haemorrhage. Trauma patients should have the cervical spine assessed for injury before any manipulation is undertaken. The pupils should be examined for size and light reflex. Pinpoint pupils occur with opiate overdoses, small pupils with brainstem lesions and dilated pupils with cocaine or amphetamine use, hypoglycaemia, post-ictal states and brainstem death. A unilateral fixed and dilated pupil occurs with an oculomotor nerve lesion, which may result from pressure exerted from intracranial haemorrhage or tumour. Fundoscopy should be performed to identify loss of retinal vein pulsation or frank papilloedema indicating raised intracranial pressure. A limited neurological examination can be performed on comatose patients; this will include assessment of tone, reflexes and the Babinski response. Unilateral increased tone, hyperreflexia and an up-going plantar response is indicative of a contralateral upper motor neurone lesion, such as a stroke, intracranial haemorrhage or tumour.

GENERAL INVESTIGATIONS

- FBC
  ↑ WCC with meningitis. Viral meningitis is associated with lymphocytosis, and neutrophilia is associated with bacterial meningitis.

- Blood glucose
  A bedside blood sugar estimation is very useful to exclude hypoglycaemia.

- Urinalysis
  Ketones will be present in diabetic ketoacidosis. The urine should also be sent for toxicology analysis if poisoning is suspected.

- U&Es
  The urea and creatinine is elevated with renal failure. Disorders of sodium levels will be readily identified.

- LFTs
  The bilirubin and transaminases are markedly elevated in liver failure.

- TFTs
  ↑ TSH, ↓ T_4 with hypothyroidism.

- Toxicology screen
  For cases of suspected poisoning and overdose, serum levels of salicylates and paracetamol will be helpful in both diagnosis and treatment. Ethanol levels should also be checked, and carboxyhaemoglobin levels if carbon monoxide poisoning is suspected.

- ECG
  An ECG is useful to diagnose arrhythmia and myocardial infarction (p. 54); either disorder may compromise the circulation.

- CXR
  May reveal pulmonary oedema or lobar consolidation due to infection or aspiration.

- X-ray cervical spine
  Exclude fracture in traumatic causes of coma.

- CT
  With a history of trauma or clinical signs which suggest head injury, a CT scan should be requested (this is in preference to a skull X-ray). Additionally, CT will reveal the presence and location of intracranial bleeding and tumours.

SPECIFIC INVESTIGATIONS

- **Lumbar puncture**
  A lumbar puncture is performed in cases of suspected meningitis and the CSF (which may be turbid) is then sent for microscopy and culture.

- **EEG**
  The EEG is indicated when the diagnosis of epilepsy is suspected. Status epilepticus, however, should be diagnosed and treated clinically. The EEG is also useful in the diagnosis of encephalitis.

- Coma is a medical or surgical emergency. The cause must be identified as rapidly as possible in order to improve the prognosis. Early brain imaging is advised once metabolic causes have been excluded.

CONFUSION

Confusion is a behavioural state of reduced mental clarity, coherence, comprehension and reasoning. The causes may be organic or psychiatric. The organic causes are listed below.

CAUSES ⚠ (ALL CAUSES OF ACUTE CONFUSION REQUIRE URGENT ASSESSMENT)

TOXINS/DRUGS
- Alcohol intoxication/withdrawal
- Drug intoxication

HYPOXIA
- Respiratory disorders
- Cardiac failure

METABOLIC DISORDER
- Hyperglycaemia/hypoglycaemia
- Electrolyte imbalance, e.g. sodium, calcium
- Thiamine (vitamin B_1) deficiency
- Vitamin B_{12} deficiency
- Folate deficiency

SYSTEMIC DISEASE
- Renal failure
- Liver failure
- Thyroid disorders

NEUROLOGICAL
- Head injuries
- Epilepsy (post-ictal)
- Stroke/TIA
- Cerebral metastasis
- Intracerebral haemorrhage

INFECTION
- Urinary tract infection
- Respiratory tract infections
- Sepsis
- Meningitis/encephalitis

MISCELLANEOUS
● Dementia
● Constipation
● Environmental changes (elderly)

HISTORY

Onset

Sudden onset of confusion may be precipitated by head injuries, epilepsy, stroke and metabolic disorders. Systemic infection, systemic disease and cerebral metastasis tend to pursue a more gradual onset.

Past medical history

Diabetes is associated with abnormalities of glucose levels, with hyperglycaemia resulting from poor diabetic control, and hypoglycaemia developing due to drug administration error, missing meals or unaccustomed exercise. A history of thyroid disorder is very relevant and confusion can result from both hyper- and hypothyroidism. The presence of carcinoma may precipitate confusion as a result of cerebral metastasis or the development of hypercalcaemia. Encephalopathy is a feature of both liver failure and thiamine deficiency. Renal disease can lead to confusion from uraemic encephalopathy or as a result of electrolyte disorders. Hypoxia may result from cardiac failure and respiratory disease. There may be an underlying history of chronic cognitive impairment prior to the acute presentation, and this is important to elicit.

Drug history

Both the use and abrupt withdrawal of benzodiazepines, barbiturates, steroids and illicit drugs can result in confusion. A drug history is especially important in the elderly, as many drugs may precipitate confusion. Alcohol intoxication and withdrawal may cause confusion.

Associated symptoms

Confusion with associated motor weakness may be due to a stroke, intracerebral haemorrhage or cerebral metastasis. Sensory deficits may result from thiamine and vitamin B_{12} deficiencies. The elderly are particularly susceptible to confusion precipitated by respiratory or urinary tract infections and may complain of pyrexia or cough with purulent sputum, or dysuria, frequency, malodorous urine, pyuria and haematuria, respectively. Occasionally, myocardial infarction may present as confusion in the elderly.

EXAMINATION

Temperature

The presence of pyrexia is suggestive of an infective aetiology and a focus for this should be sought.

General

The mental state should be assessed and level of consciousness documented by a GCS score. Careful inspection may reveal scalp lacerations, bleeding or haematoma to suggest the presence of head injury. The antecubital forearm veins and groins may have evidence of needle punctures with intravenous drug abuse.

Systemic examination

Examination of the systems is required to identify general features suggestive of cardiac, respiratory, liver, renal and thyroid diseases.

Neurological examination

The cranial nerves are examined, and the presence of nystagmus may be due to acute alcohol intoxication, phenytoin toxicity, barbiturate overdose or cerebellar disease from chronic alcohol abuse. When nystagmus is associated with ocular palsies and ataxia, it is suggestive of Wernicke–Korsakoff syndrome, caused by thiamine deficiency. Isolated cranial nerve abnormalities may also result from meningitis. The motor system is examined and unilateral upper motor neurone weakness may be due to stroke or cerebral metastasis. Sensory neuropathy can result from diabetes, renal failure, alcoholism, carcinoma, thiamine and vitamin B_{12} deficiency. With subacute combined degeneration of the cord from vitamin B_{12} deficiency, there is predominant involvement of the posterior columns, with loss of vibration, proprioception and light touch. Classically, loss of ankle jerks and an extensor plantar response accompany this.

GENERAL INVESTIGATIONS

- **Blood glucose**
  Hypoglycaemia/hyperglycaemia.
- **Oxygen saturation**
  ↓ with cardiac or respiratory disorder.
- **ABGs**
  Hypercapnia with respiratory disease. Hypoxaemia.
- **Infection screen**
  Sputum, urine and blood cultures.
- **Toxicology screen**
  Plasma and urine for alcohol or specific drug/toxin.
- **FBC**
  Macrocytic anaemia with vitamin B_{12}, folate or thyroid deficiency. WCC ↑ indicate likely infection. Thick blood film if malaria is suspected.
- **U&Es**
  ↓ or ↑ sodium, ↑ urea and creatinine with renal failure.
- **LFTs**
  ↑ bilirubin and transaminases with liver failure.

- Serum calcium
  ↑ or ↓.
- TFTs
  Hypothyroidism (myxoedema). Hyperthyroidism.
- B_{12} assay
  ↓ with subacute combined degeneration of the cord.
- Serum folate
  ↓ conditions causing folate deficiency.
- ECG
  To screen for silent myocardial infarction.
- CXR
  Bronchial or lobar consolidation – pneumonia.

SPECIFIC INVESTIGATIONS

- CT or MRI head
  Cerebral metastasis. Stroke. Head injuries.
- EEG
  Epilepsy.
- Lumbar puncture
  Meningitis.

- Acute confusion requires immediate investigation to exclude metabolic causes. A low threshold for brain imaging is mandatory, as urgent treatment may be required. Delay in treatment may have devastating consequences, such as in stroke or meningococcal meningitis.

CONSTIPATION

Constipation is a common complaint that results from decreased frequency of abnormally firm motions. It must be considered relative to the patient's normal bowel habit. Absolute constipation in the absence of both bowel motions and flatus. Acute constipation due to acute intestinal obstruction (p. 232) may require admission to hospital, whereas changes in bowel habit may be investigated in the outpatient setting.

CAUSES

CONGENITAL

- Hirschsprung's disease

ACQUIRED

OBSTRUCTION
- Diverticular disease
- Colonic carcinoma ⚠
- Iatrogenic Ileus
- Extrinsic compression, e.g. pregnancy, ovarian tumours

PAINFUL ANUS
- Fissure-in-ano
- Perianal abscess ⚠
- Strangulated haemorrhoids ⚠
- Post-haemorrhoidectomy

ADYNAMIC BOWEL
- Paralytic ileus
- Neurological disorders (i.e. multiple sclerosis)
- Spinal cord injury

ENDOCRINE
- Diabetes (autonomic neuropathy)
- Hyperparathyroidism

DRUGS
- Codeine phosphate
- Morphine
- Tricyclic antidepressants
- Atropine
- Laxative abuse

OTHER
- Dietary changes (i.e. low-fibre diet, dehydration)
- Anxiety/depression
- Starvation

HISTORY

Congenital

Hirschsprung's disease usually presents with constipation from birth. Gross abdominal distension may eventually occur. The condition may not be picked up until well into the teens or even early adult life.

Acquired

Obstruction

There may be rapid onset of constipation, although the onset is usually gradual, with the patient complaining of colicky abdominal pain, bloating, weight loss, lethargy and occasionally spurious diarrhoea. Constipation may occur from pressure from adjacent organs, e.g. with pregnancy, ovarian cyst or large fibroids. Diverticular disease with or without stricture may cause constipation.

Painful anus

Patients may become constipated from any anal disorder that results in pain on defecation. The most common cause is fissure-in-ano, and other causes include strangulated haemorrhoids (the patient often giving a past history of haemorrhoids), perianal abscess and haemorrhoidectomy.

Adynamic bowel

Paralytic ileus may follow abdominal surgery or abdominal inflammatory conditions. It may also arise following spinal fractures or prolonged bedrest, especially in the elderly. The patient's main complaint is usually of a distended abdomen.

Endocrine

Check for a history of diabetes, as diabetic autonomic neuropathy *per se* can result in constipation. Myxoedema results in constipation, and there may be associated symptoms of cold intolerance, coarse hair and skin changes. Hypercalcaemia (e.g. hyperparathyroidism) is associated with constipation and symptoms include nocturia, nausea, vomiting, abdominal pain and mental disturbances.

Drugs

Take a careful drug history. Chronic laxative abuse may make the bowel 'lazy' and result in constipation.

Other

Patients with anxiety or depression may complain of constipation. Symptoms of depression include a change in sleep pattern, waking early and having difficulty getting back to sleep. With irritable bowel syndrome, the patient may complain of constipation or diarrhoea, or both alternating. A change in diet alone can also cause constipation in patients deliberately trying to lose weight or in those with conditions associated with reduced food intake. Generalised disease, which affects the appetite, particularly results in constipation.

EXAMINATION

Obstruction

There will be a distended abdomen with obstructive high-pitched tinkling bowel sounds. The rectum will usually be empty on digital rectal examination. With a diverticular stricture, there may be tenderness in the left iliac fossa. With malignancy, a mass may be palpable in the abdomen.

Painful anus

Inspection of the anus may reveal a chronic fissure-in-ano, strangulated haemorrhoids or a perianal abscess. With fissure-in-ano, digital rectal examination will be extremely painful, if not impossible. Patients who are post-haemorrhoidectomy may become constipated if appropriate medication has not been given.

Adynamic bowel

The abdomen will be distended, and this is often a painless distension. Bowel sounds will be absent. There may be signs of recent surgery. A full neurological examination should be carried out if the cause of the ileus is not apparent.

Endocrine

With diabetes, there will usually be other complications of diabetes. In myxoedema, check carefully for other signs, e.g. coarse and dry hair, large tongue, hoarse voice, slow relaxing reflexes.

For any patient with constipation, a digital rectal examination must be carried out. The rectum may be completely empty with obstruction, or contain rock-hard faecal masses with functional constipation.

GENERAL INVESTIGATIONS

- FBC, ESR
  Hb ↓ anaemia associated with bowel carcinoma. WCC ↑ diverticulitis. ESR ↑ carcinoma.

- U&Es
  Urea ↑ with dehydration with obstructive causes.

- LFTs
  Albumin ↓ in starvation.

- AXR
  Obstruction – dilated bowel.

SPECIFIC INVESTIGATIONS

- Serum calcium & magnesium
  Hyperparathyroidism.

- TFTs
  T_4 ↓, TSH ↑ in myxoedema.

- **Blood glucose**
  Diabetes – diabetic autonomic neuropathy.
- **Colonoscopy**
  Tumours. Biopsy.
- **Sigmoidoscopy**
  Tumour – biopsy. Hirschsprung's disease, biopsy – absence of ganglion cells.
- **Barium enema**
  Tumours. Diverticular disease.
- **US**
  Intra-abdominal masses (i.e. tumours, ovarian cysts, fibroids, pregnancy).
- **MRI**
  Spinal trauma. Spinal disease.

- **In a patient presenting with constipation, a digital rectal examination is mandatory.**
- **Constipation is common in the elderly. If it is accompanied by weight loss, rectal bleeding or mucus discharge, carcinoma is a likely diagnosis.**
- **Hirschsprung's disease does not always present at birth. It may not be picked up until the child is well into their teens. Consider the diagnosis in a child with constipation, a persistently swollen abdomen and an empty rectum on digital examination.**

CONVULSIONS

A convulsion is a series of involuntary violent contractions of voluntary muscles.

CAUSES

NEUROLOGICAL

- Epilepsy
- Febrile convulsions

TRAUMATIC

- Head injuries ⚠

METABOLIC

- Hypoxia
- Hypo and hyperglycaemia
- Electrolyte abnormalities, e.g. calcium, sodium
- Uraemia

VASCULAR ⚠

- Ischaemic stroke
- Subarachnoid haemorrhage
- Intracranial haemorrhage

INFECTIVE ⚠

- Meningitis
- Encephalitis
- Cerebral abscess

NEOPLASTIC

- Brain tumours

TOXIN/DRUG-INDUCED

- Alcoholism/withdrawal
- Amphetamines, cocaine, antipsychotics, 'ecstasy'

OTHER

- Functional seizures
- Neurosurgery

HISTORY

Event

When evaluating patients with convulsions, it is also important to exclude the causes of syncope (p. 410). An accurate description from an observer is invaluable for documentation and may help in differentiating the forms of epileptic seizures. A prodrome or aura may be associated with the onset of a seizure.

Precipitating factors

The history should start with precipitating factors, e.g. causes such as trauma, surgery or drug overdose. Flashing lights may precipitate a seizure in patients with a past history of epilepsy.

Headache

Convulsions associated with headaches may be due to trauma, subarachnoid haemorrhage, meningitis or raised intracranial pressure from a tumour. Patients with subarachnoid haemorrhage may also complain of sudden onset of blinding headache. The headache associated with meningitis is often accompanied with neck stiffness and photophobia. In the presence of raised intracranial pressure, the headache tends to be worse in the mornings and on coughing or sneezing. It may be associated with nausea or vomiting. For a fuller description, see p. 207.

Associated neurology

Pre-existing neurological impairment before the onset of convulsions has important implications. A stroke, subarachnoid haemorrhage or intracranial bleed may precipitate neurological impairment preceding a convulsion. Chronic progressive impairment preceding a seizure may be a result of tumour growth. In the post-ictal period, transient motor weakness may accompany epilepsy (Todd's paresis). Permanent neurological deficit can be induced by cerebral anoxia from prolonged seizures.

Past medical and drug history

Co-existing disease such as diabetes will predispose to abnormalities of serum glucose concentrations. A drug history should be obtained and specific enquiries undertaken regarding illicit drug use. Alcohol consumption should be documented. In epileptics, poor drug compliance may lead to seizure control failure.

EXAMINATION

Temperature

The presence of pyrexia usually suggests an infective aetiology, such as meningitis or cerebral abscess. Examination should also be undertaken to look for the primary focus, such as otitis media or mastoiditis.

Convulsions may result as a complication of a pyrexia alone, especially in children.

General examination

A general examination is performed to look for the presence of head injury and also any damage resulting as a consequence of the convulsion.

Neurological examination

The primary aim of a neurological examination following a convulsion is to determine the presence of residual neurological deficit. The neurological assessment should include mental state and higher cortical function. If an abnormality is detected, the location may be determined by clinical examination to allow focussed investigation. However, neurological abnormalities present immediately after a seizure, may resolve completely. Todd's paresis may occur post-ictally.

GENERAL INVESTIGATIONS

- **Blood glucose test strips**
  Rapid assessment for hypoglycaemia and hyperglycaemia.
- **FBC**
  WCC ↑ meningitis, encephalitis, cerebral abscess.
- **U&Es**
  ↑ or ↓ sodium, ↑ urea and creatinine – renal failure.
- **Serum calcium**
  ↑ or ↓ calcium.
- **Blood glucose**
  ↑ or ↓ glucose.
- **ABGs**
  Hypoxia.
- **CT or MRI head**
  Especially in the presence of neurological deficit. Cerebral tumours – alterations in brain density. Skull fractures. Intracranial bleeding – high-density signal during the first two weeks. Subarachnoid haemorrhage – high signal (blood) in the subarachnoid space. Strokes – infarction appears normal in the first 24 hours.

SPECIFIC INVESTIGATIONS

- **Toxicology screen**
  Drug use.
- **EEG**
  Epilepsy.
- **Lumbar puncture**
  Meningitis/encephalitis.

- Metabolic causes of convulsions must be excluded immediately. Brain imaging is indicated if the cause is not easily identified, as delay in treatment may result in a poor prognosis.

COUGH

Cough is a reflex explosive expiration that prevents aspiration and promotes the removal of secretions and foreign particles from the lung.

Figure 12 CT of thorax showing a left lower lobe non-small-cell lung cancer revealed as a peripheral cavitating mass (arrow). The patient presented with cough and haemoptysis.

CAUSES

ACUTE

● Inhaled foreign body ⚠
● Respiratory tract infection

CHRONIC

PRODUCTIVE

● COPD (mucoid/purulent)
● TB (bloodstained) ● *(common where TB is endemic)*
● Bronchiectasis (purulent)
● Pulmonary oedema (pink, frothy)

- Lung cancer (bloodstained) (Fig. 12)
- Pulmonary embolism (bloodstained) ⚠

NON-PRODUCTIVE
- Asthma
- Post-nasal drip
- Gastro-oesophageal reflux
- Drugs (ACE inhibitors)
- Sarcoidosis
- Pulmonary fibrosis (idiopathic or acquired)

HISTORY

Onset and duration

The onset of a cough may be acute or chronic (usually defined as a cough that has persisted for more than 3 weeks). Sudden onset of an unrelenting bout of violent coughing may be due to an inhaled foreign body. If this is large enough to occlude the airway, coughing abruptly ceases and is supervened by cyanosis and eventually unconsciousness.

Sputum

The frequency, quantity and appearance of expectorated sputum can be very helpful in the differential diagnosis. Cough continuously productive of purulent sputum is suggestive of COPD and bronchiectasis. Expectorated bloodstained sputum tends to be a complaint of patients with bronchogenic carcinoma, pulmonary embolism and TB.

Smoking history

Smoking alone may cause a chronic cough; however, a long smoking history predisposes to bronchogenic carcinoma and COPD.

Associated symptoms

Episodic (or even seasonal) wheezing with shortness of breath is common with asthma. This should be differentiated from the monophonic wheeze, which is suggestive of intraluminal obstruction from foreign bodies or tumour.

Most of the respiratory causes of coughing tend to be accompanied by shortness of breath, but sudden onset of dyspnoea may result from aspiration or pulmonary embolism. Shortness of breath that is worse on recumbency is suggestive of pulmonary oedema; however, asthma may also be worse at night. Weight loss can be a prominent feature with lung tumours and TB.

Pleuritic chest pain may be experienced with pulmonary emboli and pneumonia, retrosternal burning chest pain precipitated by posture suggests gastro-oesophageal reflux disease, and the associated cough is due to aspiration of refluxed material. Frequent clearing of the throat due to nasal discharge or a history of allergy with rhinitis may result in post-nasal drip and precipitate coughing.

EXAMINATION

Temperature

The presence of pyrexia usually indicates an infective aetiology; the temperature may also be raised with pulmonary embolism.

Inspection and palpation

With COPD, the chest may be barrel-shaped. Patients suffering with lung cancer or TB may appear cachectic. Cyanosis is a feature of pulmonary embolism and COPD. The fingers should be inspected for clubbing (p. 56), which is associated with bronchial carcinoma and bronchiectasis. The JVP is raised in congestive cardiac failure. The supraclavicular nodes may be palpable with respiratory tract infections, TB and lung cancer.

Auscultation

On auscultation, coarse crepitations are a feature of bronchiectasis and pulmonary oedema. Fine crepitations are associated with pulmonary fibrosis. Auscultatory features of bronchial carcinoma are non-specific and may manifest as a pleural effusion (dull to percussion, absent breath sounds, decreased vocal resonance) or segmental collapse of the lung. Widespread wheezing is suggestive of asthma, and a fixed inspiratory wheeze may be heard with bronchial luminal obstruction.

GENERAL INVESTIGATIONS

- **Sputum cultures**
  If a productive cough is present, sputum should be sent for cultures. This will include TB-specific cultures and Ziehl–Neelsen staining.
- **Peak flow**
  Bedside determination of peak expiratory flow rate is useful in the diagnosis of asthma (low peak flow).
- **WCC**
  A raised WCC is a non-specific indicator of infection, as it may also be raised with pulmonary embolism.
- **CXR**
  Very useful and may reveal areas of consolidation with infection. Dilated bronchi with persistent areas of infection are suggestive of bronchiectasis. Apical pulmonary consolidation with calcification and hilar lymphadenopathy is characteristic of TB. The presence of pulmonary oedema is appreciated by bilateral patchy shadowing; this may be accompanied by other radiological features of cardiac failure, including cardiomegaly, upper lobe diversion of the pulmonary veins, bilateral pleural effusions and Kerley B lines (1–2 cm horizontal lines

SECTION A

in the periphery of the lung fields). Bronchial carcinoma may present as a hilar mass, peripheral mass or with collapse and consolidation of the lung due to airway obstruction. Bilateral hilar lymphadenopathy is suggestive of sarcoidosis.

■ **Respiratory function tests**
Formal respiratory function tests can be used to diagnose airway obstruction (asthma, chronic bronchitis and bronchiectasis), and flow volume loops may reveal fixed airway obstruction.

SPECIFIC INVESTIGATIONS

■ **CT Pulmonary Angiography**
Indicated when the diagnosis of pulmonary embolism is suspected (especially where CXR is normal).

■ **CT thorax**
Useful for the diagnosis and staging of lung cancer; it is also specific for the diagnosis of bronchiectasis. High-resolution CT is required if pulmonary fibrosis is suspected.

■ **pH studies**
24-hour pH monitoring may be required when a diagnosis of gastro-oesophageal reflux disease cannot be made on the history alone.

- Persistent cough, weight loss and hoarseness in a smoker are ominous signs. Arrange a CXR to exclude malignancy.

- An unrelenting bout of violent coughing of sudden onset may be due to an inhaled foreign body. If this is large enough to occlude the upper airways, coughing may cease abruptly and cyanosis and unconsciousness ensue. Cricothyroidotomy may be life-saving.

- Ask about foreign travel, especially to countries where TB is endemic.

CYANOSIS

Cyanosis is the abnormal blue discoloration of the skin and mucous membranes, resulting from the presence of reduced oxygenated haemoglobin in the blood. It is not synonymous with hypoxaemia, which may be present (e.g. anaemia) without cyanosis.

CAUSES

CENTRAL CYANOSIS

DECREASED OXYGEN SATURATION
- Severe respiratory disease
- Pulmonary oedema ⚠
- Pulmonary embolism ⚠
- Congenital cyanotic heart disease

ABNORMAL HAEMOGLOBIN
- Methaemoglobinaemia
- Sulphaemoglobinaemia

PERIPHERAL CYANOSIS
- All causes of central cyanosis
- Cold exposure
- Raynaud's phenomenon
- Arterial occlusion ⚠
- Venous occlusion
- Acrocyanosis

HISTORY

Central cyanosis

Onset

Cyanosis due to congenital heart disease causing anatomical right to left shunts may have been present from birth or the first few years of life. Immediate onset of cyanosis may be due to pulmonary emboli or cardiac failure. Acute onset of cyanosis may be precipitated by pneumonia and asthma. Patients with COPD develop cyanosis over many years. Accompanying polycythaemia may exacerbate cyanosis in these patients.

Chest pain

Cyanosis associated with pleuritic chest pain may be due to pulmonary emboli or pneumonia. Dull, aching chest tightness is experienced by patients who develop cyanosis from pulmonary oedema as a complication of myocardial infarction.

Dyspnoea

Sudden onset of dyspnoea can occur with pulmonary emboli and pulmonary oedema, while conditions such as asthma may produce a more gradual onset.

Past medical history and drug history

Any co-existing respiratory disease is significant, as cyanosis can result from any lung disease of sufficient severity. Consumption of drugs such as metoclopramide and sumatriptan may precipitate methaemoglobinaemia and sulphaemoglobinaemia, respectively.

Peripheral cyanosis

General history

Acrocyanosis is a condition in which the hands are persistently blue and cold; it is not associated with pain. Raynaud's phenomenon is the episodic three-colour change that occurs, with arterial vasospasm (white), cyanosis (blue) and reactive hyperaemia (red). It may be idiopathic or be associated with connective tissue diseases and drugs such as beta blockers.

Peripheral cyanosis may also result from acute arterial occlusion and is accompanied by pain and mottling of the skin. Iliofemoral deep venous thrombosis can produce a painful blue leg, termed phlegmasia cerulea dolens.

EXAMINATION

Temperature

Pneumonia and pulmonary emboli may be associated with pyrexia.

Inspection

It is often difficult to detect minor degrees of cyanosis. Central cyanosis produces a blue discoloration of the mucous membranes and digits; peripheral cyanosis produces blue discoloration only of the digits. Episodic peripheral cyanosis may be due to Raynaud's disease, and this may be associated with small areas of infarction on the fingertips. The presence of clubbing may be due to congenital cyanotic heart disease. Classically, patients with COPD appear cyanosed with a poorly expanding barrelled chest. The JVP is elevated with congestive cardiac failure.

Respiratory examination

Poor chest expansion occurs with COPD and asthma. Unilateral impairment of expansion may occur with lobar pneumonia; in addition, dullness to percussion is experienced over the area of consolidation. Localised crepitation may be auscultated with lobar pneumonia, but is more widespread with bronchopneumonia, pulmonary oedema and chronic bronchitis. Air entry is poor with COPD and asthma. Bronchial breathing may be auscultated over an area of consolidation, and additional sounds, such as wheezing, may be heard with asthma.

GENERAL INVESTIGATIONS

- **Oxygen saturation**
  Saturation is usually below 85% with cyanosis (unless methaemoglobinaemia, where saturation is normal).
- **ABGs**
  ↓ pO_2 all severe lung disease.
- **FBC**
  Hb ↑ chronic cyanosis. WCC ↑ pneumonia and pulmonary embolism.
- **ECG**
  Features of myocardial infarction (p. 54). Non-specific abnormalities with pulmonary emboli.
- **CXR**
  Pneumonia, pulmonary infarct, cardiac failure (p. 53).

SPECIFIC INVESTIGATIONS

- **Sputum and blood cultures**
  Pneumonia.
- **CT pulmonary angiography or V/Q scan**
  Pulmonary embolus.
- **Echocardiography**
  Cardiac failure.
- **Hb spectroscopy**
  Methaemoglobinaemia, sulphaemoglobinaemia.
- **Arterial CT/MRI**
  Acute arterial occlusion.
- **Duplex Doppler or venography**
  Acute venous occlusion.

- **The sudden development of cyanosis is an emergency, and causes for this, such as pulmonary embolus and pulmonary oedema, must be identified immediately.**
- **Arterial occlusion as a cause of peripheral cyanosis must also be recognised and acted on urgently.**

SECTION A

DEAFNESS

Deafness is loss of hearing and may be divided into 'conductive' and 'sensorineural'.

CAUSES

CONDUCTIVE DEAFNESS

ACQUIRED
- Ear wax
- Otitis externa
- Otitis media (including glue ear)
- Labyrinthitis
- Otosclerosis
- Foreign body
- Perforation of the tympanic membrane (TM)
- Barotrauma
- Cholesteatoma

CONGENITAL
- Atresia of the meatus

SENSORINEURAL DEAFNESS

ACQUIRED
- Presbyacusis (age-related sensorineural hearing loss)
- Noise-induced trauma
- Meniere's disease
- Ototoxicity (e.g. aminoglycosides, aspirin, furosemide and cytotoxic agents)
- Stroke
- Head injuries
- Infection (e.g. mumps, herpes zoster, meningitis
- Acoustic neuroma (vestibular schwannoma)
- Brain tumours

CONGENITAL
- Infections (e.g. maternal rubella, toxoplasmosis and CMV)
- Genetic (e.g. Alport syndrome)

HISTORY

Hearing loss can occur solely or in conjunction with other symptoms. It is important to consider the following.

Duration

Childhood deafness, may result from maternal rubella infection or arise as a complication of childhood infection (meningitis, toxoplasma or CMV infection). The duration of symptoms may coincide with the introduction of ototoxic drugs during pregnancy.

Onset

Deafness usually occurs if a foreign body perforates the tympanic membrane or disrupts the chain of ossicles. Sudden onset of deafness may also result from trauma, vascular abnormalities or Ménière's disease. Conversely, gradual development of deafness occurs with otosclerosis, tumours and age.

Pain

Deafness associated with ear pain may be a result of infection including otitis externa, otitis media or herpes zoster. Severe pain is experienced with both direct trauma perforating the tympanic membrane and barotrauma, which can result from a 'slap on the ear' or extreme activities including scuba diving.

Precipitating factors

Sensorineural deafness can result as a complication of mumps or from prolonged exposure to high noise levels due to occupation (e.g. airport or factory workers).

Associated symptoms

Tinnitus in combination with episodic deafness and vertigo can occur with Ménière's disease. When tinnitus occurs with deafness alone, consider otosclerosis, noise exposure, ototoxic drugs or acoustic neuroma.

Drug history

Ototoxic drugs can easily be determined from a drug history.

EXAMINATION

Examination of the ear

On visual inspection, the vesicles of herpes zoster or presence of otitis externa may be obvious. With otitis externa, the skin appears erythematous with scaling and exudation. Tenderness will be elicited by movement of the pinna or compression of the tragus.

More detailed otoscopic examination will identify ear wax, foreign bodies, osteoma or even exostosis, occluding the external auditory canal. In a patent ear canal, the tympanic membrane may be visualised as a 'white cone of light' reflex. Traumatic perforations may be seen as a tear of the tympanum, accompanied with blood. Otitis media can be visualised as bulging, air bullae, erythema or frank perforation of the tympanic membrane.

Assessment of hearing

Gross hearing tests of the vestibulocochlear nerve can be performed with conversational voice, whispered voice or even measuring how far away from the ear the ticking of a watch can be heard.

Rinne's test is performed with a 512-Hz tuning fork, placed on the mastoid. AC conduction is normally better than BC. Weber's test is performed holding the base of the struck tuning fork against the centre of the forehead. Normally, the sound is heard equally in both ears (see Table).

Deafness	Rinne's test	Weber's test
Sensorineural	AC > BC	Sound heard in good unaffected ear
Conductive	BC > AC	Sound heard in deaf affected ear

General examination

A complete neurological examination may also be performed. Nystagmus and a positive Romberg's test may be present with Ménière's disease; rarely, acoustic neuromas may affect the facial nerve, producing unilateral facial paralysis; and motor or sensory deficits resulting from brain tumours. Examination should also include the nose and throat, as nasopharyngeal sepsis may be a factor predisposing to middle ear infection.

GENERAL INVESTIGATIONS

- Pure tone audiometry
  Allows accurate measurements of hearing levels with bone and air conduction.
- Swab of ear discharge
  In cases of possible infection (i.e. otitis externa).

SPECIFIC INVESTIGATIONS

- Speech audiometry
  Impaired speech discrimination in the 50–80% range occurs with conductive deafness, and 0–50% range with sensorineural causes.
- Electric response audiometry
  Assessment of hearing in babies, e.g. otoacoustic emission test, which may lead to auditory brainstem response if abnormal.
- CT Ear
  Rule out petrous or basal skull fracture.
- MRI brain
  Acoustic neuroma or brain tumour.

- Progressive unilateral deafness accompanied by tinnitus, vertigo or neurological symptoms/signs should prompt urgent investigation to exclude acoustic neuroma.
- Sudden hearing loss alone (<3 days) needs urgent assessment.

DIARRHOEA

Diarrhoea is an increased frequency of abnormally loose motions. The diagnosis of diarrhoea must be related to the patient's normal bowel habit.

Figure 13 Small bowel enema showing Crohn's disease. *A stricture is seen in the terminal ilium (arrow).*

CAUSES

INFECTIVE ENTERITIS

Non-specific, Bacterial
- *Campylobacter* spp ● *(rare in tropical Africa)*
- *Salmonella* spp ● *(rare in tropical Africa)*
- *Escherichia coli*
- *Clostridium difficile*
- Staphylococci
- *Shigella* spp
- *Vibrio cholerae*
- *Yersinia enterocolitica* ● *(common in the Indian sub-continent)*

Viral, Fungal, Protozoal
- *Cryptosporidium* spp

- *Giardia lamblia* ● *(more common in children worldwide)*
- *Entamoeba histolytica*

INFLAMMATORY
- Ulcerative colitis
- Crohn's disease (Fig. 13)

MALABSORPTION
- Coeliac disease
- Blind loop syndrome
- Short bowel syndrome
- Radiation

NEOPLASTIC
- Carcinoma
- Villous adenoma

OTHER INTESTINAL
- Diverticular disease ● *(rare in rural Africa and Asia)*
- Irritable bowel syndrome
- Faecal impaction – overflow diarrhoea
- Ischaemic colitis
- Ileocolic fistula

GASTRIC
- Post-vagotomy (vagotomy rarely performed nowadays)

PANCREATIC
- Chronic pancreatitis
- Cystic fibrosis
- Carcinoma
- Pancreatic resection

ENDOCRINE
- Diabetes
- Thyrotoxicosis
- Carcinoid syndrome
- Zollinger–Ellison syndrome
- VIPoma
- Medullary thyroid cancer

DRUG-INDUCED
- Antibiotics
- Laxatives

● Proton pump inhibitors
● Sorbitol (in sugar-free foods)
● Magnesium-containing antacids
● Cytotoxic agents

OTHER

● Anxiety
● Diet

HISTORY

Infective enteritis

There is usually colicky abdominal pain and diarrhoea. The diarrhoea may be bloody. Cholera presents with cramping abdominal pain, vomiting and severe diarrhoea, described as 'rice water' stools. There may be fever, rapid dehydration, collapse and death. In infective enteritis, check for ingestion of any unusual food or whether anyone else has been affected in the family. Check for a history of foreign travel (traveller's diarrhoea). *C. difficile* is the most important cause of hospital-acquired diarrhoea. Over 80% of infection occurs in those over 65 years of age, affecting particularly those who have been treated with broad spectrum antibiotics. Infection ranges from mild to severe diarrhoea to more, unusually, pseudomembranous colitis.

Inflammatory bowel disease

Both Crohn's disease and ulcerative colitis present with frequent diarrhoea with blood, and occasionally mucus and pus, associated with colicky abdominal pain. The patient may be toxic and febrile, with abdominal pain and distension if toxic dilatation of the colon has occurred.

Malabsorption

In addition to diarrhoea, there may be offensive stools, which are fatty and float, i.e. steatorrhoea. Has the patient had any previous surgery for resection of the bowel to suggest short bowel syndrome, or any bypass surgery to suggest blind loop syndrome? Is there any history of abdominal radiotherapy?

Neoplastic

Carcinoma may cause diarrhoea associated with colicky abdominal pain and the passage of blood and mucus per rectum (PR). The diarrhoea may be spurious, liquefied stools only passing through an area of obstruction, with faecal masses behind the obstruction. Loose watery mucus passed frequently may be associated with a villous adenoma, the patient complaining of weakness associated with hypokalaemia due to the passage of excessive mucus rich in potassium.

Other intestinal

Diverticular disease may cause diarrhoea. The condition usually occurs in the older patient. The patient will also complain of associated colicky abdominal pain and pain usually in the left iliac fossa. Irritable bowel syndrome may cause similar symptoms to diverticular disease but occurs in the younger patient. Faecal impaction may result in spurious diarrhoea, while an ileocolic fistula associated with diverticular disease or rectosigmoid carcinoma is also associated with diarrhoea. Ischaemic colitis usually presents in an elderly patient with colicky abdominal pain, diarrhoea and passage of dark-red blood PR.

Gastric

Check for a history of gastric surgery. Destruction of the pylorus or section of the vagus nerve may result in diarrhoea, often associated with dumping. Vagotomy is rarely, if ever, performed nowadays.

Pancreatic lesions

These may result in diarrhoea or steatorrhoea. Check for a history of cystic fibrosis. The patient may have chronic pancreatitis, in which case, there may be chronic back pain associated with epigastric pain and weight loss. Check for a history of pancreatic surgery. Patients with carcinoma of the pancreas may also present with diarrhoea.

Endocrine disorders

Diabetes is associated with an increased incidence of diarrhoea. Check for a history of thyroid disease. The patient may complain of sweating, anxiety, tremor and have obvious eye signs. The patient may also have noticed a goitre. Carcinoid syndrome may present as flushing (especially after alcohol, coffee and certain foods), asthma and loud bowel sounds, e.g. borborygmi. Patients with Zollinger–Ellison syndrome may have a past history of recurrent peptic ulceration, with haematemesis or melaena, in addition to diarrhoea. VIPoma is rare but presents with severe watery diarrhoea associated with potassium loss, with weakness due to hypokalaemia. Check whether the patient has a goitre, as diarrhoea may be associated with medullary carcinoma of the thyroid. Symptoms and signs of hyperparathyroidism and phaeochromocytoma may also be present (MEN syndrome).

Drugs

Take a careful drug history, especially for recent antibiotics, laxative abuse, proton pump inhibitors, sorbitol (in sugar-free foods), the ingestion of magnesium-containing antacids or recent cytotoxic agents.

Other

Anxiety and dietary changes may lead to diarrhoea. A careful history should be taken, particularly looking at any recent changes in the diet.

EXAMINATION

Infective enteritis

The patient may be dehydrated or collapsed. Check for tachycardia and hypotension. There may be abdominal tenderness and distension. Digital rectal examination may reveal blood and pus on the examining glove.

Inflammatory bowel disease

There may be little to find except for mild, localised tenderness. In toxic dilatation, there will be fever, malaise, abdominal distension, vomiting and localised tenderness. Perforation may occur with peritonitis. An abdominal mass may be palpable with Crohn's disease.

Neoplastic

There may be abdominal distension if obstruction has occurred. There may be a palpable abdominal mass. Digital rectal examination may reveal a carcinoma or a villous adenoma.

Other intestinal

With diverticular disease, there may be little to find other than tenderness in the left iliac fossa. The findings are similar in irritable bowel syndrome. With faecal impaction, rock-hard faecal masses may be felt on digital rectal examination. There may be little to find with an ileocolic fistula. With ischaemic colitis, there will be tenderness and guarding in the left side of the abdomen. Rectal examination will reveal dark-red blood.

Gastric

Other than a scar and history of gastric surgery, there may be nothing else to find on examination.

Pancreatic

With pancreatic carcinoma, there may be epigastric tenderness or a palpable mass in the epigastrium.

Endocrine

With thyrotoxicosis, there will be tachycardia, sweating, brisk reflexes, eye signs and a goitre. With carcinoid syndrome, there may be hepatomegaly and signs of tricuspid incompetence and pulmonary stenosis. In Zollinger–Ellison syndrome, there may be little to find on examination. With VIPoma, other than weakness due to hypokalaemia, there may also be little to find on examination. With medullary carcinoma of the thyroid, there will be a palpable goitre.

GENERAL INVESTIGATIONS

- **FBC, CRP/ESR**
  Hb ↓ bleeding. WCC ↑ infection. ESR ↑ inflammation, tumour.
- **U&Es**
  Creatinine/urea ↑ dehydration. Potassium ↓ severe diarrhoea, villous adenoma.
- **LFTs**
  Alkaline phosphatase ↑ with liver metastases.
- **Stool culture and microscopy**
  Infective causes. Microscopy for parasites.
- **Abdominal X-Ray**
  Inflammatory bowel disease (toxic mega colon)
- **Sigmoidoscopy**
  Carcinoma, inflammatory bowel disease, villous adenoma, pseudomembranous colitis.
- **Barium enema**
  Tumours, colitis, diverticular disease.
- **Colonoscopy**
  Tumours, colitis (extent and severity), diverticular disease.

SPECIFIC INVESTIGATIONS

- **TFTs**
  T_4 ↑, TSH ↓ in thyrotoxicosis.
- **24-hour urine**
  5HIAA↑in carcinoid.
- **Ultrasound**
  Carcinoid. Liver metastases.
- **Serum gastrin**
  Zollinger–Ellison syndrome.
- **Serum calcitonin**
  Medullary carcinoma of the thyroid.
- **Serum vasoactive intestinal peptide**
  Raised in VIPoma.
- **Faecal fats**
  Malabsorption.
- **Duodenal/jejunal biopsy**
  Malabsorption – coeliac disease.
- **Small bowel enema**
  Crohn's disease.

- Acute diarrhoea in adults is most likely to be due to infection.
- Do not forget to ask about foreign travel.
- It is important to distinguish diarrhoea from steatorrhoea and faecal incontinence.
- Do not be caught out by overflow diarrhoea in the elderly. Always do a PR.
- Chronic diarrhoea in association with weight loss suggests serious underlying disease.

DIZZINESS

Spatial disorientation may be expressed by the patient as dizziness, vertigo or feeling 'light-headed'. True vertigo, however, is not experienced as a sensation of movement but as tilting or sloping of the environment, often characterised as the room spinning around them.

CAUSES

EPISODIC

- Ménière's disease*
- Benign paroxysmal positional vertigo (BPPV)
- Arrhythmia
- Postural hypotension
- Migraine/Vestibular migraine
- Hyperventilation
- Drugs (antihypertensives, antidepressants)
- Hypoglycaemia
- Posterior circulation TIAs ⚠
- Anxiety
- Seizures (partial)
- Carbon monoxide poisoning (e.g. faulty heating)
- Persistent postural-perceptual dizziness (PPPD)

CONSTANT

ACUTE ONSET

- Labyrinthitis*
- Vestibular neuronitis
- Acute alcohol or recreational drug intoxication
- Head injuries*
- Posterior circulation CVA

GRADUAL ONSET

- Diabetes mellitus
- Hypothyroidism
- Multiple sclerosis
- Aortic stenosis
- Cerebellopontine angle tumour* (e.g. acoustic neuroma, cholesteatoma) ⚠
- Ototoxicity – aminoglycosides (i.e. gentamicin), chemotherapeutic drugs*
- Infections – HIV, syphilis, Lyme disease

*Indicates causes accompanied by audiological symptoms.

HISTORY

General

A clear history is crucial to assess if emergency management is indicated. The causes above are listed according to speed of onset and duration of symptoms. Conditions that are accompanied by additional audiological symptoms, such as tinnitus or hearing loss are marked with an asterisk,*.

Precipitating factors

Causes of dizziness that are precipitated by movements of the head include BPPV, labyrinthitis and head injuries. Patients with BPPV complain of short episodes of dizziness accompanying changes in the position of the head. Labyrinthitis may result as a complication of systemic viral infection. Postural dizziness precipitated by rising from a lying position may be caused by orthostatic hypotension, commonly secondary to antihypertensive drugs.

Associated symptoms

Dizziness may be precipitated by arrhythmia, with patients complaining of associated palpitations. It may also be experienced with migraine attacks, and patients may complain of associated unilateral throbbing headache, nausea, vomiting and photophobia. Ménière's disease is diagnosed with a history of episodic severe vertigo, with continuous tinnitus and hearing loss. Patients with vertebrobasilar insufficiency from cervical spondylosis may complain of dizziness with extension of the neck, although this term is becoming increasingly outdated. With posterior circulation TIAs, sudden onset of dizziness is caused by ischaemia of the lateral brainstem or cerebellum. This may be accompanied by syncope, nausea, vomiting, visual field defects and diplopia. Severe and sudden vertigo, nausea and vomiting may result from a cerebellar stroke (infarction or haemorrhage). Patients with anxiety disorders may experience attacks of dizziness, tinnitus and tremor, with or without accompanying hyperventilation. Certainly, hyperventilation alone is sufficient to precipitate dizziness. Vertigo is also a prominent feature of multiple sclerosis when demyelination occurs in the brainstem; this may be accompanied by dysarthria and cranial nerve palsies, common with younger age. Tumours of the cerebellopontine angle tend to present gradually, dizziness may be mild, and this may be accompanied by numbness, facial paralysis, hearing loss and reduced balance.

Drug history

Numerous drugs have ototoxic effects; perhaps the most commonly known are aminoglycosides and furosemide.

EXAMINATION

Assessment of nystagmus, hearing and positional testing provide the most information when determining the cause of dizziness and assessing for red flags.

Multidirectional nystagmus results from diffuse cerebellar disease, while unidirectional nystagmus occurs either with ipsilateral cerebellar disease (multiple sclerosis, posterior circulation TIA/CVA) or contralateral vestibular disease (Ménière's, labyrinthitis, acoustic neuroma). Conversely, on lateral (horizontal) gaze, nystagmus of the abducting eye, with failure of adduction of the opposite eye, is due to internuclear ophthalmoplegia, classically caused by brainstem demyelination.

Hearing is assessed with Rinne's and Weber's tests (see p. 88 for cases of sensorineural hearing loss). Hearing loss accompanied by trigeminal and facial nerve palsy may be due to tumour arising at the cerebellopontine angle.

Specific positional tests, such as the Dix-Hallpike test, are performed to assess the integrity of the vestibulo-ocular and labyrinthine pathways. Patients with BPPV usually complain of vertigo and exhibit delayed horizontal nystagmus that fatigues on repeated testing.

A complete neurological examination is then undertaken including cranial nerve examination, and cerebellar examination may be indicated. Signs such as homonymous hemianopia can result from posterior circulation infarcts and brainstem lesions such as demyelination. Stroke may give rise to combinations of ipsilateral cranial nerve palsies and motor or sensory deficits of the face. In addition, pale optic discs due to optic atrophy may be seen in multiple sclerosis. Patients with cerebellar disease will exhibit an intention tremor when performing the finger–nose test, as well as exhibiting a broad-based ataxic gait, nystagmus, dysdiadochokinesis and dysarthria.

When a cardiovascular cause is suspected, the pulse is assessed for irregularities of rhythm, which may suggest atrial fibrillation. Blood pressure is measured both lying and standing to screen for postural hypotension, and potential sites for emboli, such as the cardiac valves and the carotid blood vessels, are auscultated for murmurs and bruits, respectively. Severe aortic stenosis may lead to dizziness with an urgent referral indicated.

GENERAL INVESTIGATIONS

Most causes of dizziness can be diagnosed on history and clinical examination, but common investigations may include.

- ■ FBC
  WCC ↑ infection.
- ■ ESR
  ↑ CVA, malignancy, infection, inflammation.
- ■ Urinalysis
  Raised glucose detectable in diabetes.
- ■ LFTs
  May be abnormal in alcohol abuse.
- ■ Thiamine
  Reduced in chronic alcohol abuse.

SPECIFIC INVESTIGATIONS

- **24-Hour ECG**
  To screen for arrhythmia.
- **Audiometry (pure-tone audiometry)**
  Allows assessment and classification of any accompanying hearing loss.
- **Carotid Doppler**
  To evaluate patency of the vessel and to screen for the presence of plaque (TIAs).
- **Echocardiography**
  To evaluate for valvular heart disease (i.e. aortic valve).
- **Tilt-table testing**
  To assess for orthostatic hypotension.
- **CT head**
  Stroke, cerebellar haemorrhage, evaluation of severe head injuries.
- **MRI brain**
  Acoustic neuroma and other cerebellopontine angle tumours, demyelination with multiple sclerosis.
- **EEG**
  To detect seizure activity.

- Dizziness accompanied by sudden onset and/ or presence of additional symptoms should be investigated immediately and include:
  - Neurological signs and symptoms
  - Unilateral hearing loss
  - Vertical nystagmus
  - New headache
  - Severe tinnitus
  - Loss of consciousness
  - Palpitations

DYSPHAGIA

Dysphagia means difficulty in swallowing and should be distinguished from pain on swallowing. Dysphagia may be associated with ingestion of solids or liquids, or both. Pain on swallowing is odynophagia, which in itself does not interfere with the act of swallowing.

Figure 14 Barium swallow showing oesophageal stricture caused by a carcinoma. The barium swallow reveals an irregular narrowing at the distal oesophagus with 'shouldering,' where the contrast tapers into the stricture (see arrow).

CAUSES

CONGENITAL

● Oesophageal atresia ⚠

ACQUIRED

IN THE LUMEN
● Food bolus
● Foreign body

IN THE WALL
● Gastro-oesophageal reflux
● Carcinoma (Fig. 14) ⚠
○ Irradiation
○ Scleroderma
● Caustic stricture
● Candidiasis
● Achalasia
● Plummer–Vinson syndrome
● Chagas' disease ● *(South America)*

OUTSIDE THE WALL
● Goitre
● Paraoesophageal (rolling) hiatus hernia
● Mediastinal tumours/lymphadenopathy
◐ Pharyngeal pouch
● Enlarged left atrium (mitral stenosis)
● Thoracic aortic aneurysm ⚠
● Dysphagia lusoria

NEUROMUSCULAR DISORDERS
● CVA ⚠
◐ Bulbar palsy
◐ Guillain–Barré syndrome
◐ Motor neurone disease
● Myasthenia gravis

OTHERS
◐ Globus

HISTORY

Congenital

Oesophageal atresia

This may be associated with maternal polyhydramnios. The newborn baby will show dribbling of saliva, inability to swallow feeds, production of frothy mucus, choking attacks, cyanotic attacks and chest infections.

Acquired

In the lumen

There may be a history of ingestion of a foreign body such as a coin (children) or false teeth or chicken bone (elderly). Occasionally, the history may not be forthcoming. In the case of a food bolus, it is unusual for this to cause dysphagia without there being some form of underlying stricture.

In the wall

With a caustic stricture, there is usually a history of caustic ingestion, except in psychiatric patients, where the history may not be apparent. There will be a sudden onset of pain and dysphagia, which may improve with appropriate treatment, only to recur after several months due to a stricture. Patients with inflammatory stricture due to gastro-oesophageal reflux associated with a hiatus hernia will have a history of retrosternal burning pain and acid reflux, which is worse on recumbency or bending down. The dysphagia is usually of gradual onset, and the patient may localise the site of dysphagia to the level of the lower end of the sternum. Oesophageal candidiasis may cause dysphagia, and this usually occurs in the immunocompromised patient. Achalasia is a disorder where there is degeneration of the oesophageal myenteric plexus, resulting in loss of peristaltic contraction in the oesophagus and failure of the lower oesophageal sphincter to relax in response to swallowing. It usually presents between 30 and 50 years of age. The dysphagia may be intermittent, and then gets progressively worse. Fluid regurgitation at night may result in aspiration pneumonitis. With carcinoma, the dysphagia is usually of rapid onset. Initially, it is for solids, then for fluids. There may be associated weight loss, anorexia and symptoms of anaemia. There may be a history of achalasia or Barrett's oesophagus. Dysphagia with food sticking at the upper end of the oesophagus in a middle-aged woman may suggest Plummer–Vinson syndrome. This is due to a web in the upper oesophagus (post-cricoid web). The condition is pre-malignant. A history of radiotherapy to chest or mediastinum may suggest an irradiation stricture. With scleroderma, the patient may have noticed changes in the skin, around the lips, in the fingers (sclerodactyly) or may have a past history of Raynaud's phenomenon. Chagas' disease is extremely rare and is associated with degeneration of the myenteric plexus associated with trypanosomal infection. The symptoms are identical to those of achalasia.

Outside the wall

The presence of a large goitre will be obvious. With the pharyngeal pouch, patients are usually of middle age or elderly. They may have noticed a swelling, usually in the left posterior triangle of the neck. They may also have dysphagia localised behind the manubrium associated with the pouch pressing on the oesophagus. On lying down, there is regurgitation of food with coughing. The patient may also have halitosis. With bronchial carcinoma, there may be direct pressure on the oesophagus from the tumour or via secondary spread to the mediastinal lymph nodes. There may be a history of bronchial carcinoma or the patient may present with haemoptysis. With dysphagia from mediastinal lymphadenopathy, the patient may have noticed enlarged swellings at other sites, e.g. axilla or groin.

Dysphagia from pressure of an enlarged left atrium may be associated with mitral stenosis, and there may be a past history of this. With a paraoesophageal (rolling) hernia, the dysphagia may be intermittent, due to a full stomach pressing on the adjacent oesophagus. Hiccups may occur due to irritation of the diaphragm.

Neuromuscular

There will usually be a history of Guillain–Barré syndrome, poliomyelitis, motor neurone disease, myasthenia gravis or a CVA.

Others

Globus is a subjective feeling of a lump or foreign body in the throat. The term 'globus hystericus' was previously used because it was felt to be psychogenic, but it is now considered that a globus sensation may still indicate organic pathology. Investigation is required to exclude the true causes of dysphagia.

EXAMINATION

With oesophageal atresia, an orogastric tube is passed, and it will arrest at the site of the obstruction.

In many cases of dysphagia, there will be nothing to find on examination. A goitre is usually an obvious swelling that moves on swallowing. With a pharyngeal pouch, there may be a palpable swelling low down in the posterior triangle of the neck (usually left), which gurgles on palpation. With carcinoma, there may be signs of weight loss, a palpable liver due to metastases, or cervical lymphadenopathy due to metastases. Koilonychia, angular cheilitis and glossitis are clinical features associated with Plummer–Vinson syndrome. With irradiation stricture, there may be changes in the skin consistent with previous radiotherapy. With scleroderma, there may be calcinosis of the subcutaneous tissue, Raynaud's phenomenon, sclerodactyly and telangiectasia. With dysphagia, due to an enlarged left atrium in mitral stenosis, there may be signs of mitral stenosis, e.g. peripheral cyanosis, malar flush, left parasternal heave, tapping apex beat, opening snap and mid-diastolic murmur best heard at the apex. A variety of neurological abnormalities will be associated with dysphagia of neuromuscular origin.

GENERAL INVESTIGATIONS

- **FBC, ESR**
  Hb ↓ associated with carcinoma but may also occur with oesophagitis associated with peptic strictures. Anaemia may also be associated with Plummer–Vinson syndrome. ESR ↑ in malignancy and scleroderma.

- **U&Es**
  Dehydration.

- **LFTs**
Alkaline phosphatase ↑ in liver secondaries.

- **CXR**
Foreign body if radio-opaque. Air-fluid level in achalasia.
Gastric air bubble in chest in paraoesophageal hernia. Hilar
lymphadenopathy. Bronchial carcinoma. Widened mediastinum
with aortic aneurysm. Large left atrium (double shadow behind
the heart) – mitral stenosis.

- **ECG**
Left atrial hypertrophy.

SPECIFIC INVESTIGATIONS

- **Barium swallow**
Pharyngeal pouch (never OGD, as it may perforate the pouch),
stricture, achalasia, external compression.

- **OGD**
Foreign body. Food bolus. Candidiasis. Benign versus malignant
stricture. Plummer–Vinson syndrome – post-cricoid web.
Biopsy – benign lesion versus malignant lesion, absence of
myenteric plexus in achalasia.

- **CT**
May help identify extrinsic compression. Goitre. Mediastinal
nodes. Spread of malignancy. Tumour staging. Aortic aneurysm.
Dysphagia lusoria (abnormally placed arteries causing external
compression).

- **Recent onset of progressive dysphagia in the elderly
is due to carcinoma of the oesophagus until proved
otherwise.**

- **It is unusual for dysphagia to occur due to a food
bolus alone.**

- **Patients with a long history of oesophagitis who
develop dysphagia may have a stricture or carcinoma.**

DYSPNOEA

Dyspnoea is the subjective awareness of breathing discomfort.

Figure 15 A pneumothorax, visible on the right side. Note the absence of lung markings at the periphery. The lung edge is visible (arrow).

CAUSES

SUDDEN (SECONDS TO MINUTES) ⚠

- Pneumothorax (Fig. 15)
- Chest trauma
- Aspiration
- Pulmonary oedema
- Pulmonary embolism
- Anaphylaxis

ACUTE (HOURS TO DAYS)

- Asthma
- Respiratory tract infection
- Pleural effusion
- Lung tumours
- Metabolic acidosis ⚠

CHRONIC (MONTHS TO YEARS)

- Chronic airflow limitation (COPD)
- Anaemia
- Arrhythmia
- Valvular heart disease
- Cardiac failure
- Cystic fibrosis
- Idiopathic pulmonary fibrosis
- Chest wall deformities
- Neuromuscular disorders
- Pulmonary hypertension

HISTORY

Many cardiac or respiratory diseases of sufficient severity produce dyspnoea. When considering chronic respiratory causes, you may relate them anatomically to diseases of the pulmonary vasculature, airways, interstitium and chest wall. When approaching a patient with dyspnoea, it is important to ensure that the ABCs are attended to before continuing with the diagnostic process.

Onset

The speed of onset is a useful indicator of the disease process. Classification by speed of onset narrows the differential diagnosis in urgent clinical situations.

Precipitating factors

An obvious precipitating factor may be present, such as trauma causing either fractured ribs or a pneumothorax. Aspiration of a foreign body may be determined from the history; however, aspiration of vomit is more difficult, as it usually occurs in patients with decreased consciousness levels or who have lost the gag reflex. Dyspnoea on recumbency is caused by cardiac failure; occasionally, patients may complain of waking up at night gasping for breath (paroxysmal nocturnal dyspnoea). Dyspnoea associated with asthma may be associated with particular allergens, e.g. grass pollen, house dust mites. A history of severe allergy should lead to the consideration of anaphylaxis. Stressful events can precipitate asthma attacks but may also cause anxious patients to hyperventilate.

Relieving factors

Dyspnoea resulting from cardiac failure may be relieved by sitting upright, and, when due to asthma, by beta agonists.

Associated factors

Cough productive of (green, yellow, rusty) sputum indicates the presence of a chest infection. This may be the primary cause, or it may exacerbate dyspnoea in patients with an existing condition such as asthma, COPD or cardiac failure. Bloodstained sputum may result from a chest infection (especially TB), pulmonary embolism or a tumour. Wheezing may result from asthma or aspiration of a foreign body (if aspirated into the lower airways).

EXAMINATION

Inspection

Cyanosis, which is observed from the fingertips (peripheral) or in the mucous membranes (central), is an indicator of severe underlying disease. Decreased consciousness level may indicate a life-threatening situation. However, it may also be the presenting feature of patients with a metabolic acidosis (diabetic ketoacidosis). Kyphosis severe enough to cause dyspnoea should be evident on general inspection. Patients with COPD may appear barrel-chested and cyanosed or thin and tachypnoeic (with pursed-lip breathing), accompanied by the prominent use of the accessory musculature.

The respiratory rate *per se* may not be very specific, but extremes may be indicators of severity of the underlying disease. The respiratory rate should be carefully counted and not just estimated.

The hands should be inspected for clubbing, as it is associated with bronchial carcinoma and idiopathic pulmonary fibrosis (p. 56).

Pulse

A change in rate or regularity of rhythm may indicate an arrhythmia as a precipitating factor (usually in pre-existing heart or lung disease). The rate itself is not, however, very specific to the underlying aetiology.

JVP

Acute elevation of the JVP suggests tension pneumothorax, pulmonary embolism, cardiac tamponade or tricuspid regurgitation (prominent *v* waves). Chronic elevation results from congestive heart failure or any chronic lung disease with right heart failure (cor pulmonale).

Temperature

An elevated temperature may occur with a chest infection and pulmonary embolism.

Trachea

The trachea deviates away from the side of a tension pneumothorax, pleural effusion and any large mass. It deviates to the side of a collapsed segment, which can result with obstruction of the bronchial lumen from a tumour or foreign bodies.

Expansion

May be reduced on the side of an area of consolidation (infection), pneumothorax and effusion. It may be reduced bilaterally in patients with COPD.

Percussion

The area overlying consolidation, effusion or collapse is dull to percussion. Hyper-resonance is often described on the affected side of a pneumothorax; however, a 'relative dullness' of the unaffected side is the usual initial finding.

Auscultation of the precordium

Auscultation may reveal murmurs associated with valvular heart disease. The presence of a third heart sound is consistent with cardiac failure, and quiet heart sounds may be due to an overexpanded chest from COPD.

Breath sounds

Localised reduction in the intensity of breath sounds occurs over areas with consolidation or collapse of the lung; however, it may be reduced generally with asthma and COPD.

Added sounds

Wheezing may be appreciated in a localised area following intraluminal airway obstruction from an inhaled foreign body or tumour. Generalised wheezing usually occurs with asthma. When a history of pre-existing asthma is not evident, then consider anaphylaxis. Localised crepitations may be auscultated over areas of pulmonary consolidation. Extensive bilateral crepitations occur with idiopathic pulmonary fibrosis (fine inspiratory), pulmonary oedema and bronchopneumonia.

GENERAL INVESTIGATIONS

- **FBC**
  Hb ↓ points to anaemia as the primary cause or as an exacerbating factor of underlying disease. Hb ↑ (polycythaemia) may be seen in chronic lung disease. WCC ↑ usually indicates infection, but it can also occur with other conditions, such as pulmonary embolism.

- **Peak expiratory flow rate**
  This simple bedside test allows you to evaluate airflow limitation. A reduced flow rate may indicate asthma or chronic airflow limitation.

- **ECG**
  Arrhythmias are readily appreciated on the ECG; atrial fibrillation or supraventricular tachycardia may precipitate dyspnoea in patients with pre-existing heart or lung disease. However, an arrhythmia may be a manifestation of the underlying cause, such as myocardial infarction, pulmonary embolism and hypoxia. ST segment elevations occur with myocardial infarction and are also a non-specific finding in pulmonary embolism. Right bundle-branch block may occur in the presence of longstanding lung disease.

- **Pulse oximetry**
  Although low saturation *per se* is not very discriminatory, acute severe impairment of oxygen saturation is associated with pulmonary embolus and pneumothorax. Post-exercise desaturation is helpful if opportunistic pneumonia is suspected.

- **ABGs**
  Useful to quantify severity of the disease and subtype of respiratory failure. Normal levels of oxygenation, however, are not useful to exclude respiratory or cardiac disease. Low levels of bicarbonate indicate metabolic acidosis and should lead to the investigation of the underlying cause, such as diabetic ketoacidosis. An alkalosis (high pH) with low pco_2 and high po_2 points to hyperventilation. CO_2 retention may result from chronic lung disease (type II respiratory failure) or may indicate the need for ventilation with co-existing hypoxia in asthmatics.

- **Serum cardiac markers**
  Cardiac troponin is elevated with myocardial infarction in the setting of acute left ventricular failure.

- **CXR**
  Hyperinflation of the lungs (if the hemidiaphragm is below the 7th rib anteriorly or the 12th rib posteriorly) is a feature of COPD, and may also result from asthma. Areas of consolidation are seen on a plain film; however, radiographic changes of a chest infection may lag behind in time with the clinical findings. The presence of cardiac failure is appreciated by cardiomegaly, upper lobe diversion of the pulmonary veins, bilateral pleural effusions, Kerley B lines (1–2 cm horizontal lines in the periphery of the lung fields) and patchy pulmonary oedema. A pneumothorax may be diagnosed by identifying the line of the pleura and the absence of lung markings beyond it. Bronchial carcinoma may present as a hilar mass, peripheral opacity or collapse and consolidation of the lung due to airways obstruction.

SPECIFIC INVESTIGATIONS

- **Sputum and blood cultures**
  Should be taken if an infective aetiology (pneumonia, lung abscess) is suspected, preferably before antibiotics are administered.

- **Respiratory function tests**
  Apart from physiological measurements of the lung, spirometry allows classification of restrictive or obstructive lung defects. It can also provide information regarding severity of the disease and the response to inhaled bronchodilators. Flow volume loops can indicate fixed airways obstruction (plateau in the expiration phase), which can result from foreign body or intraluminal tumour. Restrictive pattern of ventilatory impairment is characterised by a normal FEV1 to FVC ratio and a reduced vital capacity. It is characteristic of pulmonary fibrosis, infiltrative lung disease and

restriction of chest wall motion. Obstructive pattern of ventilatory impairment is characterised by a reduced FEV1 to FVC ratio and a normal vital capacity. It is characteristic of asthma, COPD, bronchiectasis and cystic fibrosis.

■ Bronchoscopy
Bronchoscopy should be performed if aspiration of a foreign body is suspected, the procedure can be both diagnostic and therapeutic. Intraluminal bronchial carcinomas may be visualised and biopsied. Bronchoscopy also allows collection of specimens for culture in the diagnosis of pneumonia.

■ CT thorax/pulmonary angiogram
The majority of pulmonary emboli may be diagnosed by CT pulmonary angiography. In addition, complete visualisation of the thorax by CT is useful to evaluate masses of unknown aetiology, and for staging of bronchial carcinoma. High-resolution CT is useful to screen for features of idiopathic pulmonary fibrosis.

■ Echocardiography
An echocardiogram is indicated if cardiac failure or valvular heart disease is suspected. A large pulmonary embolus can be diagnosed by a finding of right heart failure and elevated pulmonary artery pressures. Elevated pulmonary artery pressures can also be caused by pulmonary hypertension causing dyspnoea. Although a proportion are idiopathic, known causes are congenital heart disease, any severe lung disease and recurrent pulmonary emboli.

- **Cyanosis associated with dyspnoea is an ominous sign. Emergency admission and treatment is required.**

- **Pneumothorax is more common in asthmatics. If an asthmatic suddenly becomes short of breath, consider pneumothorax as a possible diagnosis.**

- **Sudden onset of breathlessness in an elderly patient may be due to LVF. This may be the result of a myocardial infarction.**

- **Always remember an inhaled foreign body as a possible cause of acute dyspnoea.**

EAR DISORDERS

Ear disorders are common in general, with earache being a frequent complaint. It may represent ear disease or referred pain from the oral cavity or pharynx. Causes of deafness are dealt with on p. 86, with many differentials overlapping.

Figure 16 Acute otitis media (AOM). There is inflammation (e.g. hyperaemia) of the tympanic membrane, which is also bulging due to pus within the middle ear.

CAUSES

LOCAL

EXTERNAL EAR
- Trauma
- Boils
- Dermoid/epidermoid cyst
- Malignancy (e.g. basal cell carcinoma, squamous cell carcinoma)

EXTERNAL AUDITORY MEATUS
- Otitis externa
- Boils
- Malignancy
- Osteomas/exostosis
- Chondrodermatitis nodularis helicis

MIDDLE EAR

- Acute otitis media (AOM) (Fig. 16)
- Chronic otitis media
- Mastoiditis

REFERRED PAIN

- Dental problems (e.g. severe gum disease)
- Pharynx
  - Tonsillitis
  - Pharyngitis
  - Foreign body
  - Quinsy
- Carcinoma of the posterior third of the tongue
- Laryngeal cancer

NEUROLOGICAL

- Herpes zoster
- Glossopharyngeal neuralgia

HISTORY

Local

External ear

Trauma may cause subperichondrial haematoma. This is usually caused by a shearing injury with the patient presenting with bruising and swelling. If the swelling is not drained, repeated trauma occurs, and this will lead to the condition of 'cauliflower ear', often seen in rugby players. Avulsion of the ear is rare but may occur in major trauma. Occasionally, cellulitis and swelling of the ear may occur due to bites. Enquire whether there has been any recent ear-piercing, as dermoid cysts may result. Ulcers may arise on the pinna as a result of malignant disease, the most common being squamous cell carcinomas (SCC) and rodent ulcers (BCC).

External auditory meatus

The patient may complain of irritation, discharge, pain and occasionally deafness. Inflammation may spread out onto the pinna. It may also occur in those who swim frequently at public baths. With a furuncle (boil) in the external auditory meatus, the patient will present with extreme pain and throbbing sensation. The pain is made worse by inserting an auriscope into the meatus.

There may be a history of a foreign body inserted into the external auditory meatus. The patient is most commonly a child. Seeds or pips may have been inserted into the ear. In adults, it is often matchsticks, cotton-wool buds or paperclips that have been inserted to remove wax from the ear. There is usually pain and discharge. Malignant disease of the external auditory meatus is rare. When advanced, it may cause intractable pain, bloodstained discharge and may invade the middle ear, facial nerve or the temporomandibular joint (e.g. acoustic neuroma).

Middle ear

Acute otitis media usually occurs in children. There may be a preceding history of the common cold, tonsillitis or adenoiditis. In adults, there may be a history of sinusitis, trauma, air-travel or temporal bone fracture. The patient presents with severe earache, often with deafness, appearing flushed and ill. Chronic otitis media can result from AOM and presents with a history of deafness, discomfort in the ear, tinnitus and occasionally problems with the balance. Acute mastoiditis is a complication of otitis media but is rare nowadays because of antibiotics. This presents with pain, discharge (creamy and profuse), deafness and swelling behind the ear.

Referred pain

Check for a history of dental problems (e.g. abscesses). In the elderly, there may be carcinoma of the posterior third of the tongue. Check for a history of tonsillitis or pharyngitis or difficulty in swallowing due to quinsy. Occasionally, a foreign body lodged in the pharynx may be responsible. Other malignant disease of the pharynx or larynx may cause referred pain. Check for a history of dysphagia.

Neurological

Herpes zoster oticus may give rise to lesions of the external auditory meatus, pinna and sometimes the palate, with ear pain often being the first feature. Glossopharyngeal neuralgia presents with very severe pain radiating from throat to tongue and into the ear.

EXAMINATION

Local

External ear

With trauma, there may be obvious subperichondrial haematomas. Bites will result in cellulitis and swelling of the ear. Dermoid cysts usually follow ear-piercing and present as lumps in the lobe of the ear adjacent to the area of piercing. Malignant disease will usually present as an ulcer, either with a typical appearance of a BCC or with the everted edges of an SCC.

External auditory meatus

There is often inflammation at the entry to the meatus. The meatus itself is tender, and there is moist debris, oedema and redness of the ear canal on examination with an auriscope. A furuncle (boil) is extremely painful. Examination with the auriscope will reveal a tender boil or even pus in the external auditory meatus. A foreign body is usually obvious on examination with the auriscope, as is malignancy.

Middle ear

With acute otitis media, the patient is usually flushed and ill, often with a temperature of 39–40°C. Examination of the tympanic membrane shows redness, fullness bulging of the drum and a disruption of the light reflex. There may be signs of perforation with otorrhoea, with a mucoid, purulent or bloodstained discharge. Chronic otitis media shows fluid in the middle ear (glue ear), with discoloration and often retraction of the tympanic membrane. Tuning-fork tests will reveal conductive deafness. In acute mastoiditis, the child is usually ill with a high pyrexia. There is tenderness over the mastoid process with post-auricular swelling. The tympanic membrane may be red, bulging or perforated with discharge.

Referred pain

Examine for dental problems. Examine the posterior third of the tongue for carcinoma. Inspect the throat using adequate light and with a tongue depressor, looking for tonsillitis, pharyngitis, quinsy, foreign body or malignancy.

Neurological

With herpes zoster, there will be vesicles in the meatus, on the pinna and sometimes on the palate and fauces. This will have been preceded by severe otalgia. With glossopharyngeal neuralgia, there may be a trigger area in the throat in the same way as there is a trigger area that may initiate trigeminal neuralgia.

GENERAL INVESTIGATIONS

The majority of ear disorders can be diagnosed on clinical examination alone.

- Hb, FBC, ESR
  Hb ↓ malignant disease. WCC ↑ acute otitis media. Acute mastoiditis. ESR ↑ malignancy and infection.

- Ear swab
  C&S. Otitis externa. Otitis media with discharge. Furuncle. Recurrent tonsillitis.

- Biopsy
  Malignant disease of the pinna and external auditory meatus. Carcinoma of the posterior third of the tongue.

- Skull X-ray
  Opacity and coalescence of the air cells in mastoiditis.

- CT ear
  Malignancy. Mastoiditis.

- MRI ear
  Inner ear pathology.

- Referred pain to the ear is not uncommon. In the elderly, it may represent referred pain from a carcinoma of the posterior third of the tongue, the nasopharynx or larynx.
- Beware the patient with middle ear infection who develops headache, confusion or neurological signs. Middle ear infection may progress to cause meningitis or a cerebral abscess in rare cases.

EYE DISORDERS

Most eye disorders tend to present as 'red eye'. It is the most common ophthalmic complaint encountered by general practitioners.

Figure 17 Acute infection of an eyelash follicle (stye).

CAUSES

EYELIDS

- Stye (hordeolum internum/externum) (Fig. 17)
- Xanthelasma
- Blepharitis
- Meibomian cyst (chalazion)
- Entropion (in-turning of the eyelid)
- Ectropion (out-turning of the eyelid)

EYE

SURFACE
- Trauma
- Foreign body

CONJUNCTIVA
- Subconjunctival haemorrhage
- Conjunctivitis
  - Bacterial
  - Viral

- Allergic
- Chlamydia

SCLERA

- Episcleritis
- Scleritis

CORNEA

- Corneal abrasion
- Corneal ulceration (keratitis)
  - Viral (herpes simplex keratitis)
  - Bacterial
  - Fungal
  - Amoebic
  - Parasitic

IRIS AND CILIARY BODY

- Anterior uveitis

INTRAOCULAR

- Acute angle-closure glaucoma
- Endopthalmitis

HISTORY

Pain

Sudden onset of unilateral eye pain and lacrimation may be due to a foreign body. Patients with infective conjunctivitis tend to complain of a soreness rather than true pain, whereas patients with allergic conjunctivitis (hayfever, acute allergy or atopy) tend to complain of itching rather than pain. Patients with blepharitis complain of a foreign body sensation or grittiness. More severe pain is experienced with corneal abrasions, ulcers, angle-closure glaucoma, herpes zoster ophthalmicus, uveitis and scleritis. Patients with the last two conditions experience exacerbation of pain on palpating the globe. A stye is a suppurative inflammation of an eyelash follicle which can either be internal or external. It is common and extremely painful. A meibomian cyst is a retention cyst from a resolving infection of the meibomian gland. This may resolve spontaneously or leave a pea-size swelling, which may require drainage. Entropion is the rolling inwards of the lid margin. The eyelashes irritate the conjunctiva and cornea, causing a painful, red eye. The opposite condition is known as ectropion and usually results in a watery eye. Subconjunctival haemorrhages are usually spontaneous and, although they may present with impressive chemosis (soft-tissue swelling) often alarming to patients, they are not usually painful and resolve spontaneously. Endopthalmitis occurs following surgery, with a red, painful eye and loss of vision.

Visual disturbance

Impairment of vision can occur with corneal ulceration, anterior uveitis and acute angle-closure glaucoma. This is usually associated with photophobia. In addition, patients with glaucoma may perceive halos around lights due to corneal oedema and reduced visual acuity.

Discharge

Documenting the presence, amount and colour of any discharge originating from the eye is important. A purulent discharge is associated with bacterial and chlamydial conjunctivitis, with a clear discharge with allergic and viral conjunctivitis.

Past medical history

A history of atopy or hayfever may be present in patients with allergic conjunctivitis. Previous herpes infection on the face may be the only clue with dendritic corneal ulceration. Conjunctivitis, urethritis and arthritis form the triad of Reiter's syndrome, caused by *Chlamydia trachomatis* infection. A history of contact lens use is important, as patients may develop sight-threatening infections acutely and may need to be referred to exclude a corneal ulcer.

Scleritis is a deeper and more severe inflammatory process than episcleritis. It tends to be associated with connective tissue diseases, such as rheumatoid disease and SLE.

Uveitis is associated with inflammatory bowel disease, reactive arthritis psoriasis, ankylosing spondylitis and sarcoidosis. Orbital congestion may be seen in patients with thyroid disorders. Xanthelasma are fatty plaques in the skin of the eyelids. Extensive or multiple xanthelasma may indicate abnormalities of cholesterol metabolism, diabetes or arterial disease.

EXAMINATION

Visual acuity should be assessed with correcting spectacles or pinhole, and documented with reference to a Snellen chart. Conditions that present with visual impairment are corneal ulceration, uveitis and glaucoma. Patients with these conditions should be referred urgently to an ophthalmologist. The eyelids should be carefully inspected. Swelling of the eyelid with redness may indicate a stye. There may be a bead of pus apparent at the infected hair follicle. The eyelid should be everted to inspect for a meibomian cyst and foreign bodies. Papillae (conjunctival elevations with a vessel in the centre) are seen with allergic conjunctivitis, and follicles (collections of lymphocytes) may be visible with viral or chlamydial infection. Ectropion and entropion are usually obvious: in the former, the lower eyelid is everted, and in the latter, it is inverted, the eyelashes scratch the conjunctiva and cornea giving rise to a red, watery eye. A similar effect is produced by trichiasis, which is caused by irregular pointing lashes. Xanthelasma are fatty plaques deposited in the skin of the eyelids. They look like masses of yellow opaque fat. They are not painful or tender.

Inspection is then undertaken to identify the presence of any foreign bodies on the surface of the eye. Areas of erythema should be carefully assessed. Diffuse erythema, maximal in the fornices, is a feature of conjunctivitis. Localised areas of segmental erythema may be due to episcleritis, but if it is maximal near the limbus (junction of cornea and conjunctiva), it may be a focal keratitis. Scleritis produces a brawny, red discoloration, while a deep crimson-red area is observed with a subconjunctival haemorrhage. Marked erythema adjacent to the iris is known as a ciliary flush and occurs with anterior uveitis and glaucoma.

Attention is then focussed on to the cornea. Ulceration of the cornea may not be visible without fluorescein staining. Infection may extend to the anterior chamber, and a collection of pus (hypopyon) can present as a white fluid level in anterior uveitis. Loss of brightness of the cornea occurs with glaucoma due to corneal oedema, as well as a dull hazy appearance.

The pupil is then examined, and the resting position noted. A constricted pupil may result from ciliary spasm with uveitis and a fixed, semi-dilated position with glaucoma.

Fluorescein staining should be performed, and the eye is then viewed with a blue-filtered light: corneal abrasions or ulcerations glow green.

GENERAL INVESTIGATIONS

- Eye swab
  Microscopy and C&S for infective organisms, e.g. stye and bacterial, viral and chlamydial conjunctivitis.

- Rose bengal staining
  To assess for dead and damaged conjunctival and corneal cells. It is useful in outlining a dendritic ulcer with herpes simplex infection.

- Blood glucose
  Infections are often associated with diabetes, as are xanthelasma.

SPECIFIC INVESTIGATIONS

- Slit-lamp examination with intraocular pressure measurements
  ↑ glaucoma (but not all cases), uveitis.

- Corneal scrape
  For infective lesions.

- A unilateral painful, red eye often warrants urgent assessment by a clinician.

- If there is a history of a foreign body, always check for high-speed injuries, e.g. metal fragments. Urgent specialist referral is required to exclude an intraocular foreign body.

- Fluorescein staining should be performed in the assessment of painful disorders of the eye to exclude corneal ulceration.

ERECTILE DYSFUNCTION

Erectile dysfunction is failure in the adult male to sustain an adequate erection. Erectile dysfunction leads to and can be caused by psychological problems, often with relationship breakdown. Psychological causes of impotence are common, but the most common organic disease is diabetes mellitus.

CAUSES

ENDOCRINE

- Diabetes mellitus
- Hyperlipidaemia
- Hypogonadism
- Hypothyroidism
- Cushing's syndrome
- Metabolic syndrome
- Addison's disease

VASCULAR

- Diabetic vascular disease
- Aortoiliac disease (Leriche's syndrome)

NEUROLOGICAL

- Spinal lesions
- Neuropathies (e.g. diabetes)
- Spina bifida
- Pelvic surgery (damage to nervi erigentes)

DRUGS

- Antihypertensives
- Antidepressants
- Alcohol
- Beta-blockers
- Oestrogens
- Cocaine
- Smoking

LOCAL PAINFUL CONDITIONS

- Phimosis
- Peyronie's disease
- Short frenulum

SYSTEMIC DISEASE

- Malignancy
- Hypertension
- Cirrhosis
- Chronic renal failure
- Parkinson's disease

PSYCHOGENIC

- Depression

OTHER

- Ageing

HISTORY

Is there a gradual versus sudden onset of symptoms? Does the patient experience erections at any time, especially early morning? And on ones own? Is there a history of premature ejaculation? History of peripheral vascular disease, especially buttock claudication (Leriche's syndrome)? History of neurological disease? Take a full drug history, including any recreational drugs. Check for a history of diabetes, hypothyroidism, Addison's disease or Cushing's disease. Pelvic surgery, e.g. with damage to the nervi erigentes. Check for any local, painful conditions of the penis. History of chronic renal failure: nausea, lethargy, nocturia, peripheral oedema, pulmonary oedema, dyspnoea, vomiting, hiccups, convulsions. Is there a clear history of stress to account for the onset of impotence? Any major life events or change in partner? Any change in libido?

EXAMINATION

Vascular

Check all the pulses in the lower limb. Listen for bruits in the chest, abdomen and pelvis.

Neurological

Carry out a full neurological examination.

Endocrine

There will usually be a clear history of diabetes. Check for peripheral neuropathy and consider diabetic foot examination. Check for hypothyroidism: weight gain, dislike of cold weather, hoarse voice, lethargy, constipation. Check for Cushing's syndrome – thin skin, cushingoid facies, abdominal striae, obesity, buffalo hump, hypertension. Check for Addison's disease – weakness, weight loss, pigmentation of palmar creases and buccal mucosa, hypotension. Examine the testes for hypogonadism. Check for development of male secondary sexual characteristics.

Local painful conditions

Examine the penis for phimosis, Peyronie's disease or short frenulum.

Systemic disease

Check for chronic renal failure: pallor of skin, peripheral oedema, pericarditis, pleural effusions, hypertension. Check for cirrhosis, liver palms, spider naevi, ascites, leuconychia, flapping tremor, testicular atrophy, Dupuytren's contracture.

GENERAL INVESTIGATIONS

History and examination suggests the diagnosis in most cases.

- **FBC, ESR**
  Hb ↓ anaemia, e.g. chronic renal failure and malignancy. ESR ↑ malignancy.
- **U&Es**
  Creatinine raised in chronic renal failure.
- **Lipids**
  Assess for dyslipidaemia.
- **LFTs**
  Abnormal in cirrhosis.
- **Blood glucose**
  Diabetes mellitus.
- **TFTs**
  ↑ TSH ↓ T_4 in hypothyroidism.
- **Doppler studies**
  Peripheral vascular disease. Penile-brachial pressure index <0.6 suggests a vascular cause.
- **Serum testosterone**
  Low in hypogonadism. Test between 9 and 11am.

SPECIFIC INVESTIGATIONS

- **Nocturnal penile tumescence study**
  Erection versus no erection.
- **Intracorporeal injection of papaverine**
  If no abnormality of arterial inflow, this should cause an erection. If there is excessive venous leakage, the penis remains flaccid.
- **MRI or CT head**
  Pituitary abnormality.
- **Arteriography**
  May show vascular lesion, especially isolated narrowings of the internal iliac arteries.
- **Serum prolactin**
  Hypoprolactinaemia.

- **Serum FSH and LH**
  Low in pituitary dysfunction.
- **Serum prolactin**
  Hyperprolactinaemia.
- **ACTH stimulation test**
  Addison's disease.
- **24-Hour urinary cortisol assay**
  Cushing's syndrome.
- **Dexamethasone supression test**
  Cushing's syndrome.

- **Loss of libido may be an early manifestation of significant psychogenic causes (e.g. depression).**
- **Admit to hospital if there is evidence of priapism.**

FACIAL PAIN

Most patients are able to distinguish between pain arising from the cranium, which is termed headache, and that of the face, which is covered here under the heading of facial pain.

Figure 18 Facial herpes zoster. *The visible vesicular skin eruptions are in the distribution of the ophthalmic division of the trigeminal (5th) cranial nerve.*

CAUSES

LOCAL

SINUS
- Sinusitis
- Carcinoma ⚠

EAR
- Otitis media
- Otitis externa

EYE
- Optic neuritis

MASTOID
- Mastoiditis

TEETH AND SALIVARY GLAND
- Dental abscess
- Periodonitis
- Sialadenitis

SKIN
- Herpes zoster (Fig. 18)
- Post-herpetic neuralgia
- Cellulitis
- Candidiasis

JOINTS
- Temporomandibular (TMJ) dysfunction

PAROTID GLAND
- Mumps
- Parotitis
- Tumour (most common tumour type)

GENERAL
- Migraine
- Cluster headache
- Trauma
- Trigeminal neuralgia
- Temporal arteritis ⚠
- Tumour
  - Nasopharyngeal carcinoma (associated with EBV)
    - *(common in Chinese populations)*
- Chronic paroxysmal hemicrania

HISTORY

In the majority, facial pain originates from local structures. Therefore when formulating a differential diagnosis, consider the conditions affecting the anatomical structures of the face.

Site

The site of pain is perhaps the most useful feature when discriminating between the causes. Although local tenderness may direct the clinician to the affected site, do not forget to consider referred pain from adjacent structures. Pain in the region of the ear may be referred from the skin, teeth, tonsils, pharynx, larynx or neck. Tenderness over the maxilla may be due to sinusitis, dental abscess or carcinoma.

Character

Patients with trigeminal neuralgia often describe paroxysms of sharp, severe pains in the distribution of the trigeminal nerve or its major divisions triggered by light touch and emotion. A dull aching pain is associated with infections of structures such as the teeth, mastoid and ear.

Precipitating factors

Pain precipitated by food or chewing action may be due to a dental abscess, salivary gland disorder, salivary duct disorder, temporomandibular joint disorder or jaw claudication due to temporal arteritis. Pain arising from most structures is aggravated by touch; however, with trigeminal neuralgia, even the slightest stroking of the skin (i.e. non-painful stimuli) is sufficient to produce intense pain (allodynia).

Associated symptoms

Complaints of otorrhoea and hearing loss should direct the clinician to infections affecting the ear or mastoid. Nasal obstruction and rhinorrhoea occur with maxillary sinusitis and carcinoma of the maxillary antrum. These latter may be accompanied by unilateral epistaxis. Swelling of the cheek may be experienced with dental abscesses and maxillary carcinoma. Proximal muscle pain, stiffness and weakness may accompany temporal arteritis due to associated polymyalgia rheumatica. Paraesthesia in the distribution of the trigeminal nerve often precedes the rash of herpes zoster.

EXAMINATION

Inspection

A thorough inspection of the face, salivary glands, ear, nose and throat may produce a wealth of information. This involves the use of specific equipment, such as the otoscope and nasal speculum. Unilateral erythema and vesicles in the distribution of the trigeminal nerve may be striking with herpes zoster infection but may not be present in the early stages of the disease. Localised areas of erythema or swelling may also correspond to the site of infection, such as the sinus, ear, mastoid and parotid gland. Post-auricular swelling and downward displacement of the pinna may be observed with mastoiditis, which should be urgently treated. Maxillary swelling and erythema can be caused by dental abscess or maxillary carcinoma. With otitis media, injection or perforation of the tympanic membrane may be visualised with an otoscope. Nasopharyngeal masses indicating nasopharyngeal carcinoma may be seen on direct inspection of the nose and throat, and facial paralysis may be seen with infiltration of the facial nerve by tumours of the parotid gland.

Palpation

Gentle stroking of the skin of the face will precipitate severe pain with trigeminal neuralgia. Tenderness may be elicited over the frontal bone with frontal sinusitis and over the maxilla with maxillary sinusitis. With dental abscesses, pain is elicited over the maxilla or mandible. Mastoid tenderness occurs with mastoiditis or otitis media, and parotid tenderness can result from either mumps or parotitis. Tenderness along the course of the superficial temporal artery is suggestive of temporal arteritis. Movement of the pinna itself produces pain with otitis externa.

Palpation of the superficial lymph nodes of the neck may reveal lymphadenopathy in the distribution of the lymph drainage of structures affected by infection or carcinoma.

GENERAL INVESTIGATIONS

■ FBC
Hb ↓ malignancy. WCC ↑ infection.

■ ESR and CRP
Malignancy and temporal arteritis.

■ X-rays
X-rays of the sinuses show mucosal thickening with air-fluid levels in sinusitis. Occasionally, total opacification is seen with sinusitis and mastoiditis on mastoid films. In carcinoma of the sinuses, there may be complete opacification of the sinus and destruction of the adjacent bone. CT is often needed to reveal the extent of invasion.

SPECIFIC INVESTIGATIONS

■ CT
Carcinoma of the sinuses, nasopharyngeal carcinoma, parotid conditions. Extent of tumour and degree of invasion will be apparent.

■ MRI
Tumours – assess extent and invasion.

■ Sialography
Parotid conditions, e.g. duct stones, sialectasis.

■ FNAC
Parotid tumours.

■ Temporal artery biopsy
Temporal (giant cell) arteritis may reveal skip lesions.

- Temporal arteritis as a possible cause of facial pain requires emergency investigation and treatment. Other features include jaw claudication, scalp tenderness and visual disturbance associated with a raised ESR and/or CRP. In patients with visual disturbance, urgent review by an opthamologist is needed.

- Unremitting facial pain should be investigated thoroughly to exclude malignancy.

FACIAL SWELLINGS

Facial swelling is a common presenting complaint. It may be generalised or localised. Many cases are due to trauma or infection, but it may be a sign of systemic disease.

Figure 19 Pleomorphic adenoma (benign) of the parotid gland. A swelling is seen in the typical position below the earlobe between the posterior border of the ramus of the mandible and the upper end of sternomastoid.

CAUSES

TRAUMATIC
- Insect bites
- Facial fractures

INFECTIVE
- Dental infection (e.g. abscesses)
- Sinusitis
- Parotitis (bilateral: mumps)
- Cellulitis/Erysipelas
- Actinomycosis

NEOPLASTIC
- Sinuses
- Parotid (Fig. 19)

●   Jaw

●   Mediastinal tumours

VASCULAR

●   Superior vena cava thrombosis ⚠

●   Cavernous sinus thrombosis ⚠

ENDOCRINE

●   Cushing's syndrome

●   Congenital hypothyroidism

●   Severe hypothyroidism (myxoedema)

●   Acromegaly

DRUG-INDUCED

●   Steroids

OTHER

●   Allergic reactions ⚠

●   Angioedema (without anaphylaxis)

●   Paget's disease

●   Renal failure

HISTORY

Traumatic

Usually there is a history of trauma. Swelling may be severe, with bruising and closure of the palpebral fissures. Insect bites may cause swelling due to allergy or infection.

Infective

Cellulitis is rare unless peri-orbital in origin. Erysipelas is an uncommon skin infection caused by streptococci. Pain and redness are apparent usually over the cheek. Pyrexia and malaise may occur. Dental infections are common (see Jaw pain and swellings, p. 242) and are often initially localised, but the side of the face may swell. There is severe associated throbbing pain. Sinusitis presents with constant unilateral pain over the frontal or maxillary sinuses. There is usually puffiness of the skin overlying the sinus. Parotitis presents with pain and swelling over the gland. If this is due to obstruction in the duct, the swelling occurs during eating, when the patient salivates and regresses afterwards. Bilateral parotitis occurs with mumps. Actinomycosis is a slow growing soft skin infection invading adjacent structures.

Neoplastic

Neoplasia may affect the parotids, sinuses and jaw. There is usually localised swelling with carcinoma of the sinuses. The patient complains of a blocked nose and a bloodstained discharge, which may be foul-smelling.

With neoplastic lesions of the jaws, there is usually deep-seated boring pain in relation to the swelling. Mediastinal tumours compress the superior vena cava and may cause suffusion of the face and facial oedema.

Vascular

Superior vena caval thrombosis may occur, although this is rare. There is cyanotic suffusion of the face with facial oedema. Cavernous sinus thrombosis usually presents following a history of infection of the face or in the sinuses. The patient complains of pain in the eye and forehead, with swelling around the eye and a protruding eye. The swelling may eventually involve the whole of the side of the face. Double vision occurs as a result of cranial nerve involvement. This can be life threatening and needs immediate hospital referral.

Endocrine

Cushing's syndrome presents with swelling of the face (moon face) with a typical red appearance. Facial swelling is also seen in acromegaly. The patient will usually complain of an increase in shoe size and large hands. There may also be a hoarse voice, protrusion of the jaw and cardiac failure. Congenital hypothyroidism is associated with a puffy swollen face and with enlargement and protrusion of the tongue. Severe hypothyroidism produces characteristic non-pitting oedematous changes in the skin of the face, with puffiness around the eyes, giving rise to a characteristic clinical appearance.

Drugs

History of steroid therapy (i.e. steriod-induced Cushing's syndrome).

Other

Allergic reactions to drugs, especially antibiotics or blood transfusions may result in periorbital or facial oedema. Take a careful drug history. Angioedema chiefly affects the eyelids and lips. Recurrent attacks of sudden onset of burning and irritation. A family history suggests the diagnosis. Paget's disease often presents with painful enlargement of the skull, femur and clavicles and bowing of the tibia. Puffiness around the eyelids usually indicates renal failure. Pre-eclampsia is seen in pregnancy of >20 weeks gestation with associated hypertension and protein in the urine. This can lead to seizures.

EXAMINATION

Traumatic

Fractures are usually obvious. Check pupillary reaction, and test the cranial nerves. Insect-bite puncture wounds may be obvious, but often they are not. There is often surrounding cellulitis and oedema.

Infective

Erysipelas presents as a red, tender area with well-demarcated margins raised above the surrounding normal skin. The patient is usually pyrexial. Dental abscesses are usually obvious, with local tenderness and oedema.

Sinusitis is largely diagnosed from the history, with localised tenderness and swelling. With parotitis, the gland is swollen and tender if infection has occurred, with, occasionally, redness over the skin. It may be unilateral or bilateral. Examine the orifice of the parotid duct for stone or stenosis.

Neoplastic

Neoplasia of the parotid usually presents as an enlarged, irregular, firm or hard swelling. Test the integrity of the facial nerve, which may be affected by carcinoma. Carcinoma of the maxillary sinus may present with swelling over the sinus. Superior vena cava obstruction presents with facial oedema and cyanotic suffusion of the face. Examine the chest. Jaw swellings are considered on p. 242.

Vascular

Superior vena cava thrombosis presents in a similar way to obstruction. With cavernous sinus thrombosis, there will be oedema, redness and swelling around the orbit, spreading onto the face. Exophthalmos will be present with visual loss. Test cranial nerves III, IV, V and VI. The patient will usually be very unwell.

Endocrine

In Cushing's syndrome, there will be moon face, and usually other features such as striae, buffalo hump, proximal myopathy. In congenital hypothyroidism, there is a broad, flat face, the eyes are wide apart and the tongue protrudes from the mouth. In acromegaly, there is a large face with overgrowth of the soft tissues of the face, nose, lips and tongue. The patient will have large hands and a large protuberant jaw (prognathism).

Drugs

Steroid therapy gives an appearance similar to Cushing's syndrome.

Other

In allergic reactions, there is often swelling of the eyes, lips and face, with urticaria of other areas on the body. Laryngeal oedema and bronchospasm may occur. Angioedema is usually diagnosed from the history. Examination will reveal swellings of the eyelids and lips, with burning and irritation. In Paget's disease, there is an enlargement of the skull, with the vault of the skull bulging outwards above the eyes. Deafness may occur. Occasionally, there is compression of the cranial nerves. Test the cranial nerves. High output cardiac failure may be present.

In renal failure, the swelling usually occurs around the eyes. There may also be peripheral oedema and hypertension. There is usually a bronze-lemon tinge to the skin in chronic renal failure.

GENERAL INVESTIGATIONS

■ FBC, ESR
  Hb ↓ malignancy. WCC ↑ infection, e.g. sinusitis, cavernous sinus thrombosis. ESR ↑ infection, malignancy.

- U&Es
  Urea and creatinine ↑ in renal failure.

- Skull X-rays
  Fractures. Sinusitis for opaque sinus. Malignancy for opaque sinus and erosion of bone. Bone tumours. Paget's disease. Pituitary fossa assessing for acromegaly, Cushing's disease.

- CXR
  Mediastinal tumour primary bronchial carcinoma with inappropriate secretion of ACTH leading to Cushing's syndrome).

- Swab
  C&S – infection, e.g. erysipelas, insect bites.

SPECIFIC INVESTIGATIONS

- Hand X-ray
  Acromegaly.

- CT
  Acromegaly. Cushing's disease. Fractures. Mediastinal tumours. Carcinoma of the sinuses. Parotid tumours. Cavernous sinus thrombosis.

- Sialography
  Parotid conditions, e.g. stone in parotid duct.

- TFTs
  Hypothyroidism.

- Plasma cortisol
  Cushing's syndrome.

- Glucose tolerance test with growth hormone assay and serum insulin-like growth factor 1 (IGF-1)
  Acromegaly.

- Localised swelling with complaint of a blocked nose or a bloodstained nasal discharge may be suggestive of carcinoma of the sinuses.

- Parotid swelling with facial palsy suggests a malignant parotid tumour with involvement of the facial nerve (compared with pleomorphic [benign] adenoma).

- Sudden generalised swelling of the face, lip and tongue suggests an allergic reaction and is life-threatening.

FACIAL ULCERS

Most facial ulcers are serious. Malignant facial ulcers are common in patients who work outdoors and are exposed to ultraviolet light. Lesions of the lips have been dealt with elsewhere (p. 293) and will not be included here.

Figure 20 The larger nodular lesion on the cheek is a typical basal cell carcinoma. Note the pearly, rolled appearance of the lesion which is beginning to ulcerate. The smaller lesion lateral to the basal cell carcinoma is a benign naevus.

CAUSES

TRAUMATIC

- Physical
- Chemical
- Irradiation
- Dermatitis artefacta
- Bites

NEOPLASTIC

- Basal cell carcinoma (rodent ulcer) (Fig. 20) ● *(rare in tropical Africa)*
- Squamous cell carcinoma ▲
- Malignant melanoma ▲

- Herpes simplex
- Herpes zoster ⚠
- Keratoacanthoma
- Syphilis (i.e. chancre, gumma)
- Leishmaniasis ● *(common in tropical and subtropical areas)*

- Pyoderma gangrenosum

HISTORY

A history of trauma should be sought. In the case of the face, anaesthesia may have arisen following surgery to the trigeminal ganglion for trigeminal neuralgia. Syringobulbia is a rare cause of facial anaesthesia. This may be as minor as scratching a spot or trauma caused during the puncturing of skin for anaesthetic or aesthetic purposes. Self-inflicted injury resulting in dermatitis artefacta may be suspected when other causes have been excluded. Has the patient had radiotherapy in the past to suggest irradiation causes? Check for a history of bites, insect, animal or human, which may become infected and ulcerate.

Malignant ulcers are usually on exposed areas of the face. Check the patient's occupation. Malignancy is more common in outdoor workers exposed to ultraviolet light. Most rodent ulcers occur above a line drawn from the angle of the mouth to the lobe of the ear. Their incidence increases with age. Malignant ulcers are usually painless, unless they become infected. They may be pigmented, and there may be a history of a change in a pre-existing mole to suggest malignant melanoma. These changes include: change in size; change in colour, with deepening pigmentation; bleeding or ulceration; itching; inflammatory 'halo'; satellite nodules; palpable regional lymph nodes.

Infection may be due to herpes simplex, which may spread from around the lips or nose. The patient will complain of an itchy, burning red area, on which vesicles form, and then crust over and ulcerate. Herpes zoster may arise in the distribution of the trigeminal nerve. Pain precedes malaise and fever by a few days. Vesicles develop later and may ulcerate. Syphilis is rare and may give rise to either a chancre or gumma (see Lip lesions, p. 293). Leishmaniasis is spread by sandflies, and there would be a history of travel to India, Africa, the Middle East or the Mediterranean. There would be a history of bite leaving an itchy papule, leading to an ulcer. Keratoacanthoma may be due to a virus. It resembles a squamous cell carcinoma, from which it needs to be carefully distinguished. It occurs in adults as a rapidly growing lump, with a central core filled with keratin. It usually takes 2–3 weeks to grow and often resolves spontaneously over several months. A history of inflammatory bowel disease will suggest pyoderma gangrenosum.

EXAMINATION

Benign ulcers

These usually have a sloping edge. Check the face for normal sensation to pain and temperature.

Malignant ulcers

Basal cell carcinomas (rodent ulcers) usually have a raised, rolled, pearly margin. They may become very large and erode deeply and locally. They do not metastasise, and therefore local lymph nodes should not be enlarged unless the lesion becomes infected. Squamous cell carcinoma presents as an ulcerated lesion with an everted edge. Metastasis occurs to local lymph nodes, and these may be palpable. Care should be taken to distinguish a squamous cell carcinoma from a keratoacanthoma, which is a benign, fast-growing, self-limiting papule surmounted by a keratin plug (it resembles a small volcano with a crater). Malignant melanomas vary in colour from pinkish-brown to black. They may develop a purplish hue due to a rich blood supply. There may be a brownish-pink 'halo' around the lesion, or there may be 'satellite' nodules. The local lymph nodes may be enlarged. Early metastases may occur to the liver, and therefore patients should be examined for hepatomegaly.

Infective

The characteristic lesions of herpes simplex will be seen around the lips and nose. In immunosuppressed patients, these lesions may coalesce and become infected. Ophthalmic herpes zoster will be recognised by its characteristic distribution in the ophthalmic division of the trigeminal nerve. It may affect the cornea. A syphilitic chancre begins as a macule, becoming a painless, hard ulcer, which is very infectious. It develops rapidly and is associated with enlargement of the local lymph nodes. A gumma occurring on the face is uncommon. It appears as a punched-out ulcer with a wash-leather base. Cutaneous leishmaniasis (oriental sore) develops at the site of a sandfly bite, commencing as an itchy papule, from which the crusts may separate, leaving an ulcer with deep perpendicular edges. Pyoderma gangrenosum presents with a nodule or pustule, which ulcerates with tender, reddish-blue necrotic edges.

GENERAL INVESTIGATIONS

- **FBC, CRP, ESR**
  WCC & CRP ↑ infected ulcer. ESR ↑ malignancy, syphilis.

- **LFTs**
  Alkaline phosphatase may be raised with liver secondaries, e.g. malignant melanoma.

- **Swab**
  C&S from infected ulcer. Dark-ground illumination microscopy for *Treponema pallidum*.

■ Biopsy
   Benign versus malignant. Keratoacanthoma versus squamous cell
   carcinoma. In the case of malignant melanoma, excision biopsy is
   required.

SPECIFIC INVESTIGATIONS

■ VDRL
   Syphilis.
■ Aspiration of lesion
   Leishmaniasis – protozoal organism may be seen by microscopy in
   aspirates from fluid at the edge of the ulcer.
■ Viral culture
   Herpes simplex, herpes zoster (rarely needed – diagnosis usually
   obvious clinically).
■ Antibody titres
   Herpes simplex, herpes zoster (rarely needed – diagnosis usually
   obvious clinically).

- Facial ulcers in the elderly, and those with outside
  occupations, are likely to be malignant. Rodent ulcers
  are the most common.

- Ophthalmic herpes zoster will be recognised by its
  characteristic distribution in the ophthalmic division
  of the trigeminal nerve. Corneal ulceration may occur.
  Urgent treatment is required.

FAECAL INCONTINENCE

Faecal incontinence implies loss of voluntary control of passage of faeces from the anus. Any disease process that interferes with rectal sensation or affects function of the anorectal musculature may produce incontinence. However, incontinence may still occur with normal sphincters and pelvic floor, for example in severe diarrhoea.

CAUSES

NORMAL SPHINCTERS AND PELVIC FLOOR

- Severe diarrhoea, e.g. infection, irritable bowel syndrome, inflammatory bowel disease
- Faecal impaction ('overflow' diarrhoea)

ABNORMAL SPHINCTERS AND/OR PELVIC FLOOR

CONGENITAL
- Anorectal anomalies, meningomyelocele

ACQUIRED

Traumatic
- Iatrogenic
  - Internal sphincter surgery, e.g. anal dilatation or sphincterotomy
  - Fistula-in-ano surgery
  - Obstetric – traumatic childbirth
- Pelvic fractures
- Impalement

Neurological
- Multiple sclerosis
- Spinal injuries ⚠ (if acute onset)
- Spinal tumours
- Peripheral neuropathy
- Stroke
- Dementia

Other
- Rectal prolapse
- Extensive anorectal carcinoma
- Fistula-in-ano
- Radiotherapy

HISTORY

Is there a history of trauma, e.g. pelvic fractures, impalement injuries? Probably the commonest cause of faecal incontinence is gastroenteritis. The history will be obvious. A history of inflammatory bowel disease may be elicited. Other important factors to elicit in the history are recent anorectal surgery; recent difficult childbirth – long duration of labour, forceps delivery, forceful delivery, perineal tears, episiotomy; predisposition to peripheral neuropathy, e.g. diabetes mellitus, vitamin B_{12} deficiency, alcoholism or medication. A history of constipation may suggest faecal impaction. A history of a recent stroke, dementia or neurological illness will usually be obvious. Associated symptoms of altered sensation, urinary retention and severe lower back pain may indicate a diagnosis of cauda equina syndrome.

EXAMINATION

Soiling of the underwear may be apparent at examination. Digital rectal examination will demonstrate any reduction in anal tone and the inability to sustain a voluntary contraction. It may be possible to feel the defect in the anorectal ring. Faecal impaction may well also be obvious on digital rectal examination. Is there any evidence of trauma or infection? Rectal prolapse may be apparent or descend during straining. Look for evidence of a fistula-in-ano or extensive anorectal cancer. Full neurological examination will often be necessary.

GENERAL INVESTIGATIONS

- FBC, ESR
  Macrocytic anaemia may be associated with vitamin B_{12} deficiency (peripheral neuropathy).
- LFTs
  Deranged in alcoholism, which may be a cause of peripheral neuropathy.
- Blood glucose
  Neuropathy of diabetes mellitus.
- Sigmoidoscopy
  Biopsy.
- Proctoscopy
  Biopsy.

SPECIFIC INVESTIGATIONS

- Endoanal US
  May show defect in anorectal musculature.
- Anorectal manometry
  May demonstrate cause of incontinence.

SECTION A

- EMG
- MRI
  Defects in anorectal musculature. Pelvic malignancy. Spinal tumours.

- Faecal incontinence is common in frail, elderly people.
- Faecal incontinence is a feature of many neurological diseases. Up to 50% of patients with multiple sclerosis may experience faecal incontinence.
- Onset of faecal incontinence with associated recent spinal injury is concerning for cauda equina syndrome and should be investigated urgently.

FINGER LESIONS

Finger lesions form part of the wider subject of hand deformity. (See hand deformity chapter.) Lesions of the fingers are those which can result in hand function impairment. Painful finger lesions are dealt with on p. 147.

Figure 21 Boutonnière deformity. This common deformity is seen in rheumatoid arthritis, resulting from the rupture of the central slip of the extensor tendon over the proximal interphalangeal joint. The lateral slips of the extensor tendon mechanism are displaced to the sides and maintain the deformity.

CAUSES

CONGENITAL
See chapter on hand deformity

ACQUIRED

TRAUMATIC/DEGENERATIVE
- Dupuytren's contracture
- Trigger finger
- Implantation dermoid
- Pyogenic granuloma
- Mallet finger
- Swan-neck deformity

- Boutonnière deformity (Fig. 21)
- Heberden's/Bouchard's nodes
- Mucous cyst
- Calluses over knuckles (bulimia)

METABOLIC
- Gouty tophi
- Ectopic calcification

CONNECTIVE TISSUE DISEASE
- Calcinosis in CREST (Calcinosis, Raynaud's phenomenon, oesophageal dysmotility, sclerodactyly, and telangiectasia) syndrome

NEOPLASTIC
- Subungual melanoma
- Chondroma

HISTORY

Congenital

These lesions will be recognisable at birth. They may be associated with other congenital abnormalities.

Acquired

Traumatic/degenerative

Dupuytren's contracture

In the early phases, the patient may merely complain of a nodule in the palm near the base of the ring finger. Eventually, the patient complains of being unable to extend fully the metacarpophalangeal (MCP) joint at the ring, and later, the little finger. It affects the patient's grip. The patient complains of difficulty dressing – either poking themselves in the eye while brushing hair or catch the finger on a trouser pocket. There may be a family history. Check also for a history of epilepsy, alcoholic liver disease or diabetes.

Implantation dermoid

Cysts occur where skin is forcibly implanted into the subcutaneous tissue as a result of injury. There is likely to be a history of injury, often minor, e.g. pinprick. Implantation dermoid used to be common in women who sewed – hence the use of protective thimbles. The patient complains of small painful swellings on the finger tips.

Pyogenic granuloma

Pyogenic granuloma is a common inflammatory lesion of the skin, which arises in response to minor penetrating foreign bodies such as splinters or thorns. Pyogenic granulomas are solitary, reddish-blue, fleshy nodules. The surface may be ulcerated, in which case, the lesion may be clinically indistinguishable from amelanotic malignant melanoma.

Trigger finger
The patient complains that the finger 'jumps' or 'clicks' as it moves. It may get stuck in the flexed position. There is usually no history of injury.

Mallet finger
This results from injury to the extensor tendon of the terminal phalanx. There is usually a history of injury. It occurs if the tip of the finger is forcibly flexed during active extension (stubbed).

Swan-neck/Boutonnière deformity
The patient complains of deformity of the distal finger.

Heberden's/Bouchards nodes
The patient complains of swelling close to the distal finger joints, i.e. swelling and deformity of the knuckles. This is a feature of hand osteoarthritis.

Mucous cyst
The patient complains of a swelling, often a result of a fluid-filled sac over the dorsum of the distal Interhalangeal (DIP) joint. It may discharge.

Calluses over knuckles
Calluses over the knuckles (Russell's sign) may arise in bulimics due to repeated self-induced vomiting over a long period of time. The condition arises from the patient's knuckles making contact with the incisor teeth during the act of inducing the gag reflex at the back of the throat with the fingers.

Metabolic

Gouty tophi
Deposits of uric acid occur in joints or soft tissues, and the patient complains of swellings on the fingers.

Ectopic calcification
The patient complains of hard, whitish, subcutaneous swellings. There may be a history of hyperparathyroidism, hypercalcaemia or chronic renal failure.

Connective tissue disease

CREST syndrome
The patient complains of white deposits in the pulps of the fingers.

Neoplastic

Subungual melanoma
This occurs as a pigmented lesion beneath the nail. There is no history of trauma as with a subungual haematoma, which may also appear pigmented when the bruise organises. A melanoma does not grow out with the nail. Eventually, the melanoma may lift the nail and ulcerate.

Chondroma
The patient notices a bony, hard swelling along the finger. It may occur beneath the nail and result in deformity of the nail (subungual exostosis).

EXAMINATION

Congenital

Congenital anomalies of the fingers will be obvious at birth. With camptodactyly, there is painless flexion deformity at the proximal interphalangeal (PIP) joint of the little finger. Check for other associated congenital anomalies.

Acquired

Traumatic/degenerative

Dupuytren's contracture
Examination may reveal only a firm painless nodule in the palmar fascia near the base of the ring finger. Puckering of skin of the palm may be obvious. Eventually, the MCP joint and PIP joint become flexed. The DIP joint remains extended. Check for signs of diabetes or liver disease. Occasionally, the condition is associated with Peyronie's disease of the penis.

Implantation dermoid
Examination reveals small firm spherical swellings in the subcutaneous tissues of the finger tips.

Trigger finger
The patient may be able to demonstrate how the finger sticks and then snaps out in extension. Thickening of the tendon and the tendon sheath may be felt over the head of the metacarpal bone.

Mallet finger
The distal phalanx of the affected finger remains flexed at about 20° when the patient tries to straighten the finger.

Swan-neck deformity
There is hyperextension of the PIP joint and flexion of the distal interphalangeal joint.

Boutonnière deformity
This is the opposite of swan-neck deformity. Flexion of the PIP joint occurs, with hyperextension of the DIP joint. It develops when the PIP joint pokes through a rupture of the centre of the extensor expansion.

Heberden's/bouchard's nodes
In Heberden's nodes, there are bony swellings on the dorsal surface of the fingers just distal to the DIP. In Bouchard's nodes, these swellings are located near the PIP.

Mucous cyst
Swelling on the dorsum of the DIP joint. Discharge may be apparent. May be a groove in the nail due to pressure on the nailbed.

Metabolic

Gouty tophi
Swellings, often multi-lobulated, occur on the fingers. They contain toothpaste-like infiltrates of uric acid crystals.

Ectopic calcification
Firm to hard, yellow-white deposits of calcium occur in the subcutaneous tissues.

Connective tissue disease

CREST syndrome
Small, hard, subcutaneous nodules in the finger pulps and on the dorsal aspects of the fingers. Sclerodactyly can present as tight, thickened skin.

Neoplastic

Subungual melanoma
A subungual melanoma is seen as a brown lesion with an indistinct edge. Occasionally, it may be quite extensive and have lifted the nail.

Chondroma
This is a painless, hard swelling on the bone. The surface of it is usually smooth. It may occur under the nail and lift the nail.

GENERAL INVESTIGATIONS

The diagnosis of most of these lesions is made on clinical history and examination alone.

- **FBC, ESR**
  Hb ↓, ESR ↑ in disseminated malignancy from subungual melanoma.
- **Blood glucose**
  Diabetes (Dupuytren's).
- **LFTs**
  Cirrhosis (Dupuytren's).
- **Serum calcium**
  Hypercalcaemia – ectopic calcification. Hyperparathyroidism.
- **Serum uric acid**
  Gout.
- **Rheumatoid factor**
  Rheumatoid arthritis – swan-neck deformity and Boutonnière deformity.
- **Finger X-ray**
  Heberden's and Bouchard's nodes. Chondroma. Mucous cyst – degenerative/osteoarthritic changes in the DIP joint. Ectopic calcification. Calcinosis. Erosion of phalangeal bone with gouty tophi.
- **Biopsy**
  Biopsy to distinguish pyogenic granuloma from amelanotic malignant melanoma. Excision biopsy for malignant melanoma.

- Subungual melanoma needs to be carefully distinguished from subungual haematoma. Check for a history of trauma. A subungual haematoma grows out with the nail, whilst a subungual melanoma does not.

FINGER PAIN

A painful finger is a common presenting symptom. This may vary from an obvious local lesion to part of a generalised disease, e.g. rheumatoid arthritis. Impairment of the function of even a single finger may grossly impair the overall function of the hand.

Figure 22 Raynaud's phenomenon. There is severe blanching of the tip of the left middle finger. The phase of pallor is followed by a phase of cyanosis followed by a sudden vasodilatation with a painful tingling red digit.

CAUSES

TRAUMATIC

- Subungual haematoma
- Fractures ⚠

INFLAMMATORY/INFECTIVE

- Paronychia
- Pulp space infection ⚠
- Tendon sheath infection – especially if open ⚠

NEOPLASTIC

- Glomus tumour
- Bone tumour

DEGENERATIVE
- Rheumatoid arthritis

VASCULAR
- Chilblains
- Small vessel disease
  - Raynaud's phenomenon (Fig. 22)
  - Buerger's disease
  - Emboli ⚠

METABOLIC
- Gout

AUTOIMMUNE
- Scleroderma

NEUROLOGICAL
- Carpal tunnel syndrome
- Cervical lesions

HISTORY

Traumatic

There will be a history of trauma, often a crushing injury. Subungual haematoma results from 'trapping' of the nail. It is extremely painful, as a bruise comes up between the nail and the nailbed.

Inflammatory/infective

Paronychia

This presents as a painful, tender spot close to the nail. It throbs and may keep the patient awake. There may be a history of picking the skin around the nail. Pus may exude from the side of the nail.

Pulp space infection

This occurs in the pulp space of the fingertip. There may be a history of penetrating injury, e.g. a prick with a sharp object. There is pain, redness and swelling, and the finger throbs.

Tendon sheath infection

There may be a history of a direct puncture wound, or there may be a preceding pulp space infection, which has extended into a tendon sheath. The patient presents with a red, swollen and painful finger held in slight flexion at the IP and MCP joint.

Neoplastic

Glomus tumour

This is a rare lesion. The patient complains of severe pain every time the nail is touched, the most common site being below the nail.

Degenerative

Rheumatoid arthritis

Women are more commonly affected than men. The usual symptoms are pain, swelling and stiffness of the fingers. General malaise may occur. The patient may complain of deformities of the fingers.

Vascular

Chilblains

The simplest vascular problem that affects the fingers is chilblains. Women are more affected than men. The patient complains of a swelling on the side or backs of the fingers, which develops rapidly after exposure to cold. The lesion is painful and itches. The lesions are usually multiple and occur most commonly in winter.

Small vessel disease

Ischaemia results in sudden onset pain, discoloration, ulceration or frank gangrene. There may be a history of Raynaud's phenomenon, Buerger's disease, diabetes or scleroderma. There may be cardiac disease, peripheral vascular disease or a cervical rib to suggest embolism. With Raynaud's phenomenon, there are often the characteristic changes of sudden onset of pallor induced by exposure to the cold, followed by cyanosis, followed by sudden vasodilatation with a painful, tingling, red digit.

Metabolic

Gout

Gout usually affects the first MTP joint but may affect any joint. The patient will complain of sudden onset of pain, swelling and redness in relation to a joint. There may be a previous history of gout. There may be a family history. An attack may be precipitated by trauma, starvation, infection, diuretics, cytotoxic or immunosuppressive drugs. Gouty tophi may be present.

Autoimmune

Scleroderma

Females are affected more than males. There may be thickening of the fingers. The patient may also complain of Raynaud's phenomenon and splits and ulcers of the fingertips. There may be a change in facial appearance, and the patient may complain of dysphagia.

Neurological

Carpal tunnel syndrome

The patient will complain of pain, paraesthesia in the thumb, index and middle fingers. Worse in bed at night. Relieved by hanging the arm out of bed.

Cervical lesions

The patient may complain of pain or tingling in the fingers. There may be a history of cervical spondylosis or other previous problems with the cervical spine.

EXAMINATION

Traumatic

Deformity, redness and swelling to suggest a fracture will be obvious. 'Trapping' of the nail or a blow to it will cause a collection of blood under the nail. The diagnosis is usually obvious from the history, and the patient will be in considerable pain.

Inflammatory/infective

Paronychia

The skin at the base and side of the nail is red, shiny and bulging. A bead of pus may be seen discharging from under the nail.

Pulp space infection

There is swelling and redness over the pulp of the finger. A pus-filled blister may be seen. If the tension is not rapidly relieved, it may either discharge into the tendon sheath or may cause pressure necrosis and osteomyelitis of the distal part of the terminal phalanx.

Tendon sheath infection

The finger is acutely painful and held in slight flexion. It is red and swollen and exquisitely tender along the line of the tendon sheath.

Neoplastic

Glomus tumours

These are rare. They are angioneuromyomas. If the tumour occurs under the nail (most common site), there is a small purple-red spot below the nail.

Primary and secondary tumours

These are rare. There is palpable bony swelling, which may or may not be tender.

Degenerative

Rheumatoid arthritis

The finger joints enlarge and become fusiform. Joint deformities occur, with ulnar deviation at the wrist and hyperextension of the proximal interphalangeal joints. There is wasting of muscles of the hand.

Vascular

Chilblains

These usually occur on the dorsum and side of the fingers. The skin over the swelling is reddish-blue. The swellings are oedematous and may burst and ulcerate. There are usually chilblains on the ankles and feet as well as on the fingers.

Small vessel disease

In ischaemic patients, there may be pallor, cyanosis or even frank gangrene of a finger. Ischaemic ulcers may be apparent on the fingertips. The pulp of the fingers may be wasted. Palpate for a cervical rib. Check the pulse for atrial fibrillation (emboli).

Metabolic

Gout

Acute inflammation of a joint occurs, the skin being tense, shiny, hot and red over the joint. The presence of gouty tophi locally or elsewhere, e.g. on the ears, suggests the diagnosis.

Autoimmune

Scleroderma

The skin of the hands has a thickened, white, waxy appearance. The fingers appear swollen with thickened skin, while the pulps of the fingers may be wasted. Small subcutaneous nodules, which are hard, may be palpable. These are due to calcinosis. Look for other signs of scleroderma, e.g. the skin of the face looks tight and shiny and is puckered around the mouth. There may be multiple telangiectasias over the face. Evidence of weight loss due to dysphagia may be present.

Neurological

Carpal tunnel syndrome

Wasting of the thenar muscles. The reduction of sensation in distribution of the median nerve in the hand occurring in advanced cases. Pressure over the carpal tunnel may reproduce symptoms.

Cervical spondylosis

Check sensation in the fingers. Check also the range of neck movements and the reflexes in the upper limbs.

GENERAL INVESTIGATIONS

- **FBC, ESR, CRP**
  Hb ↓ anaemia of chronic disease, e.g. rheumatoid arthritis. WCC and CRP ↑, e.g. tendon sheath infection. ESR ↑, e.g. rheumatoid arthritis.

- **U&Es**
  Urea and creatinine raised in chronic renal failure, which may be associated with gout or scleroderma.

- **Serum uric acid, serum calcium, serum phosphate**
  Gout, pseudogout.

- **Blood glucose**
  Diabetes – important to consider especially in infective causes.

- **ECG**
  Atrial fibrillation – emboli.

- **Hand X-ray**
  Rheumatoid arthritis. Bone lesions. Pulp space infection – pressure necrosis with osteomyelitis of the distal part of the terminal phalanx. Calcium deposits in connective tissue in CREST syndrome.

- **CXR with thoracic inlet**
  Cervical rib – Raynaud's phenomenon, emboli.

- **Cervical spine X-ray**
  Cervical spondylosis with referred pain.

SPECIFIC INVESTIGATIONS

- **Rheumatoid factor**
  Rheumatoid arthritis.

- **Autoantibody screen**
  Autoimmune disease.

- **Cold agglutinins**
  Raynaud's disease.

- **Echocardiography**
  Cardiac disease – embolism.

- **Arteriography**
  Arterial lesions. Mural thrombus from aneurysms leading to emboli. Peripheral vascular disease.

- Referred pain to the fingers is not uncommon. This is usually due to cervical spondylosis or carpal tunnel syndrome. Always carry out a full neurological examination.

- Infection of the fingers and restriction of movement may represent a tendon sheath infection. Antibiotics and urgent referral are required.

FOOT AND ANKLE DEFORMITIES

The deformity will often be apparent at birth but occasionally does not present until the child starts walking. A deformity of the foot and ankle is normally referred to as 'talipes'. Other terms may qualify the word talipes, e.g. varus (inverted heel), valgus (everted heel) and equinus (foot plantar-flexed). Deformities of the toes are dealt with under toe lesions (p. 426).

CAUSES

CONGENITAL

- Talipes congenital talipes equinovarus (congenital clubfoot)
- Metatarsus adductus (intoeing)
- Pes planus (flatfoot)
- Pes cavus (high-arch foot)
  - Idiopathic
  - Neuropathic
  - Spastic dysplasia
  - Spina bifida (including spinda bifida occulta)
  - Cerebral palsy
  - Poliomyelitis
  - Charcot–Marie–Tooth disease (hereditary motor and sensory neuropathy)
  - Friedreich's ataxia
- Acquired talipes equinovarus (causes listed below)

UPPER MOTOR NEURONE LESION

- Cerebrovascular accident
- Traumatic brain injury
- Spastic paresis

LOWER MOTOR NEURONE LESION

- Spina bifida
- Poliomyelitis
- Meningitis
- Amyotrophic lateral sclerosis
- Cerebellar lesions
- Friedreich's ataxia

MUSCULAR DISEASE

- Muscular dystrophy
- Volkmann's ischaemic contracture

HISTORY

Talipes equinovarus

Apparent at birth, occurring in 2/1000 live births. The child is born with clubfoot, which is picked up on routine postnatal examination.

Metatarsus adductus

Common cause of intoeing in children, presenting when the child is walking. Only the forefoot is adducted and not the hindfoot.

Pes planus

All children are flatfooted, and the arches are not fully developed until the age of ten. The parents may notice an abnormality of gait and perhaps rapid and uneven wear and tear of the shoes. Pain is rare.

Pes cavus

There is accentuation of the longitudinal arch of the foot. There may be pain and discomfort. Again, the condition may be noted by the child's parent, with no specific cause found. Alternatively, there may be a history of spina bifida, cerebral palsy poliomyelitis or rarely Friedreich's ataxia, for which there will be a family history. Charcot–Marie–Tooth disease begins at puberty, with foot drop and weakness in the legs.

Acquired talipes

There are a variety of causes of upper and lower motor neurone lesions, giving rise to acquired talipes. Check for a history of spastic paresis, cerebrovascular accident, spina bifida and poliomyelitis. There may be a family history of Friedreich's ataxia. With Volkmann's ischaemic contracture, there will be a history of ischaemia of the calf muscles, (e.g. from supracondylar fracture of the femur, with popliteal artery damage).

Trauma

There will usually be an obvious history of trauma or burns causing contractures.

EXAMINATION

Talipes equinovarus

This will usually be apparent in the newborn. There is an equinus deformity, i.e. the hindfoot is drawn up with a tight Achilles tendon; varus deformity – the sole faces inwards; and adduction of the forefoot – the inner border of the forefoot is concave and points upwards.

Metatarsus adductus

The hindfoot is normal with a normal-sized heel; however, the forefoot is adducted.

Pes planus

The longitudinal arch is flattened, and the medial border of the foot rests on the ground.

Pes cavus

The high arch is clearly visible. The toes are clawed due to hyperextension of the MTP joints and flexion of the IP joints. The patient cannot straighten the toes. Callosities usually develop under the metatarsal heads. Check for spina bifida, spina bifida occulta (hairy patch over lumbar spine), poliomyelitis. With Charcot–Marie–Tooth disease, there will be foot drop and also atrophy of the peroneal muscles. With Friedreich's ataxia, there will be other signs, e.g. ataxia, dysarthria and nystagmus.

Acquired talipes

Examine for upper motor neurone and lower motor neurone lesions. Volkmann's ischaemic contracture will demonstrate firmness and wasting of the calf muscles together with clawing of the foot.

Trauma

The deformity will depend on the type and severity of the trauma. Scarring and contractures from burns will be obvious.

GENERAL INVESTIGATIONS

The diagnosis of nearly all of the above conditions is made on history and clinical examination.

- Foot X-rays
  AP and lateral views may help with assessment.
- CT foot
  For detailed assessment of underlying tissue
- Hip ultrasound
  In cases with suspected hip involvement

- **Foot deformities are rare. Orthopaedic or neurological referral is usually required, especially if there is a history of pain, unilateral signs, limping/falls or delayed developmental milestones.**

SECTION A

FOOT PAIN

Pain in the foot is a common presenting complaint. The majority of causes are related to injury, overuse or conditions causing inflammation.

Figure 23 Foot pain due to chronic limb ischaemia with distal gangrene.

CAUSES

TRAUMATIC

- Fractures
  - March fracture

INFECTIVE

- Cellulitis – esp if suspected necrotising fascitis ▲
- Osteomyelitis ▲
- Pyogenic arthritis

INFLAMMATORY

- Rheumatoid arthritis
- Plantar fasciitis
- Reiter's disease
- Osteochondritis of the navicular bone (Köhler's disease)
- Osteochondritis of the metatarsal head (Freiberg's disease)

VASCULAR

- Ischaemia (Fig. 23) especially if acute ▲
- Ulcers

METABOLIC

- Gout/pseudogout

DEGENERATIVE

- Osteoarthritis
- Flatfoot

OTHER

- Corns and callosities
- Referred pain, e.g. disc lesions, neuropathies
- Metatarsalgia
- Morton's metatarsalgia
- Plantar warts

HISTORY

Traumatic

History of trauma, e.g. heavy object falling on foot, crush injuries. Fatigue or march fractures may occur with prolonged walking, e.g. as in soldiers marching or in hikers. It usually affects the second or third metatarsal bones. Track and field athletes are particularly susceptible to stress fractures.

Infective

Patients usually presents with pain, redness and swelling over the area affected. Cellulitis may occur following a puncture wound, e.g. standing on a nail, insect bite. The history will usually be apparent. Osteomyelitis is rare but may follow blood-borne infection or local infection, especially in diabetics. Pyogenic arthritis is rare and affects the joint.

Inflammatory

The foot is commonly involved in rheumatoid arthritis. Deformities are multiple and eventually severe. There are usually signs of rheumatoid arthritis elsewhere. Plantar fasciitis causes pain under the heel. The patient is often middle aged. It may also be associated with Reiter's disease. The pain is often worse on standing after a period of rest. Osteochondritis may affect the second metatarsal head (Freiberg's disease) or the navicular bone (Köhler's disease). Pain, tenderness and swelling occur in relation to the particular bone.

Vascular

There may be a history of intermittent claudication progressing to ischaemic rest pain. The patient complains of severe pain in the foot, usually in bed at night, which is relieved by hanging the foot out of bed. The patient may also complain of ulcers and discoloration of the foot. Gangrene may be apparent. Check for a history of smoking, diabetes.

Metabolic

Gout classically affects the first MTP joint, but other joints of the foot may be affected. There is acute onset of pain, redness and swelling.

There may be a previous history. Attacks may be precipitated by trauma, surgery, infection or drugs, e.g. diuretics. There may also be a history of leukaemia, polycythaemia and cytotoxic or immunosuppressive therapy.

Degenerative

Osteoarthritis, flatfoot or other foot deformities (p. 153) may cause foot pain. Hallux rigidus, i.e. primary osteoarthritis of the MTP joint of the great toe, causes pain and stiffness.

Other

Metatarsalgia causes pain under the metatarsal heads. It is most common in middle-aged women. Excessive standing triggers the symptoms. Morton's metatarsalgia is caused by a digital neuroma. It most often affects the nerve running between the third and fourth metatarsal heads. It is commonest in women aged 40–50 years. Sharp intermittent pains shoot into the toes, usually occurring only when shoes are worn. Plantar warts are painful. The patient will usually have noticed the wart. They are common in the region of the metatarsal head, great toe and heel. Corns and callosities over pressure points may be painful. They are often associated with deformities of the foot. Referred pain to the foot may occur due to spinal lesions. A history of backache or weakness in the limb may be relevant.

EXAMINATION

Traumatic

Pain, tenderness, swelling, deformity or crepitus will be present with fractures. With march fractures, there may be localised tenderness and oedema on the dorsum of the foot.

Infective

Cellulitis, osteomyelitis and pyogenic arthritis will be associated with fever, malaise and swelling, redness and tenderness of the foot.

Inflammatory

Rheumatoid arthritis may be associated with signs elsewhere, e.g. hands. In the foot, there may be pes planus, hallux valgus, clawing of the toes and subluxation at the MTP joints. With plantar fasciitis, there is usually localised tenderness over the undersurface of the os calcis. With Reiter's disease, there may be urethritis and conjunctivitis. Freiberg's disease and Köhler's disease present with swelling and tenderness over the relevant bone.

Vascular

Look for signs of chronic limb ischaemia (i.e. ulcers/gangrene, intermittent claudication, rest pain) and acute limb ischaemia (i.e. pain, pallor, cold, pulseless, parathesia, paralysis).

Metabolic

With gout/pseudogout, there will be swelling, redness and tenderness of the affected joint. The first MTP joint is typically affected, gouty tophi may be present elsewhere.

Degenerative

Osteoarthritis presents with pain and stiffness, e.g. hallux rigidus. Flatfoot and other deformities may be apparent (p. 153).

Other

In metatarsalgia, there is tenderness under the metatarsal heads. Callosities may be present under the metatarsal heads. In Morton's metatarsalgia, squeezing the forefoot may produce the symptoms. Plantar warts (verruca plantaris) are usually obvious. They present as flat, hyperkeratotic lesions, which seem to have been pushed into the skin of the sole of the foot. In contrast to callosities, pressure over them causes pain. If referred pain is suspected, a full neurological examination should be carried out.

GENERAL INVESTIGATIONS

- **FBC, ESR, CRP**
  Hb ↓ anaemia of chronic disease, e.g. rheumatoid arthritis. WCC/CRP ↑ infection, e.g. cellulitis, osteomyelitis. ESR ↑ rheumatoid arthritis.

- **Serum uric acid, calcium, phosphate**
  Gout/pseudogout.

- **Blood glucose**
  Diabetes.

- **Foot X-ray**
  Fractures (march fractures may not be apparent until callus forms, therefore need repeat X-rays). Osteomyelitis – normal in early stages, osteoporosis, subperiosteal new bone, sequestration. Rheumatoid arthritis. Osteoarthritis. Osteochondritis – dense fragments of bone. Foot deformities.

SPECIFIC INVESTIGATIONS

- **Blood culture**
  Osteomyelitis.

- **Bone scan**
  Osteomyelitis.

- **CT**
  Vertebral lesions – referred pain.

- **MRI**
  intervertebral disc lesions – referred pain.

- **Duplex ultrasound Doppler**
  Arterial or venous peripheral vascular disease.

■ Arteriography
Vascular disease. Site of disease. Small vessel versus large vessel disease.

- Sudden onset of pain in the foot in an arteriopathy or in a patient with atrial fibrillation is likely to be due to ischaemia. Examine the pulses. Urgent referral is usually required.

- Systemic illness and fever with localised severe bone pain may suggest osteomyelitis or septic arthritis. Risk factors include diabetes and immunosuppression. Urgent investigation is required.

- Pain with no obvious signs, especially lack of localised tenderness, may suggest neuropathy or an L5/S1 nerve lesion.

FOOT ULCERS

Ulcers on the feet are common. The majority of them are of vascular or neuropathic origin.

Figure 24 Chronic penetrating ulcers in a 60-year-old man with diabetes.
The deep ulcer beneath the head of the first metatarsal is characteristically surrounded with a thick keratin margin, and the ulcer on the medial side of the foot has an exposed tendon in its base.

CAUSES

VASCULAR

LARGE VESSEL DISEASE
- Arteriosclerosis
- Embolism ⚠

SMALL VESSEL DISEASE
- Diabetes
- Raynaud's disease
- Embolism ⚠
- Vasculitis, e.g. SLE, rheumatoid arthritis, scleroderma
- Buerger's disease

NEUROPATHIC

PERIPHERAL NERVE LESIONS
- Diabetes (Fig. 24)
- Peripheral nerve injuries
- Leprosy • (in endemic areas)
- Alcoholism

SPINAL CORD LESIONS
- Spina bifida
- Tabes dorsalis
- Syringomyelia

NEOPLASTIC
- Squamous cell carcinoma
- Malignant melanoma

TRAUMATIC
- Ill-fitting footwear

INFECTIVE
- Madura foot • (endemic in Africa, India)

HISTORY

Vascular

Ischaemic ulcers are common in the elderly. They are painful and do not bleed much. They show no signs of healing. There is often a history of intermittent claudication and rest pain. Check for a history of diabetes. In the younger patient, diabetes, Buerger's disease or Raynaud's disease may be responsible. Check for a history of cardiac disease, which may suggest embolism leading to ischaemic ulceration. Proximal arterial disease, e.g. aneurysm, may also cause emboli.

Neuropathic

These are painless ulcers occurring over pressure points. Patients may give a history of neuropathy. They may describe a feeling, as though they are walking on cotton wool. Check for a history of diabetes and peripheral nerve lesions. Spinal cord lesions may also be present. In diabetes, ulceration may be associated with both ischaemia and neuropathy.

Neoplastic

Malignant ulcers may occur on the foot. Squamous cell carcinoma is rare, but malignant melanoma is not infrequent, especially on the sole of the foot. The patient may have noticed the pigmented lesion, which has changed, with bleeding, itching and ulceration. The patient may also have noticed a lump in the groin, suggesting lymph node secondaries.

Traumatic

Foot ulcers may be caused by minor trauma, e.g. ill-fitting shoes. However, there is usually a history of an underlying predisposing condition, e.g. poor circulation, steroid therapy, neuropathy.

Infective

Pure infective ulcers on the foot are rare. Infections may occur with *Nocardia* species in tropical countries, causing Madura foot. Check for a history of foreign travel.

EXAMINATION

Vascular

Ischaemic ulcers are found on the tips of the toes and over the pressure areas. The edge is usually punched out, and healing does not occur. The base may contain slough or dead tissue. Occasionally, tendons are seen in the base of the ulcer. Pulses may be absent. Check for atrial fibrillation, which may be associated with embolism as a cause of ischaemic ulceration.

Neuropathic

Neuropathic ulcers are deep, penetrating ulcers. They occur over pressure areas, but the surrounding tissues are healthy and have good circulation. The ulcers themselves are painless. Examine the surrounding tissues for blunting of sensation, e.g. absence of pinprick sensation. Pulses are usually present. Carry out a full neurological examination looking for peripheral nerve injuries or evidence of spinal cord lesions.

Neoplastic

Squamous cell carcinomas have an everted edge, often with necrotic material in the base of the ulcer. The edge of the ulcer is hard. Check for inguinal lymphadenopathy. Ulcers associated with malignant melanoma tend to vary from brown to black, although they may be amelanotic. Bleeding and infection may make the surface of the tumour appear wet, soft and boggy. Check for inguinal lymphadenopathy and hepatomegaly.

Traumatic

Traumatic ulcers tend to occur either at pressure points, due to ill-fitting footwear, or at a site of injury. They usually have sloping edges and granulation tissue developing in the base. Always check the circulation, as most traumatic foot ulcers readily heal unless there is an abnormality of the circulation.

Infective

Infective ulcers by themselves are rare. Secondary infection may occur on any type of ulcer. With Madura foot, there may be ulceration and bone destruction with little systemic illness.

GENERAL INVESTIGATIONS

- **FBC, ESR, CRP**
  Hb ↓ malignant disease. WCC & CRP ↑ infection. ESR ↑ malignancy.
- **Blood glucose**
  Diabetes.
- **Swab**
  Microscopy – fungal infection. C&S.
- **Doppler**
  Identify absent pulses in acute ischaemia. Assess ABPI.

SPECIFIC INVESTIGATIONS

- **Antibody screen**
  Connective tissue disease.
- **Dulplex ultrasound**
  Assess for arterial and venous disease.
- **MR/CT arteriography**
  Ischaemic ulceration. Large versus small vessel disease.
- **CT/MRI spine**
  Spinal cord lesions.
- **Biopsy**
  Benign versus malignant.
- **Nerve conduction studies**
  Neuropathic ulcers.

- **A painful ulcer is likely to be infective or have an arterial aetiology.**
- **A painless ulcer is likely to be neuropathic.**
- **Neuropathic ulcers are deep and penetrating and likely to occur over pressure areas.**

GAIT ABNORMALITIES

Disorders of gait may be structural or neurological. When assessing gait, it is important to observe the whole patient and not merely the feet.

CAUSES

STRUCTURAL

- Pain – antalgic gait
- Length discrepancies – short leg gait
- Weak hip abductors – Trendelenburg or waddling gait
- Femoral anteversion – intoe gait

NEUROLOGICAL

- Stroke – hemiplegic gait ⚠
- Parkinson's disease – festinant gait
- Multiple sclerosis – scissoring gait
- Peripheral neuropathy – sensory ataxia
- Cerebellar disease – cerebellar ataxia ⚠
- Peroneal nerve palsy – foot drop gait
- Cerebral palsy – scissoring gait
- Frontal lobe lesions – apraxic gait ⚠

HISTORY

Duration

An abnormality of gait that has been present since birth is usually due to a structural cause or cerebral palsy. Discrepancies of leg length may originate from disorders affecting joint articulation, bone length or from soft-tissue contractures surrounding the joints. Most of the neurological causes of gait abnormalities result from acquired lesions of the central or peripheral nervous systems.

Associated symptoms

Pain is the underlying cause for the antalgic gait. Patients will be able to direct you to the site of origin of the pain. Loss of motor function such as paralysis of dorsiflexion of the foot causing the foot drop gait may indicate peroneal nerve palsy. More extensive paralysis of the arm and leg with the hemiplegic gait may occur with stroke. Paraesthesia, sensory loss or impairment of joint position sense is suggestive of peripheral neuropathy. Patients with sensory apraxia suffer from proprioceptive impairment and have great difficulties walking in the dark when visual cues are lost. A concomitant resting tremor is associated with Parkinson's disease and an intention tremor results from cerebellar disease.

Past medical and drug history

A previous history of trauma to the lower limb may be significant as fractures of the long bones predispose to length abnormalities on healing. Fractures of the fibular neck may disrupt the common peroneal nerve causing foot drop. Frontal lobe contusions may result from severe head injuries. Diabetes, carcinoma and vitamin B deficiencies are associated with peripheral neuropathies. Alcoholism, multiple sclerosis and drugs such as phenytoin are associated with cerebellar impairment. Direct questioning should be undertaken for previous strokes and Parkinson's disease.

EXAMINATION

The clinical examination is divided into three sections. The initial examination of a gait disorder is to determine a structural or neurological cause. If a structural lesion is suspected, then it is followed by an orthopaedic examination. Conversely, a neurological examination is performed if a neurological lesion is suspected. Once the disorder of gait is defined, the clinical examination should then be tailored to determine the underlying cause.

The asymmetrical gait

The gait is first assessed for symmetry. Apart from the hemiplegic gait, the remaining unilateral gait disorders are structural. The normal gait consists of four phases: these are (1) the swing, (2) heel strike, (3) stance and (4) toe-off. The antalgic gait or painful limp is characterised by a decrease in time spent in the stance phase. The Trendelenburg gait is characterised by a downward tilt of the pelvis when the leg is lifted forwards. It may be caused by a painful hip disorder, weakness of the contralateral hip abductors, shortening of the femoral neck or subluxation of the hip joint. With a hemiplegic gait, the leg swings in an outward arc and then back to the midline. A foot drop gait often results in the knee being lifted higher on the affected side.

The symmetrical gait

When analysing the symmetrical gait, observe movement of the whole patient. The stooped posture with small shuffling steps and reduced arm swing is characteristic of Parkinson's disease. Patients with apraxia have disjointed movements akin to 'walking on ice'; the aetiology is frontal lobe disorder, most commonly due to cortical degeneration. Attention is then brought to the movement of the legs; scissoring of the gait due to crossing of the midline when lifting the leg forwards is associated with cerebral palsy and the spastic paraparesis of motor involvement with multiple sclerosis. The movements of the feet are then noted; lifting of the knees with slapping of the foot as it contacts with the ground is descriptive of the foot drop gait. The foot is rotated inwards with femoral anteversion. The base of the gait is then analysed; a broad-based gait is characteristic of cerebellar disease and sensory ataxia. With cerebellar disease, patients are unsteady standing with their eyes open, while with sensory ataxia patients are able to stand with their eyes open but not shut (positive Romberg's test).

Orthopaedic examination

An examination of the hip, knee and ankle is required. Measurements are undertaken to determine real and apparent length of the lower limbs. The real length is the distance between the anterior superior iliac spine and the medial malleolus, and the apparent length is the distance between the xiphisternum and the medial malleolus. Any discrepancies will require individual measurements of the femur and tibia to determine the site of shortening. Thomas' test is performed to identify the presence of fixed flexion deformities of the hip that can give rise to apparent shortening. The resting position of both feet can be inspected and internal rotation due to femoral anteversion may be apparent.

Neurological examination

The mask-like facies and resting pill-rolling tremor of Parkinson's disease may be apparent on inspection, and examination of the limbs will reveal cogwheel or lead pipe rigidity. Patients with cerebellar disease will exhibit an intention tremor when performing the finger–nose test; in addition to their broad-based ataxic gait, they may also exhibit nystagmus, dysdiadochokinesia and dysarthria. With frontal lobe disorders, primitive reflexes such as the grasping (the hand of the examiner is grasped when placed or stroked along the patient's palm), sucking (sucking action is produced on stroking on side of the mouth) and palmomental reflexes (gentle stroke of the thenar eminence produces dimpling of the chin) are released. Examination of the sensory system may reveal loss of light touch, vibration and proprioception in a glove and stocking distribution with peripheral neuropathy. Unilateral upper motor neurone weakness, hyperreflexia and clasp knife rigidity are features of cortical strokes.

Specific examination

Once the diagnosis of a gait disorder is made, a specific examination is now undertaken to determine the underlying aetiology. For example, with apraxic gait due to frontal lobe disorder, a mental state examination is performed to screen for dementia, and fundoscopy is performed to screen for papilloedema, which may be indicative of raised intracranial pressure from a brain tumour.

GENERAL INVESTIGATIONS

The diagnosis of the majority of gait abnormalities is made on clinical history and examination.

SPECIFIC INVESTIGATIONS

- ■ Local X-rays
  Structural causes (i.e. fractures).
- ■ Nerve conduction studies
  Peripheral neuropathy. Peroneal nerve palsy.
- ■ CT/MRI head
  CNS causes, e.g. stroke, space-occupying lesions.

- • It is important to assess the patient in a safe environment, if necessary with an assistant to hand to prevent falls or injury.

- • Always observe the whole patient and not only the legs. The cause may be central.

- • Onset of ataxia without an obvious cause requires an urgent neurological referral.

GOITRE

A goitre is an enlargement of the thyroid gland (Fig. 25). It can result from physiological causes such as puberty (due to increased demand for thyroid hormone) which require no treatment, to frank malignant disease requiring urgent diagnosis and treatment.

Figure 25 Endemic goitre. This condition, caused by iodine deficiency, is extremely common in isolated mountainous regions. The thyroid may reach enormous size yet the symptoms are minimal and the patient is usually euthyroid.

CAUSES

SIMPLE (NON-TOXIC) GOITRE

- Simple hyperplastic goitre
- Multinodular goitre

TOXIC GOITRE

- Diffuse goitre (Graves' disease)
- Toxic nodule
- Toxic multinodular goitre

AUTOIMMUNE

- Hashimoto's thyroiditis

NEOPLASTIC GOITRE

BENIGN

- Adenoma

MALIGNANT ⚠

- Papillary
- Follicular
- Anaplastic
- Medullary
- Lymphoma

INFLAMMATORY

- de Quervain's thyroiditis
- Riedel's thyroiditis

HISTORY

Simple hyperplastic goitre

The patient presents with a swelling in the neck. Physiological causes include puberty and pregnancy. Iodine deficiency is the most common cause but is rare in the western world, where iodide is added to table salt. Where the condition is endemic (often in isolated mountainous regions such as Nepal), iodine deficiency is the usual cause.

Multinodular goitre

This is the commonest cause of goitre in western world. It is more common in women. The usual presentation is a lump in the neck, which moves on swallowing, but with a very large gland, the patient may complain of dyspnoea or dysphagia.

Toxic goitre

The patient presents with a lump in the neck. He or she may indicate a preference for cold weather, and may also complain of excessive sweating, tiredness, anxiety, increased appetite, weight loss, diarrhoea, palpitations and tremor.

Autoimmune

Hashimoto's disease presents with a firm goitre. It needs to be distinguished from lymphoma. Eventually, the patient becomes hypothyroid, and will complain of intolerance to cold weather, tiredness, a change in voice (hoarseness), weight gain, constipation, dry skin and dry hair.

Neoplastic goitre

The patient may present with diffuse enlargement of the thyroid or may have noticed a well-defined swelling in the area of the thyroid gland. Papillary carcinoma occurs in the younger patient (under 35 years) and, in addition to the goitre, the patient may have noticed lymph node swelling in the neck. Follicular carcinoma occurs in middle age (40–60 years). The patient may also complain of bone pain due to metastases. Anaplastic carcinoma occurs in the elderly. Anaplastic carcinoma may present with stridor, dyspnoea and hoarseness. There may be gross lymph node involvement. Medullary carcinoma can present at any age. Check for a family history of medullary carcinoma and symptoms related to phaeochromocytoma and hyperparathyroidism (associated MEN syndrome). Lymphoma of the thyroid is rare and may develop in pre-existing autoimmune (Hashimoto's) thyroiditis.

Inflammatory (rare)

The patient may present with a painful swelling of the thyroid associated with malaise or myalgia (de Quervain's thyroiditis). A hard mass associated with dysphagia or dyspnoea may suggest Riedel's thyroiditis.

EXAMINATION

Simple hyperplastic goitre

The patient is usually euthyroid and the goitre is smooth. Where the condition is endemic, the goiters are often asymmetrical and soft to palpation. They are composed of many large hyperplastic nodules and can reach enormous size (Fig. 25).

Multinodular goitre

The gland is usually smoothly nodular. Occasionally only one nodule may be felt – the dominant nodule in a multinodular goitre. Check for tracheal deviation when the gland is large, and percuss for retrosternal extension.

Toxic goitre

Palpation of the gland may reveal a diffuse goitre, a multinodular goitre or a solitary nodule. Check for exophthalmos, lid lag, lid retraction, warm moist palms and tremor. Check for atrial fibrillation. Examine for pretibial myxoedema. Reflexes are brisk. The goitre may have a palpable thrill or a bruit may be heard on auscultation.

Autoimmune

Hashimoto's disease presents with a diffusely enlarged, firm gland. Eventually, there may be signs of hypothyroidism. These signs include a pale, waxy skin, periorbital oedema, dry thickened skin and hair, slow pulse, large tongue, peripheral oedema and slow relaxing reflexes. Carpal tunnel syndrome may be present.

Neoplastic goitre

There may be a solitary thyroid nodule (papillary carcinoma) or a more diffuse mass (follicular carcinoma). Anaplastic carcinoma is hard and irregular and invades locally. Check for tracheal deviation. Cervical lymphadenopathy may be present with a papillary carcinoma, when the glands are usually mobile and discrete, and is invariably associated with anaplastic carcinoma, where the glands may be hard and matted. Check for recurrent laryngeal nerve palsy – has the patient got a hoarse voice or is unable to produce an occlusive cough?

Inflammatory

Subacute thyroiditis (rare). There will be a painful, swollen gland. In Riedel's thyroiditis, there is a woody, hard goitre, which infiltrates into adjacent muscle. It must be carefully differentiated from anaplastic carcinoma.

GENERAL INVESTIGATIONS

The order of investigations should be: (1) Routine blood tests (includes FBC ESR, TFTs, i.e. first 2 bullets), (2) Simple radiological investigations (includes CXR, US, CT scan), (3) Invasive investigations (includes FNAC, laryngoscopy).

- FBC, ESR
  Hb ↓ in disseminated malignancy. ESR ↑ in thyroiditis.
- TFTs
  T_4 ↑, TSH ↓ in toxic goitre. T_4 ↓, TSH ↑ in hypothyroidism.
- CXR
  Secondary deposits in thyroid carcinoma (follicular, anaplastic).
- US
  Cystic versus solid. Position of gland.
- CT scan
  Position of gland. Compression/invasion of local structures.
- FNAC
  Benign versus malignant.
- Laryngoscopy
  Involvement of recurrent laryngeal nerve.

SPECIFIC INVESTIGATIONS

- Thyroid antibodies
  Thyroid antibodies will be demonstrated in Hashimoto's disease.

- **Thoracic inlet X-ray**
  Tracheal compression.
- **Radioisotope scan**
  Hot versus cold nodule. Cold nodules may be malignant.
- **Serum calcitonin**
  Calcitonin ↑ in medullary carcinoma.
- **PTH**
  Raised in MEN syndrome.

> • Dysphagia or dyspnoea in association with a goitre requires urgent referral and may require urgent thyroidectomy.

GROIN SWELLINGS

These are common clinical problems, especially hernias. They are therefore common in clinical examinations.

Figure 26 A large left indirect inguinal hernia extending into the scrotum.

CAUSES

ABOVE THE INGUINAL LIGAMENT

- Sebaceous cyst/abscess
- Lipoma
- Direct inguinal hernia
- Indirect inguinal hernia (Fig. 26)
- Imperfectly descended testis
- Hydrocele of the cord/canal of Nuck

BELOW THE INGUINAL LIGAMENT

- Sebaceous cyst/abscess
- Lipoma
- Femoral hernia ⚠
- Lymph nodes
- Saphena varix
- Femoral artery aneurysm (true or false) ⚠
- Imperfectly descended testis ⚠

- Neuroma of the femoral nerves
- Synovioma of the hip joint
- Obturator hernia ⚠
- Psoas abscess ⚠

HISTORY

Diagnosis of most groin swellings will be based on the history and examination findings.

Sebaceous cyst/abscess

The patient will complain of a mobile lump on the skin. It may be red and inflamed and discharging. Ensure you ask about IVDU. These patients commonly present with an abscess.

Lipoma

The patient will present with a soft, painless swelling. A lipoma of the cord is often mistaken for a hernia.

Hernias

A patient with a groin hernia will present with a lump that disappears on recumbency or may be pushed back (reducible). The patient may present with a tense tender lump that cannot be reduced, accompanied by signs and symptoms of intestinal obstruction. Femoral hernia is more common in females. With hernias, there is occasionally a history of sudden straining (i.e. heavy lifting or chronic cough or trauma, following which a lump may become manifest).

Imperfectly descended testis

An imperfectly descended testis may present as a groin swelling. The patient, or, if in a young child, the mother, will have noticed absence of a testis from the scrotum. Enlargement and pain may indicate malignant change, which is more common in an imperfectly descended testis.

Hydrocele of the cord/canal of Nuck

In men a hydrocele may form around the cord or in women around the canal of Nuck. This may present as a lump in the inguinal region which does not reduce. It represents a cyst forming in the processus vaginalis.

Lymph nodes

Lymph nodes may present as swellings below the inguinal ligament. They may be discrete and firm, tender and red or matted to form a mass. The patient may have noticed a lesion on the leg. Care must be taken to elicit a full history with inguinal lymphadenopathy, as the nodes drain not only the tissues of the leg but also the penis, the scrotal skin, the lower half of the anal canal, the skin of the buttock and the skin of the lower abdominal wall, up to and including the umbilicus.

In the female, they drain the labia, the lower third of the vagina and the fundus of the uterus, via lymphatics accompanying the round ligament down the inguinal canal. A careful history should therefore be taken, of any anorectal disease, e.g. bleeding PR, or gynaecological disease, e.g. bleeding PV to suggest a carcinoma of the uterus.

Saphena varix

A saphena varix is normally associated with varicose veins lower down the leg. The patient will present having noticed a small, soft, bluish mass in the lower part of the groin.

Femoral artery aneurysm

A pulsatile expansile mass suggests a femoral aneurysm. Check for a history of arterial surgery at the groin or arteriography via the femoral artery, which may suggest the presence of a false aneurysm. A history of IVDU should also be explored.

Imperfectly descended testis

An imperfectly descended testis may descend into the upper thigh but its descent is arrested by the attachment of Scarpa's fascia to the deep fascia of the thigh.

Neuroma of the femoral nerve

This is rare and may be associated with anaesthesia or paraesthesia on the anterior aspect of the thigh and inability to extend the knee.

Synovioma of the hip joint

This is rare. The patient complains of a lump deep in the groin, which may interfere with hip movement.

Obturator hernia

This is rare. The sac passes through the obturator canal and may present in the groin deep to pectineus. A lump is rarely palpable due to the overlying pectineus. The diagnosis is not usually made until obstruction or strangulation occurs.

EXAMINATION

Sebaceous cyst/abscess

This is attached to the skin and a punctum is usually seen at the point of attachment. Sebaceous cysts are firm, spherical and mobile on the underlying tissue. They may be hot, red and tender when inflamed. A sebaceous cyst may also progress to become a firm lump (i.e. an abscess), if inflamed.

Lipoma

The lump will be soft, lobulated, mobile, being fixed neither to the skin nor to the underlying tissue. They may be distinguished from hernias, in that they are not reducible and do not have a cough impulse. A lipoma of the cord can only be confidently diagnosed at surgery.

Hernias

A hernia may be reduced and has an expansile cough impulse. They may be irreducible. Irreducible hernias may be: (1) incarcerated – imprisoned in the sac because of adhesions between contents and the wall of the sac; (2) obstructed – small bowel is caught in the sac and intestinal contents cannot pass on; (3) strangulated – in addition to being obstructed the arterial blood supply is cut off and gangrene of the contents ensues. In the last case, the lump would be tender, the overlying skin may be red and the patient will be pyrexial with a tachycardia.

It is important to distinguish between an inguinal and a femoral hernia. An inguinal hernia lies above and medial to the pubic tubercle, a femoral hernia below and lateral. An inguinal hernia may be either direct or indirect. An indirect hernia comes down the inguinal canal from the deep inguinal ring. A direct hernia comes through the posterior wall of the canal, through Hesselbach's triangle (base – inguinal ligament; lateral border – inferior epigastric artery; medial border – the lateral border of rectus abdominis muscle). Distinction between direct and indirect hernia is made by reducing the hernia and exerting pressure over the deep inguinal ring, asking the patient to cough. If the hernia sac appears medial to the fingers, it is direct. If the hernia appears only after removing the pressure over the deep inguinal ring, then it is indirect.

Imperfectly descended testis above the inguinal ligament

An imperfectly descended testis may be in an ectopic position (root of the penis, upper thigh or perineum) or along the normal line of descent. An imperfectly descended testis cannot be felt in the inguinal canal – it is usually too flabby and atrophic and cannot be palpated through the tough overlying external oblique aponeurosis. However, should it become malignant, then the hard and irregular testis can be palpated in the inguinal canal. An imperfectly descended testis may also be palpable in the upper thigh below the inguinal ligament. The scrotum will be empty on that side. The testis cannot descend more than a few centimetres into the upper thigh, as its descent is prevented by the attachment of Scarpa's fascia to the deep fascia of the thigh below the inguinal ligament. An imperfectly descended testis may also be palpable at the root of the penis or in the perineum.

Hydrocele of the cord/canal of Nuck

This is rare. There will be a smooth, palpable swelling along the line of the cord. It does not have a palpable expansile cough impulse. If gentle traction is exerted on the testis, a hydrocele of the cord will be felt to move down the canal. It may transilluminate. Findings will be similar in a hydrocele in the canal of Nuck, except there will be nothing to retract on!

Femoral hernia

This is more common in females. It lies below and lateral to the pubic tubercle. There will be an expansile cough impulse. It may be reducible. Strangulation of a femoral hernia is not uncommon, particularly one of the Richter's type. A tense, tender, irreducible swelling will be found below and lateral to the pubic tubercle.

Lymph nodes

Lymph nodes are palpable below the inguinal ligament. Classically, they are arranged into groups: (1) superficial, with subdivision into horizontal and vertical groups; and (2) deep. In practice, it is difficult to distinguish between the groups. Lymph nodes in the groin may be palpable as discrete nodules or they may be hard, irregular and matted together. This type is usually associated with malignant disease. Tender, fluctuant lymph nodes with erythema of the overlying skin are usually associated with lymphadenopathy due to an infective condition. It is important to examine all sites that are drained by these nodes, namely: (1) the skin of the leg, including examination under the toe nails; (2) the skin of the buttock; (3) the skin of the lower abdominal wall up to and including the umbilicus; (4) the skin of the scrotum, penis and glans penis; (5) the labia and lower third of the vagina; (6) the lower half of the anal canal; (7) the fundus of the uterus. It is therefore necessary not only to examine superficial structures but also to carry out a digital rectal examination and a bimanual vaginal examination.

Saphena varix

This is a soft, compressible dilatation at the termination of the saphenous vein. It has a cough impulse and disappears on recumbency. A fluid thrill is felt if the veins lower down the leg are percussed.

Femoral artery aneurysm

A femoral artery aneurysm presents as an expansile pulsatile mass in the line of the femoral artery. Look for a scar in relationship to it, which may suggest a false aneurysm.

Imperfectly descended testis below the inguinal ligament

The testis may be palpable in the upper thigh below the inguinal ligament. The scrotum will be empty on that side. The testis cannot descend more than a few centimetres into the upper thigh, as its descent is prevented by the attachment of Scarpa's fascia to the deep fascia of the thigh below the inguinal ligament.

Neuroma of the femoral nerve

It will be palpable along the course of the nerve (lateral to the femoral artery). Test the integrity of the femoral nerve (sensation on the anterior aspect of the thigh; extension of the knee joint).

Synovioma of the hip joint

There may be a palpable thickening deep in the groin in relation to the hip joint. Hip joint movements may be limited.

Obturator hernia

In a very thin patient, a lump may be felt deep in the medial aspect of the groin. More commonly, obturator hernias present with intestinal obstruction and the diagnosis is made at laparotomy.

Psoas abscess

It used to be associated with spinal TB, a cold abscess of a vertebral body discharging down the psoas sheath and presenting as a soft fluctuant swelling below the inguinal ligament. Most psoas abscesses nowadays are related to perforation of a hollow viscus retroperitoneally, e.g. the right colon into the psoas sheath.

GENERAL INVESTIGATIONS

- FBC, ESR, CRP
  Hb ↓ lymph node tumours. WCC & CRP ↑ infection in the lymph nodes, strangulated hernia. ESR ↑ lymph node tumours, infection.

- Hip X-ray
  Osteoarthritis with synovioma.

- AXR
  Intestinal obstruction associated with obstructed/strangulated hernia.

- Ultrasound +/− Duplex
  Lipoma, imperfectly descended testis, femoral artery aneurysm or false aneurysm, saphena varix, psoas abscess.

SPECIFIC INVESTIGATIONS

- Thoracolumbar spine X-ray
  Spinal abscess/TB spine or psoas abscess.

- CT/MRI scan
  Delineate and characterise a groin abscess. Psoas abscess. TB spine.

- FNAC +/− Biopsy
  Lymph node pathology.

- Herniography
  Inguinal or femoral hernia.

- An acutely painful and irreducible lump suggests a strangulated hernia. Urgent surgical treatment is required.

- Femoral hernia is more common in women and is at higher risk of strangulation.

- Undescended testis has a high risk of malignancy.

- If the cause of the swelling is thought to be lymphadenopathy, examine all regions that drain to the inguinal lymph nodes.

GYNAECOMASTIA

Gynaecomastia is enlargement of the male breast. There is an increase in the ductal and connective tissue elements of the breast. The condition should not be confused with fat in the mammary region, which may occur in obese patients and in old age with weight loss. In most cases, gynaecomastia is a result of an increase in the oestrogen–androgen ratio. In many cases, the actual mechanism is unknown or the cause is idiopathic.

Figure 27 Gynaecomastia in chronic hepatitis. Note: the patient is also jaundiced.

CAUSES

PHYSIOLOGICAL

- Puberty
- Old age
- Neonates

PATHOLOGICAL

- Chronic liver disease (Fig. 27)
- Drugs
  - Oestrogens
  - Cyproterone
  - Spironolactone

- Cimetidine
- Digitalis
- Griseofulvin
- Amphetamines
- Tricyclic antidepressants
- Cannabis

Chronic renal failure

Carcinoma of the male breast ⚠

Hyperthyroidism

Hypogonadism
- Klinefelter's syndrome
- Agenesis

Testicular tumours ⚠

Bronchial carcinoma (inappropriate secretion of hormones)

Pituitary tumours (e.g. prolactinoma)

Malnutrition

HISTORY

In newborn babies, gynaecomastia is associated with placental oestrogens and may be associated with a milky discharge from the nipple (witch's milk). A degree of gynaecomastia may occur in boys prior to puberty. This often regresses but occasionally remains and is a source of embarrassment. Senescent gynaecomastia occurs in the sixth decade or later.

Most cases of gynaecomastia present as painless or tender enlargement of one or both breasts. The majority of pathological causes of gynaecomastia are related to drugs. A careful drug history should be taken. Is there a history to suggest hypogonadism, e.g. undescended testes, bilateral torsion, Klinefelter's syndrome (XXY – tall, female distribution of fat around breast and pelvis, normal male hair distribution, atrophic testes)? Has the patient noticed any testicular swelling? Check for a history of alcoholism or hepatitis, which might suggest liver failure. Is the patient in chronic renal failure? This will usually be apparent as he will have been on some form of dialysis. Are there any signs of hyperthyroidism? Has the patient noticed any visual disturbance to suggest a pituitary tumour involving the optic chiasma?

EXAMINATION

Local

One or both breasts may be involved. Enlargement may be considerable, resembling a female breast, but this is rare; it is usually small and localised behind the areola. The swelling may be soft or hard. In the younger male, the hard enlargement is usually confined to a disc of tissue behind the areola and this usually occurs around puberty. Hard irregular enlargement in an elderly man should raise the diagnosis of carcinoma. Soft or diffuse enlargement is usually associated with drugs.

General

Examine the axillary and supraclavicular lymph nodes. Examine the testes – atrophic or enlarged (tumour). Check for signs for hyperthyroidism, liver failure or renal failure. The patient may have a CAPD tube or an arteriovenous fistula for treatment of chronic renal failure.

GENERAL INVESTIGATIONS

- **FBC, ESR**
  Hb ↓ anaemia – liver failure. ESR ↑ liver disease.
- **U&Es**
  Renal failure.
- **LFTs**
  Liver failure.
- **TFTs**
  Hyperthyroidism.
- **CXR**
  Primary tumour (bronchial carcinoma with inappropriate secretion of hormones).

SPECIFIC INVESTIGATIONS

- **Chromosome analysis**
  Klinefelter's syndrome.
- **βHCG and AFP**
  Testicular tumour.
- **Basal serum prolactin**
  Prolactinoma.
- **CT head**
  Pituitary tumour.
- **Mammography**
  Carcinoma.
- **FNAC**
  Carcinoma.

- Unilateral gynaecomastia in an adult male may be due to breast carcinoma, especially if there is a hard irregular mass behind the areola.

- In a patient with gynaecomastia, always examine the testes. There may be an underlying testicular tumour. If there is any doubt, carry out an ultrasound scan.

- Gynaecomastia associated with headache and visual disturbance may be caused by a pituitary tumour, e.g. prolactinoma.

- In a smoker with gynaecomastia and clubbing of the fingers, bronchial carcinoma is a likely diagnosis.

- Always take a full drug history, especially recreational drugs.

HAEMATEMESIS

Haematemesis is the vomiting of blood. This may be frank blood or blood altered by the action of gastric acid and digestive enzymes, i.e. 'coffee grounds'. Haematemesis is usually caused by lesions proximal to the duodenojejunal junction.

Figure 28 Endoscopic view of oesophageal varices. The bulging blue masses can be seen protruding into the oesophageal lumen.

CAUSES ⚠ (ALL PATIENTS WITH SIGNIFICANT HAEMATEMESIS SHOULD BE URGENTLY ASSESSED)

SWALLOWED BLOOD

- Epistaxis
- Haemoptysis

OESOPHAGUS

- Reflux oesophagitis
- Oesophageal varices (Fig. 28)
- Oesophageal carcinoma

STOMACH

- Peptic ulceration

- Acute gastric erosions
- Mallory–Weiss syndrome
- Carcinoma
- Leiomyoma (gastrointestinal stromal tumour – GIST)
- Hereditary haemorrhagic telangiectasia
- Vascular malformations

DUODENUM

- Peptic ulceration
- Duodenal diverticulae
- Aortoduodenal fistulae
- Invasive pancreatic tumours
- Haemobilia

BLEEDING DISORDERS

- Liver disease-associated
- Thrombocytopenia
- Haemophilia

DRUGS

- Anticoagulants
- Aspirin
- NSAIDs
- Steroids

OTHERS

- Uraemia
- Connective tissue disorders

HISTORY

Swallowed blood

Check for a recent history of epistaxis or haemoptysis.

Oesophagus

There may be a history of excess alcohol consumption or a history of other liver disease to suggest oesophageal varices. A history of retrosternal burning pain and heartburn would suggest oesophagitis. The bleeding associated with varices is often torrential; that associated with oesophagitis is minor. Check for a history of dysphagia, which can result from carcinoma.

Stomach

History of epigastric pain to suggest peptic ulceration. There may be a history of steroid or NSAID medication. Mallory–Weiss syndrome usually occurs in the younger patient who has had a large meal with a large quantity of alcohol, followed by a forceful vomit. The first vomit contains food, the second contains blood. Acute gastric erosions may occur with stressful illnesses, e.g. major surgery, acute pancreatitis, burns (Curling's ulcer) or head injuries (Cushing's ulcer). It is unusual to get a large bleed with a carcinoma. Anaemia is a common presentation, although there may be 'coffee grounds' vomit. Leiomyoma causes a moderate haematemesis. There is usually no preceding history. There will also be no preceding history with vascular malformations. Hereditary haemorrhagic telangiectasia is rare. The patient may present with a history of the condition, or it may be apparent from the telangiectasia around the lips and oral cavity.

Duodenum

Melaena tends to be a more common symptom than haematemesis with duodenal lesions. There may be a history of chronic duodenal ulceration, although often presentation may be acute with little background history. Bleeding from invasive pancreatic tumours is rare. The patient will present with malaise, lethargy, weight loss and vomiting. Haemobilia is rare. Aortoduodenal fistula is rare and usually follows repair of an aneurysm, with subsequent infection of the graft. There is massive haematemesis and melaena.

Bleeding disorders

The patient may present with a history of a bleeding disorder, e.g. haemophilia. There may be a history of spontaneous bruising or bleeding from other orifices.

Drugs

There may be a history of anticoagulant, steroid or NSAID therapy. Always question the patient carefully to see whether he or she has bought any proprietary, 'over-the-counter' preparations that may contain aspirin or NSAIDs.

Others

Uraemia may cause bleeding. Other symptoms such as dyspnoea, nausea, malaise, peripheral oedema or coma may be present. Rarely, gastrointestinal bleeding may be a presenting symptom of a connective tissue disease.

EXAMINATION

Depending upon the severity of the bleed, there may be shock. The patient will be cold, clammy, with peripheral vasoconstriction; there will be a tachycardia and hypotension.

Swallowed blood

Check for blood around the nose. Examine the chest for a possible cause of haemoptysis.

Oesophagus

There may be little to find on examination, except clinical signs of anaemia and weight loss, unless the cause is oesophageal varices. In the latter case, there may be jaundice, abdominal distension due to ascites, spider naevi, liver palms, clubbing, gynaecomastia, testicular atrophy, caput medusae, splenomegaly or hepatomegaly.

Stomach

There may be little to find on examination. There may be an epigastric mass with a carcinoma or a palpable left supraclavicular node (Virchow's node). There may be epigastric tenderness. With hereditary haemorrhagic telangiectasia, there may be telangiectasia on the lips and mucous membrane of the mouth.

Duodenum

Again, there may be little to find on examination other than epigastric tenderness. In the rare case where duodenal bleeding comes from an invasive pancreatic carcinoma, there may be a palpable mass in the region of the pancreas.

Bleeding disorders

There may be signs of bruising or bleeding from other orifices.

Drugs

The signs will depend on the severity of the bleed and the site of the lesion produced.

Others

Rarely, haematemesis may be associated with connective tissue diseases, e.g. polyarteritis nodosa. Other manifestations of polyarteritis nodosa may be apparent, e.g. neuropathies, cardiac disease or skin lesions.

GENERAL INVESTIGATIONS

- **FBC, CRP/ESR**
  Hb ↓ anaemia due to chronic bleeding, e.g. from carcinoma.
  CRP/ESR ↑ connective tissue disease.

- **U&Es**
  Urea and creatinine will be raised in uraemia. Urea may be raised due to absorption of blood from the bowel.

- **LFTs**
  Liver failure, oesophageal varices, haemobilia.

- **Clotting screen**
  Liver disease. Bleeding diatheses. Anticoagulants.

- **OGD**
  Will demonstrate most lesions, e.g. varices, oesophagitis, peptic ulcer, gastric erosions, Mallory–Weiss tear, carcinoma and rarer causes of bleeding. Biopsy may be carried out where necessary.

SPECIFIC INVESTIGATIONS

- **Angiography**
  Vascular malformations. Also may diagnose rarer distal duodenal
  causes, e.g. vascular malformations.

- **US**
  Aortic aneurysm.

- **CXR**
  Chest lesion.

- **CT**
  Aortic graft infection.

- When assessing a patient with haematemesis, it is
  important to secure intravenous access with a large-
  bore cannula and to send blood for cross-matching as
  soon as possible.

- Always take a careful drug history, especially of 'over-
  the-counter' drugs.

- Tachycardia may be the only physical sign of a
  significant GI bleed, especially in the younger patient.

- Risk stratification tools such as the Glasgow-Blatchford
  Score should always be used when taking a haemetemesis
  history.

HAEMATURIA

Haematuria is the passage of red blood cells in the urine. Care must be taken to distinguish it from other causes of discoloration of urine. All patients with haematuria must be fully investigated. If haematuria has initially been diagnosed on dipstick testing, it must always be confirmed by microscopy.

Figure 29 CT scan of the pelvis showing a transitional cell carcinoma involving the right lateral and posterior bladder wall (arrows).

CAUSES

KIDNEY

- Glomerular disease
- Carcinoma
- Stone
- Infection – pyelonephritis
- Trauma (including renal biopsy)
- Polycystic kidney
- TB ● *(common in some parts of the world where TB is endemic)*
- Embolism
- Renal vein thrombosis
- Vascular malformation

URETER

- Stone
- Neoplasm

BLADDER

- Carcinoma (Fig. 29).
- Inflammatory, e.g. cystitis, TB, schistosomiasis
- Catheter-associated
- Stone
- Trauma

PROSTATE

- Benign prostatic hypertrophy
- Carcinoma

URETHRA

- Trauma
- Stone
- Urethritis
- Neoplasm

GENERAL

- Anticoagulant therapy
- Thrombocytopenia
- Strenuous exercise
- Haemophilia
- Sickle cell disease
- Malaria ● (common where malaria is endemic)

RED URINE

- Haemoglobinuria
- Myoglobinuria
- Acute intermittent porphyria
- Beetroot
- Senna
- Rifampicin

HISTORY

Is there pain associated with haematuria to suggest infection or inflammation? Painless haematuria is usually associated with tumour or TB. Total haematuria (throughout the stream) suggests bleeding from the upper urinary tract or bladder. Initial haematuria (at the start of the stream) suggests bleeding from the urethra or the prostate. Terminal haematuria (at the end of the stream) suggests bleeding from the bladder or prostate. Check for a family history of polycystic kidney disease. There may be a history of TB elsewhere. Has there been any recent foreign travel (schistosomiasis)? Is there any pain in the loin to suggest kidney disease, or a history of ureteric colic to suggest passage of a stone or clot down the ureter? Bladder disease may be accompanied by suprapubic pain, frequency and dysuria. Catheter-associated haematuria may occur in patients with long-term indwelling bladder catheters. It is usually self-limiting. Check for symptoms of prostatism, i.e. difficulty in starting, poor stream and nocturia. Urethral injury will normally be apparent. It may occur following pelvic fractures or falling astride an object. Is the patient on anticoagulants? Is there any history of blood dyscrasia? Is there evidence of sickle cell disease or exposure to malaria? Strenuous exercise may cause haematuria. Has there been a recent renal biopsy?

Discoloration of urine may be due to a variety of causes. Haemoglobinuria may occur with haemolysis and myoglobinuria following crush injuries or ischaemia of muscle. Check for ingestion of any substance that may change the colour of the urine. Acute intermittent porphyria is extremely rare and is accompanied by abdominal pain. If the urine from a patient is allowed to stand in the light, it will become purplish-red.

EXAMINATION

Anaemia, weight loss, signs of chronic renal failure. Abdominal examination may reveal a palpable mass, e.g. hypernephroma, distended bladder. Rectal examination may reveal smooth enlargement of the prostate (benign prostatic hypertrophy) or a hard, craggy prostate (carcinoma). Feel along the course of the urethra, e.g. stone or neoplasm. Examine the chest, e.g. TB, secondary deposits from carcinoma of the kidney. Check for any localised bone tenderness, e.g. secondary deposits from carcinoma of the prostate or hypernephroma.

GENERAL INVESTIGATIONS

- FBC, CRP/ESR
  Hb ↓ gross haematuria, malignancy. Hb ↑ polycythaemia associated with hypernephroma. WCC/CRP ↑ infection. Platelets ↓ blood dyscrasias. CRP/ESR ↑ malignancy, TB.

- Urine microscopy
  Red cells (excludes haemoglobinuria and ingestion of substances that cause discoloration of urine). White cells in infection. Organisms in infection. Cytology.

- U&Es
  Renal failure.

- Clotting screen
  Anticoagulant therapy. Blood dyscrasias.

- **CXR**
  Metastases (cannonball metastases with hypernephroma). TB.
- **KUB x-ray and non-contrast CT**
  Renal calculus.

SPECIFIC INVESTIGATIONS

- **PSA**
  Prostatic carcinoma.
- **Sickling test**
  Sickle cell disease.
- **Intravenous urogram**
  Stone. Tumour. TB.
- **Ultrasound**
  Cystic versus solid. Stone. Urinary tract obstruction.
- **CT**
  Tumour (confirmation and degree of invasion). Cyst. Obstructive uropathy.
- **Cystoscopy**
  Infection. Tumour. Stone.
- **Ureteroscopy**
  Tumour. Obstruction.
- **Selective renal angiography**
  Vascular malformation. Tumour.
- **Renal biopsy**
  Glomerular disease. Tumour.
- **Prostatic biopsy**
  Carcinoma of the prostate.

- Painless haematuria suggests malignancy and requires urgent investigation.
- Dipstick testing must always be confirmed by microscopic examination of an MSU.
- A patient with microscopic haematuria associated with abnormal red cell morphology and proteinuria should be referred to a nephrologist rather than a urologist in the first instance.

HAEMOPTYSIS

Haemoptysis is the expectoration of blood or bloodstained sputum. With massive haemoptysis, the main priorities are to secure the airway and initiate emergency resuscitative measures before establishing a diagnosis.

Figure 30 Chest X-ray of a patient with widespread tuberculosis. Note the multiple small areas of consolidation (arrows).

CAUSES

RESPIRATORY

- Bronchial carcinoma
- Pneumonia
- TB (worldwide) (Fig. 30)
- Chronic obstructive pulmonary disease (COPD)
- Bronchiectasis
- Pulmonary oedema
- Goodpasture's syndrome
- Granulomatosis with polyangiitis (GPA – formerly Wegener's granulomatosis)

VASCULAR

- Pulmonary embolism ⚠
- Pulmonary hypertension – mitral stenosis
- Hereditary haemorrhagic telangiectasia

SYSTEMIC

- Coagulation disorders

HISTORY

Onset

Sudden onset of haemoptysis can occur with pulmonary embolism and acute respiratory tract infections; the remaining conditions tend to pursue chronic recurrent courses. Although the amount of blood expectorated is not very useful as a discriminating feature, small amounts of blood sufficient to stain the sputum pink are characteristic of pulmonary oedema.

Acute onset of cough with haemoptysis may occur with respiratory tract infections and pulmonary embolism. Associated sputum production may be purulent and longstanding with COPD and bronchiectasis. This is accompanied by flecks of blood when lung carcinoma, TB or mitral stenosis is present.

Dyspnoea

A long history of dyspnoea may be associated with chronic lung disease or mitral stenosis. Acute onset of dyspnoea that occurs with pulmonary embolism may be accompanied by pleuritic chest pain. Dyspnoea that is associated with pulmonary oedema may have a variable speed of onset and is often worse on recumbency.

Weight loss

Progressive weight loss is suggestive of TB or bronchial carcinoma, especially with a background of heavy smoking. Night sweats may be an additional accompanying feature of TB.

Other sites of bleeding

Other bleeding sites should be excluded as haematuria may be due to Goodpasture's syndrome. Epistaxis and haemoptysis occur together with GPA and hereditary haemorrhagic telangiectasia. Epistaxis *per se* may occasionally be confused with haemoptysis when expectorated sputum is mixed with blood originating from the nasal passages.

Past medical and drug history

A careful history is taken to identify a generalised coagulation disorder. This may be congenital, such as haemophilia, or acquired, such as with the use of anticoagulant drugs or in DIC. Previous rheumatic fever predisposes an individual to mitral stenosis. Consider Goodpasture's syndrome and GPA in the presence of co-existing renal disease.

EXAMINATION

Inspection

Cachexia is a prominent feature of carcinoma, TB and chronic lung disease. Loss of the nasal bridge and saddling of the nose may be apparent in patients with GPA. The presence of clubbing (p. 56) is associated with bronchial carcinoma, COPD and bronchiectasis. The malar flush characteristic of mitral facies may be present with mitral stenosis. Small dilated blood vessels present on the mucous membranes are features of hereditary haemorrhagic telangiectasia. The JVP may be elevated with a large pulmonary embolus or congestive cardiac failure. The chest may be hyperexpanded with decreased inspiratory movement in COPD.

Palpation

During an acute episode, tachycardia is very common. This may be due to the effort of coughing, anxiety or blood loss. The presence of an irregular heartbeat of atrial fibrillation is associated with mitral stenosis. Moreover, patients with atrial fibrillation are usually on anticoagulant therapy. Supraclavicular lymphadenopathy may be present with pulmonary infections or carcinoma. The calves should be palpated and measured for tenderness and increased girth from deep venous thrombosis, which may give rise to pulmonary emboli.

Percussion and auscultation

Localised crepitations and bronchial breathing may be audible with lobar pneumonia. Generalised coarse crepitations are suggestive of bronchiectasis, pulmonary oedema and COPD. Breath sounds tend to be decreased in intensity with COPD. Patients with bronchial carcinoma may present with a number of clinical features from the primary tumour, such as wheezing due to large airway obstruction, pulmonary collapse, pleural effusion and superior vena cava obstruction. On auscultation of the mitral area, the loud first heart sound and mid-diastolic rumbling murmur of mitral stenosis is accentuated on expiration with the patient in a left lateral position.

GENERAL INVESTIGATIONS

- Sputum analysis
  Sputum should be collected for microscopy, culture and cytology. Infective organisms may be isolated or cytological features of malignancy may be present. When TB is suspected, serial cultures should be taken from sputum, urine, bronchial washings or lung biopsy specimens during bronchoscopy.

- ECG
  Sinus tachycardia may be noted with violent coughing, anxiety and blood loss. $S_1Q_3T_3$ is indicative of right heart strain with pulmonary embolism, although non-specific ST abnormalities are more common.

- **FBC**
  Hb ↓ with chronic haemoptysis resulting in iron deficiency anaemia. Acute bleeding may not be associated with changes in the blood count until 24 hours later. WCC ↑ may be due to acute bleeding or respiratory tract infection. Monocytosis may be a feature of TB. Platelets ↓ with blood dyscrasias.

- **U&Es**
  The presence of impaired renal function with deranged urea and creatinine estimations may be due to glomerulonephritis from Goodpasture's syndrome or GPA. However, pre-renal failure may also be precipitated by acute blood loss and volume depletion.

- **Clotting screen**
  A clotting screen is performed to identify any impairment that may prolong the PT or APTT.

- **CXR**
  Bilateral patchy areas of consolidation may be seen on a chest film with bronchopneumonia and pulmonary oedema. Opacification of an entire lobe suggests lobar pneumonia, although pulmonary emboli may have a similar appearance due to the wedge-shaped shadowing of a pulmonary infarct. Recurrent fluffy shadowing may be seen with Goodpasture's syndrome and GPA, due to repeated intra-alveolar haemorrhage. The primary focus of tuberculous infection is usually in the middle to upper zones of the lung. This may resolve, with variable amounts of calcification, whereas post-primary TB tends to present with the classical apical shadow. The chest film may be normal or demonstrate hyperexpanded lung fields with COPD; however, with bronchiectasis, visibly dilated bronchi with persistent consolidation may be prominent. With bronchial carcinoma, numerous features may be seen on a chest radiograph, such as a peripheral mass, a hilar mass, collapse of a lobe or pleural effusion. The double right heart border and tenting of the left heart border are all features of enlargement of the left atrium with mitral stenosis. When pulmonary hypertension is present, there may be dilatation of the central pulmonary arteries with right ventricular enlargement.

- **Bronchoscopy**
  Fibreoptic bronchoscopy is useful for locating the site of bleeding. In addition, biopsies of the bleeding site may be sampled for pathological analysis. Multiple arteriovenous malformations will be visible with hereditary haemorrhagic telangiectasia.

SPECIFIC INVESTIGATIONS

- **Mantoux test**
  When TB is suspected, an initial dilute Mantoux test (1 in 10 000) may be performed in individuals who have not received BCG immunisation.

- **Urinalysis**
  May reveal the presence of protein and red cell casts with glomerulonephritis due to Goodpasture's syndrome and GPA.

- **Antiglomerular basement antibodies**
  Characterises Goodpasture's syndrome.

- **c-ANCA**
  GPA is associated with elevated levels.

- **Renal biopsy**
  Will aid in confirming the diagnosis in both Goodpasture's syndrome and GPA.

- **Tissue biopsies**
  Definitive tissue diagnosis can be made by biopsies from bronchoscopy, mediastinoscopy, CT-guided biopsy or surgical resection.

- **CT thorax/pulmonary angiogram**
  Very useful adjunct to the diagnosis of bronchiectasis in cases where the diagnosis cannot confidently be made on the clinical grounds and a chest film. It is also essential in the staging of lung carcinomas. The CT pulmonary angiogram is currently the investigation of choice to screen for pulmonary embolism.

- **Echocardiography**
  Allows assessment of left ventricular function with pulmonary oedema. It may also aid in the diagnosis of pulmonary embolism, as right heart failure can occur with large emboli. The integrity of the cardiac valves can be assessed, and valve stenosis with restriction of movement of the mitral valve leaflets can be visualised in mitral stenosis.

- **Haemoptysis in a smoker is an indication for a CXR, especially if associated with other features, e.g. dyspnoea, clubbing.**

- **Always consider TB, especially in the elderly, immigrants and the immunocompromised (from whatever cause).**

- **With massive haemoptysis, the main priorities are to secure the airway and initiate emergency resuscitative measures before establishing a diagnosis.**

HALLUCINATIONS

An hallucination is an apparent sensory perception of an external object when no such object is present. They may be auditory, visual, tactile, olfactory or gustatory in nature. It is to be differentiated from an illusion, which is a real perception that is misinterpreted.

CAUSES

- Fever (especially children and the elderly)
- Drugs (and drug withdrawal)
  - Marijuana
  - Cocaine
  - LSD
  - Ecstasy
  - Solvent sniffing
  - Amphetamines
  - Tricyclic antidepressant overdose
- Alcohol
  - Alcoholic hallucinations
  - Delirium tremens (alcohol withdrawal) ▲
- Extreme fatigue
- Psychiatric disorders
  - Schizophrenia
  - Bipolar disorder
  - Schizoaffective disorder
  - Post-traumatic stress disorder
- Sensory deprivation (e.g. blindness or deafness)
- Hypoxia ▲
- Severe metabolic disturbances (e.g. diabetic ketoacidosis, hypothyroidism) ▲
- Severe medical illness ▲
  - Liver failure
  - Renal failure
- Neurological disease
  - Temporal lobe epilepsy
  - Cerebral tumour
  - Post-concussional state
  - Dementia
  - Narcolepsy
- Others
  - Bereavement reaction

HISTORY

Obtain a clear history of the hallucination. Common hallucinations include hearing voices when no-one has spoken; seeing patterns, lights, beings or objects that are not there; feeling a crawling sensation on the skin. Hallucinations related to smell or taste are rare. Pure olfactory hallucinations are strongly suggestive of temporal lobe epilepsy. Enquire about recreational drugs. Auditory hallucinations are more common in psychotic conditions such as schizophrenia. Acute onset of febrile illnesses may be associated with hallucinations, especially in children and the elderly. Enquire about alcohol abuse or alcohol withdrawal. Hallucinations may be 'normal', e.g. hearing the voice of a loved one who has recently died, being part of a bereavement reaction.

EXAMINATION

Check the patient's temperature. Look for signs of infection. Look for signs of liver failure and kidney failure. Carry out a full neurological examination to exclude the possibility of a cerebral space-occupying lesion. A full mental state examination should be undertaken for possible psychiatric disorder.

GENERAL INVESTIGATIONS

- **Urinalysis**
  UTI, diabetic ketoacidosis.
- **FBC**
  WCC ↑ infection. MCV ↑ alcohol excess.
- **U&Es**
  Metabolic disturbances. Renal failure.
- **LFTs**
  Liver failure.
- **Blood sugar**
  Diabetic ketoacidosis.

SPECIFIC INVESTIGATIONS

- **ABGs**
  Hypoxia. Severe metabolic disturbances.
- **Toxicology screen**
  Drug abuse.
- **EEG**
  Temporal lobe epilepsy.
- **CT/MRI scan**
  Cerebral space-occupying lesion. Dementia.

- Hallucinations in children with febrile illness are common.
- Pure olfactory hallucinations are strongly suggestive of temporal lobe epilepsy.
- Tactile hallucinations strongly suggest acute alcohol withdrawal.

HAND DEFORMITIES

Impairment of hand function can lead to severe disability and is a common presentation.

Figure 32 Rheumatoid hand deformity. *Early changes can include synovitis of the wrist, metacarpophalangeal (MCP) joints and proximal interphalangeal joints (PIP). In advanced disease there is tendon swelling over the dorsal surfaces of the wrists, muscle wasting, ulnar deviation of the metacarpophalangeal joints, swan-neck deformity of the fingers and boutonniere deformity of the thumb.*

CAUSES

CONGENITAL

FAILURE OF FORMATION
- Absent digit
- Finger and thumb hypoplasia
- Radial club hand
- Macrodactyly

FAILURE OF SEPARATION
- Syndactyly (fusion of digits)
- Camptodactyly

DUPLICATION
- Polydactlyl

PRIMARY MUSCLE CONTRACTURES
- Arthrogryposis multiplex congenita

ACQUIRED

- Dupuytren's contracture
- Rheumatoid arthritis (Fig. 32)
- Osteoarthritis
- Trauma
- Burns
- Volkmann's ischaemic contracture
- Brachial plexus lesions
- Peripheral nerve lesions
- Spinal cord lesions
  - Poliomyelitis
  - Syringomyelia
- Multiple chondromas (Ollier's disease)

HISTORY

Congenital

These presentations will be recognisable at birth. Arthrogryposis multiplex congenita is due to non-differentiation of mesenchymal tissues, often together with a neurogenic element, the combination producing gross contractures.

Acquired

Dupuytren's contracture

In the early phases, there will be little deformity, the patient merely complaining of thickening in the palm near the base of the ring finger. Eventually, the patient will be unable to straighten the ring and little fingers. The grip is also affected. Check for a history of epilepsy, liver cirrhosis, diabetes or heavy machinery use.

Rheumatoid arthritis

By the time the hand is deformed, the patient is usually well aware of the diagnosis. There is pain and swelling of multiple joints with weakness of the hand, together with gross deformity.

Trauma and burns

There will be a clear history of previous trauma and burns.

Volkmann's ischaemic contracture

This is shortening of the long flexor muscles of the forearm due to ischaemia. There may be a history of trauma, e.g. supracondylar fracture of the humerus, a tight plaster restricting blood flow, or arterial disease, e.g. embolism. Movements of the fingers are painful and limited. There may be 'pins and needles' in the hand due to pressure on nerves. Eventually a claw hand results (permanent flexion contracture).

Spinal cord lesions

The diagnosis will usually be apparent. There may be a history of poliomyelitis.

Brachial plexus lesions

There will usually be a history of trauma, although occasionally invasion of the brachial plexus from tumours may occur (i.e. pancoast tumour).

Peripheral nerve lesions

There is usually a clear history of trauma to suggest a nerve lesion. Check for any possible causes of peripheral neuropathy, e.g. diabetes, uraemia, connective tissue disease, leprosy.

Ollier's disease

This results in deformities of the limb. The patient will complain of deformity of joints and bones and possible shortening of the limb, and will have noticed nodules along the line of bone.

EXAMINATION

Congenital

Congenital anomalies will be obvious at birth.

Acquired

Trauma and burns

A variety of deformities may be seen, depending upon the degree and type of trauma. With burns, scarring of the skin will be obvious.

Dupuytren's contracture

Examination will reveal a firm thickening in the palmar fascia near the base of the ring finger. Puckering of the skin is usually present around the flexor tendon. The MCP joint and the PIP joint are flexed with the DIP joint being extended. The ulnar digits (ring and little finger) are most commonly affected.

Rheumatoid arthritis

There is thickening of the joints, especially the MCP joint and PIP joints. There is ulnar deviation of the fingers. The wrist joint develops a fixed flexion deformity with some ulnar deviation. Swan-neck and boutonnière deformities of the fingers will be apparent. Ultimately, tendon rupture occurs and this leads to a variety of deformities.

Volkmann's ischaemic contracture

The skin of the hand is pale and the hand clawed and wasted. Extension of the fingers is limited but improves if the wrist is flexed. The forearm muscles feel hard and taut due to fibrosis.

Spinal cord lesions

For poliomyelitis the limb usually looks reddish-blue, wasted and deformed. Syringomyelia may cause a variety of hand deformities, and with upper motor neurone lesions, there may be fixed flexion of the wrist and fingers with adduction of the thumb.

Brachial plexus injuries

Upward traction on the arm may damage the lowest root (T1) of the brachial plexus, which is the segmental supply of the intrinsic muscles of the hand. The hand becomes clawed (Klumpke's paralysis). Check for a possible associated Horner's syndrome due to involvement of the cervical sympathetic chain.

Peripheral nerve lesions

With ulnar nerve lesions, it is appropriate to check for damage to the medial epicondyle and wrist. With division at the wrist, all the intrinsic muscles of the fingers (except for the radial two lumbricals – median nerve) are paralysed and the hand appears clawed. The clawing is less for the index and middle fingers because the lumbricals are intact.

In median nerve lesions at the wrist, the thenar eminence becomes wasted due to paralysis of opponens pollicis and sensation is lost over the lateral $3\frac{1}{2}$ digits. Fine movements, e.g. picking up a small object, are clumsy. With lesions at the elbow, wrist flexion is weak and the forearm muscles wasted.

Ollier's disease

Multiple lumps (chondromas) are located on the bones. This is often associated with limb shortening.

GENERAL INVESTIGATIONS

Most of the conditions described above will be obvious on clinical examination.

- **FBC, ESR**
  Hb ↓ in anaemia of chronic disease, e.g. rheumatoid arthritis.

- **CRP**
  ↑ in inflammatory disease

- **Rheumatoid factor/Anti-citrullinated protein (Anti-CCP)**
  Rheumatoid arthritis.

- **LFTs**
  Cirrhosis (Dupuytren's contracture).

- **Blood glucose**
  Diabetes. Peripheral neuropathy, Dupuytren's contracture.

- **Arm X-ray**
  Local fractures, e.g. evidence of previous supracondylar fracture of the humerus (with subsequent Volkmann's ischaemic contracture).

- **Hand X-ray**
  Rheumatoid arthritis. Ollier's disease – multiple translucent areas in the bones of the hand. Evidence of malunited fracture following trauma.

- **MRI**
  Spinal lesions, e.g. syringomyelia.

- **Nerve conduction studies**
  Brachial plexus and peripheral nerve lesions.

- The hand is a sophisticated mechanism from both motor and sensory considerations. Every attempt should be made to prevent hand deformities occurring as a result of trauma and infection.

- All hand injuries and infections resulting in reduced functional ability should be referred to a specialist hand surgeon, as expert care is necessary from the outset to preserve or restore function.

HEADACHE

When assessing a patient with headache, it is important to exclude life-threatening causes first.

Figure 33 CT scan of a subarachnoid haemorrhage due to rupture of an anterior communicating aneurysm. Blood (arrows) is seen in the subarachnoid space.

CAUSES

ACUTE HEADACHE

- Trauma
- Cerebrovascular ⚠
  - Subarachnoid haemorrhage (Fig. 33)
  - Intracranial haemorrhage/infarction
- Systemic infection
- Meningitis ⚠
- Acute angle-closure glaucoma ⚠

CHRONIC OR RECURRENT HEADACHE

- Tension headache
- Migraine (important to also consider in acute headache as may be first presentation)

- Medication overuse headache
- Cluster headaches
- Drugs, e.g. glyceryl trinitrate, nifedipine, substance withdrawal (especially alcohol)
- Cervical spondylosis
- Psychological (including anxiety and depression)
- Raised intracranial pressure ⚠ (other than IIH)
  - Tumour
  - Hydrocephalus
  - Cerebral abscess
  - Idiopathic intracranial hypertension
- Temporal arteritis ⚠
- Pre-eclampsia
- Paget's disease of bone
- Severe hypertension
- Carbon monoxide poisoning

HISTORY

Onset

Sudden onset of severe pain is usually due to a vascular cause, especially subarachnoid haemorrhage from a ruptured berry aneurysm. Cluster headache and migraine intensify over minutes and may last several hours, while meningitis tends to evolve over hours to days. Progressive severe headaches that develop over days or weeks should lead to the consideration of raised intracranial pressure from tumour or chronic subdural haemorrhage. The onset of headache may be preceded by an aura with migraine.

Site

Classically, headache from migraine is unilateral. Temporal arteritis leads to more localised pain over the superficial temporal arteries that can be accompanied by jaw claudication. Ocular pain is experienced with glaucoma, and retro-orbital pain with cluster headaches. Subarachnoid haemorrhage classically is occipital, although may present elsewhere and should not be excluded as a differential based on site alone.

Character

The intensity of pain contributes little when discriminating between the causes; however, the character of the pain may be useful. Patients with tension headache often complain of a tight band-like sensation; this is in contrast to the pain experienced with raised intracranial pressure, which is often reported to have a bursting quality. Migraine-related and temporal arteritis headaches have a throbbing character.

Precipitating factors

Headache originating from raised intracranial pressure is precipitated by changes in posture, coughing or sneezing, and is often worse in the mornings. Photophobia may be experienced by patients suffering with migraine, meningitis or glaucoma. They may prefer to lie in a darkened room when headaches arise. Certain foods such as cheese, red wine and chocolate are known to precipitate migraine. It is very common for headache to be precipitated by systemic illnesses such as a cold or influenza. Headache precipitated by touch occurs with superficial temporal artery inflammation from temporal arteritis. A drug history may elucidate the relationship between the administration of drugs with headache as a side-effect, such as glyceryl trinitrate and nifedipine. Medication overuse headache is associated with frequent use of analgesia but with refractory pain. Alternatively, headache can also result from substance withdrawal in substance-dependent patients.

Associated symptoms

Neck stiffness (meningism) is experienced with both meningitis and subarachnoid haemorrhages. Visual disturbances in the form of haloes occur with glaucoma. Flashing lights and alternations in perception of size may be reported by patients suffering with migraine, and this may be accompanied by photophobia, nausea and vomiting. Transient neurological deficits may also occur. However, progressive neurology associated with headache is more suggestive of an intracranial space-occupying lesion, such as haemorrhage, abscess and tumour. Unilateral visual loss may result as a complication of temporal arteritis, and this may be accompanied by proximal muscle pain, stiffness and weakness or tenderness. Conjunctival infection is experienced with both glaucoma and cluster headaches, along with lacrimation, which is a feature of the latter. With normal pressure hydrocephalus in adults, headaches are associated with dementia, drowsiness, vomiting and ataxia.

EXAMINATION

Temperature

Pyrexia may indicate the presence of systemic infection, meningitis or vasculitis.

Inspection

An assessment of the conscious state should be undertaken and quantified on the GCS. Impairment of consciousness is a sign of a serious underlying aetiology, such as meningitis, intracranial haemorrhage and raised intracranial pressure. Inspection of the eyes may reveal conjunctival infection with glaucoma and cluster headaches during an acute attack. With acute angle-closure glaucoma, the cornea is hazy and the pupil fixed and semi-dilated. Petechial haemorrhages classically occur with meningococcal meningitis.

Palpation

Tenderness along the course of the superficial temporal artery, with absent pulsation, is consistent with temporal arteritis.

Neurological examination

A detailed neurological examination is performed to identify the site of any structural lesion. Unilateral total visual loss can be precipitated by temporal arteritis due to ischaemic optic neuritis. Visual field defects (hemianopia) can be caused by contralateral lesions in the cerebral cortex. Fundoscopy is performed to identify papilloedema from raised intracranial pressure.

Transient hemiplegia can occur with migraine, but progressive hemiplegia is more indicative of a space-occupying lesion, such as a tumour or intracranial haemorrhage. Neck stiffness is a feature of both meningitis and subarachnoid haemorrhage. With meningitis, Kernig's sign (pain on extending the knee with the hip in a flexed position) may be present.

GENERAL INVESTIGATIONS

- FBC
  WCC ↑ meningitis, cerebral abscess and systemic infection.
- ESR and CRP
  ↑ temporal arteritis, infection, intracranial bleeding.
- U&Es
  Hypertensive headaches with renal disease.
- Alkaline phosphatase
  Elevated in Paget's disease.
- Radiology
  Cervical spine X-rays identify cervical spondylosis and cranial X-rays may reveal Paget's disease.

SPECIFIC INVESTIGATIONS

In most cases, the diagnosis can be made on clinical assessment. Features in the history and examination may guide specific investigations.

- Blood cultures
  With meningitis, systemic infection.
- CT/MRI
  Visualisation of the anatomical structures in the cranium is very useful in the presence of neurological deficit. Cerebral tumours may be visualised as high- or low-density masses. Intracranial bleeding can be identified as areas of high density during the first two weeks. An extradural haematoma presents as a lens-shaped opacity, and subdural haematoma presents as a crescent-shaped opacity. After two weeks, intracranial haematomas become

isodense and more difficult to visualise. Following subarachnoid haemorrhage, blood may be visualised in the subarachnoid space. Occasionally the offending aneurysm or arteriovenous malformation may be imaged. Enlargement of the ventricles may be an indication of hydrocephalus. Contrast-enhanced CT or MRI will increase the sensitivity to diagnose cerebral abscesses.

■ **Lumbar puncture**
A lumbar puncture may be undertaken following the exclusion of raised intracranial pressure, when there is suspicion of meningitis or subarachnoid haemorrhage. The opening pressure is recorded and the CSF obtained is inspected for consistency and colour. The consistency of the CSF is turbid with meningitis, and yellow staining of the CSF (known as xanthochromia) occurs with subarachnoid haemorrhage, owing to breakdown of haemoglobin from red blood cells. The CSF is then sent for microscopy, culture, cytology and biochemical analysis for glucose and protein. An abnormal increase in white cells may be seen on microscopy with meningitis. With bacterial or tuberculous meningitis, the glucose is low and protein content high. With viral meningitis the glucose content is normal and protein content mildly elevated. A lumbar puncture may also be helpful in cases of benign intracranial hypertension, and may be diagnostic in normal pressure hydrocephalus if performing the lumbar puncture is associated with an improvement in symptoms.

■ **Temporal artery biopsy**
Inflammation and giant cells may be seen with temporal arteritis. A normal biopsy does not, however, exclude the disease, as there may be segmental involvement of the temporal artery.

■ **Intraocular pressure measurements**
Tonometry will reveal high intraocular pressures with glaucoma.

- **Although extremely common, headache should always be investigated if there is any concern regarding sinister pathology, such as intracranial haemorrhage or malignancy.**

- **Temporal arteritis must be treated immediately with high-dose corticosteroids to avoid complete and irreversible blindness.**

HEMIPARESIS

Hemiparesis is weakness or paralysis of one side of the body; it usually arises from unilateral lesions above the midcervical spinal cord.

CAUSES ⚠ (ALL CAUSES OF ACUTE HEMIPARESIS REQUIRE URGENT ASSESSMENT)

VASCULAR

- Cerebrovascular ischaemia
- Cerebral or spinal infarction
- Intracerebral haemorrhage
- Paradoxical embolus
- Cerebral vasculitis

TRAUMATIC

- Subdural haematoma
- Extradural haematoma

OTHER

- Epilepsy (Todd's paresis)
- Multiple sclerosis
- Brain tumour
- Cerebral abscess

HISTORY

Onset

The speed of onset of hemiplegia is useful when trying to determine the underlying aetiology. Sudden onset hemiplegia is usually due to a cerebrovascular event such as a TIA, infarct or intracerebral haemorrhage. Hemiplegia developing over minutes or hours after trauma can be due to an evolving extradural or subdural haemorrhage. Although a history of trauma is usually evident, chronic subdural haematomas in the elderly may result from tearing of bridging veins without apparent trauma. Subacute hemiplegia may also result as part of a spectrum of neurological deficits caused by demyelination from multiple sclerosis. Gradual onset of hemiplegia is usually due to a tumour, although a cerebral abscess or chronic subdural haemorrhage may pursue a similar time course.

Precipitating factors

A history of trauma may be evident with extradural and subdural haemorrhages. Cerebral abscesses may result from haematogenous dissemination of bacteria from a distant site of infection, such as the lung, infective emboli from endocarditis, or more commonly from adjacent infections, such as middle ear, mastoid and paranasal sinus infections. Transient hemiplegia may also result from an epileptic seizure and this phenomenon is known as Todd's paresis. Unfortunately, the precipitating factor for the seizure may be underlying structural abnormalities such as a cerebral abscess or tumour.

Associated symptoms

Owing to the multifocal nature of demyelination, patients with multiple sclerosis may present with a host of associated symptoms, such as areas of motor deficits, sensory deficits, diplopia and monocular blindness from optic neuritis. Space-occupying lesions such as extradural haematoma, brain tumour and cerebral abscesses may also present with symptoms of raised intracranial pressure, such as headaches, classically worse in the morning, and with coughing or sneezing, nausea, vomiting and drowsiness.

EXAMINATION

The neurological examination is the key to determining the location of the lesion. Cortical lesions impinging on the motor area of the frontal lobe produce total contralateral paralysis. Similar effects can result from lesions of the internal capsule. Midbrain lesions tend to produce ipsilateral neurological deficits of the face and contralateral deficits of the limbs. Multifocal neurological deficits may be produced by demyelination or cerebral metastasis.

After determining the site of the lesion, the examination should be continued to determine the cause. Pyrexia should alert the clinician to the presence of infection, which may be caused by a cerebral abscess. The presence of facial myokymia, which is rippling of the muscles on one side of the face, is reported to be very suggestive of multiple sclerosis; cervical involvement may produce Lhermitte's sign, which is paraesthesia of the hands and feet on flexion of the neck.

Examination of the ear, mastoid and sinuses is useful to locate the site of primary infection, which may give rise to a cerebral abscess. Distant sites of infection that may precipitate cerebral abscesses are the lungs and emboli from infective endocarditis. The fingers are examined for nailfold infarcts with endocarditis and the precordium is auscultated for new or changing murmurs. The pulse is assessed for irregularity from atrial fibrillation, which is a predisposing factor for cerebral emboli. The blood pressure is measured, as hypertension is an additional risk factor for stroke. Carotid bruits from atherosclerotic plaques may be the only examination feature present with TIAs. Leg examination may reveal a deep vein thrombosis with possible paradoxical embolus.

GENERAL INVESTIGATIONS

■ FBC
   WCC ↑ infection, infarction.

- CRP/ESR
  ↑ infection, infarction, vasculitis.
- U&Es, magnesium, calcium and glucose
  Abnormal electrolytes and glucose level may precipitate a seizure.

SPECIFIC INVESTIGATIONS

- Blood cultures
  For suspected cerebral abscess.
- CT head
  Intracerebral haemorrhage, cerebral infarction, head injuries, tumour and abscess.
- MRI head and cervical spine
  Abscess, tumours, focal demyelination and periventricular plaques with multiple sclerosis.
- EEG
  Epilepsy.
- Lumbar puncture
  Exclude raised intracranial pressure first. With multiple sclerosis, there is raised CSF IgG and oligoclonal bands are present on electrophoresis.
- Ultrasound and echocardiogram
  Leg deep vein thrombosis. Evidence of valve vegetation in endocarditis or cardiac septal defect with paradoxical embolus.

- Sudden onset hemiplegia is an emergency and requires immediate investigation. A CT scan should be performed expeditiously to identify cerebral bleeds or infarction.

HEPATOMEGALY

Hepatomegaly is enlargement of the liver. The most common causes in the UK are cirrhosis, cardiac failure and secondary malignancy.

Figure 34 CT scan of the abdomen. Numerous liver metastases are seen in both the right and left lobes of the liver.

CAUSES

HEPATITIS/INFECTION

ACUTE
- Alcohol
- Viruses (Hep A/B/C, EBV)
- Bacteria (Leptospirosis, actinomycosis, pyogenic abscess)
- Protozoans (malaria, amoeba)
- Parasites (hydatid cyst, liver fluke)

CHRONIC
- Chronic active hepatitis

CONGESTION

- Congestive cardiac failure
- Constrictive pericarditis
- Budd–Chiari syndrome

INFILTRATION

- Fatty liver
- Amyloid

BILIARY TRACT DISEASE

- Extrahepatic obstruction, e.g. carcinoma of the pancreas, bile duct stricture
- Sclerosing cholangitis
- Primary biliary cirrhosis

MALIGNANCY

- Metastases (Fig. 34)
- Hepatoma
- Myeloproliferative disorders
- Myelofibrosis
- Leukaemia

METABOLIC

- Glycogen storage diseases
- Haemochromatosis
- Wilson's disease (hepatolenticular degeneration)

OTHERS

- Cryptogenic cirrhosis
- Riedel's lobe

HISTORY

Hepatitis/infection

Risk factors for infective causes include intravenous drug use, needle sharing, unsafe sexual practice (Hep B/C) and travel abroad to endemic areas. Amoebiasis occurs worldwide, and hepatitis B is prevalent in the tropics and Mediterranean areas. Hydatid disease is more common in sheep-rearing countries, e.g. Australia, Africa, Wales. Leptospirosis can result from swimming in rat-infested waters. History of alcohol abuse predisposes the patient to alcoholic cirrhosis. Chronic active hepatitis should be considered with a history of alcohol dependence, hepatitis B or hepatitis C. In the majority of hepatitis/infection cases, the patient presents with general malaise, pyrexia, weight loss and jaundice.

Congestion

History of congestive cardiac failure may be evident. With constrictive pericarditis, there is often a history of TB, but it may follow any cause of pericarditis. Budd–Chiari syndrome is hepatic vein thrombosis. A history of taking the contraceptive pill may be contributory. Tumour may also cause Budd–Chiari syndrome. It presents insidiously with portal hypertension, jaundice and cirrhosis.

Infiltration

There is usually a history of alcohol abuse with fatty infiltration. Secondary amyloidosis follows chronic infection/inflammation, e.g. rheumatoid arthritis, bronchiectasis, inflammatory bowel disease.

Biliary tract disease

There may be a history of biliary tract obstruction, e.g. carcinoma of the pancreas or stricture of the common bile duct. Sclerosing cholangitis causes jaundice and fevers and is associated with inflammatory bowel disease. Primary biliary cirrhosis is of unknown aetiology. Some 90% of the patients are female. It presents with obstructive jaundice, pruritus and hepatosplenomegaly. The patient will complain of dark urine and pale stools.

Malignancy

The chief cause is metastases from a known malignancy, which may have been treated, e.g. gastrointestinal tract or bronchus. Hepatoma is rare. With hepatoma, there may be a past history of hepatitis B infection, use of the contraceptive pill, aflatoxin exposure, or use of anabolic steroids. Myeloproliferative disease presents with tiredness, lethargy and spontaneous bruising.

Metabolic

Glycogen storage disease is rare. There is usually hepatomegaly from birth. The early features of haemochromatosis include fatigue, arthralgia and hepatomegaly. Skin pigmentation, diabetes and cardiac failure occur later.

Others

Cryptogenic cirrhosis presents with hepatomegaly without an obvious cause. Riedel's lobe is usually an incidental finding and asymptomatic. Riedel's lobe is an extension of the right lobe of the liver below the costal margin. It is a normal anatomical variation.

EXAMINATION

Remember that a liver edge that is palpable is not always enlarged and may have been pushed down by pulmonary hyperinflation, e.g. emphysema. The upper border of the liver should therefore be identified by percussion and is usually at the level of the eighth rib in the midaxillary line. The edge of the liver can be sharp or rounded and its surface smooth or nodular.

General

Carry out a general examination of the patient. Look for signs of liver failure: jaundice, flapping tremor, ascites, spider naevi, clubbing, gynaecomastia, caput medusae, leuconychia, Dupuytren's contracture, xanthoma, mental changes, coma, bruising. Look for Kayser–Fleischer rings (Wilson's disease).

Congestion

Signs of CCF. Peripheral oedema. Tense tender liver. JVP ↑. With Budd–Chiari syndrome, there will be acute ascites and right upper quadrant pain. In constrictive pericarditis, there will be right heart failure associated with ascites and the JVP rises paradoxically with inspiration.

Biliary tract disease

Deep jaundice. There may be a palpable mass associated with the primary malignancy. The gall bladder may be palpable with carcinoma of the head of the pancreas (Courvoisier's law). With primary biliary cirrhosis, there will be clubbing, xanthomata, arthralgia, hirsutism, portal hypertension and skin pigmentation.

Storage disease

With haemochromatosis, there will be signs of portal hypertension and skin pigmentation.

Malignancy

Jaundice and ascites may be present. There may be an abdominal mass representing the primary malignancy. With myeloproliferative disorders, in addition to hepatomegaly, there will be splenomegaly and lymphadenopathy.

GENERAL INVESTIGATIONS

- **FBC, CRP/ESR**
  Hb ↓ malignancy, myeloproliferative disorders. WCC ↑ infection, leukaemia. Platelets ↓ leukaemia. ESR ↑ infection and malignancy.
- **U&Es**
  ↑ Creatinine. Renal impairment often coexists with liver failure (hepatorenal syndrome).
- **LFTs**
  Liver enzymes deranged in hepatitis. Alkaline phosphatase grossly raised in obstruction. The pattern varies according to the cause of hepatomegaly.
- **Clotting screen**
  PT ↑ due to absence of clotting factors.
- **Hepatitis serology**
  Raised according to cause.

SPECIFIC INVESTIGATIONS

- Serum iron, TIBC and serum ferritin
  Abnormal in haemochromatosis.

- Blood, urine, CSF culture
  Positive in leptospirosis.

- Antibody screen
  Antimitochondrial antibodies raised in primary biliary cirrhosis.

- Bone marrow aspiration
  Myelofibrosis. Leukaemia.

- Ultrasound scan
  Cirrhosis. Secondaries. Amoebic abscess. Hydatid cyst. Riedel's lobe.

- CT
  Pancreatic lesions. Cirrhosis. Liver cysts.

- MRCP
  Ductal abnormalities, e.g. stricture, stone.

- Liver biopsy
  Establish cause, e.g. malignancy, amyloid.

- The liver edge is normally palpable in thin adults.
- A normal liver can appear enlarged if displaced downwards by lung disease, e.g. COPD.
- Remember Riedel's lobe. It can be mistaken for pathological enlargement of the liver. It is a normal anatomical variation. Its presence should be confirmed by ultrasound scan.

HICCUPS

Hiccups (hiccoughs) are the characteristic sounds produced by the involuntary contractions of the diaphragm terminated by sudden closure of the glottis. In the majority of patients, it is a self-limiting condition. The most common cause of hiccups is thought to be gastric distension after rapid ingestion of food, fluid or air. The causes of intractable persistent hiccups are listed below, with aetiology characterised by the hiccup reflex pathway.

CAUSES

PHRENIC NERVE IRRITATION

- Pharyngitis/laryngitis
- Foreign body
- Goitre
- Oesophageal carcinoma
- Lung tumour
- Thoracic surgery

DIAPHRAGMATIC IRRITATION

- Asthma
- Bronchitis
- Lower lobe pneumonia
- Empyema
- Subphrenic abscess
- Diaphragmatic hernia
- Gastric distension

GI CONDITIONS

- Gastritis
- Irritable bowel disease
- Pancreatitis

CNS CONDITIONS

- Meningitis
- Tumours
- Intracranial haemorrhage
- Brainstem stroke
- Encephalitis

OTHERS

- Diabetes
- Uraemic

- Electrolyte disturbance (hypocalcaemia, hyponatraemia)
- Hysterical
- Toxic
- General anesthesia

HISTORY

The causes of hiccups predominantly originate in the respiratory, abdominal and nervous systems; therefore the history is structured similarly.

Respiratory history

The presence of cough with purulent sputum production implies respiratory tract infection. However, patients with pneumonia tend to be more unwell and may complain of rigors with high temperatures. Following pneumonia or thoracic surgery, chronic pyrexia and pleuritic chest pains with failure of resolution of symptoms of the original infection may herald the onset of an empyema. Hiccups may (rarely) complicate routine thoracic surgery.

Abdominal history

Symptoms of rapid progressive painless dysphagia (p. 101) may be due to oesophageal carcinoma. At birth, a diaphragmatic hernia may present with respiratory distress; adults with diaphragmatic hernias may, however, be completely asymptomatic, the hernia being detected incidentally on a chest X-ray. Unremitting pyrexia, malaise and abdominal pain in patients after abdominal surgery, or following localised inflammatory conditions such as appendicitis and cholecystitis, may have developed an intra-abdominal abscess. The subphrenic region is the most common site of a collection of pus which causes nerve irritation. This is associated with intractable hiccups and pain referred to the shoulder, scapula or neck.

Neurological history

Pyrexia, headache, photophobia and neck stiffness are associated with meningitis. Patients with encephalitis tend to present with confusion, alterations in consciousness and seizures. The brainstem is an anatomically complex structure; therefore symptoms of infarction or tumour may be very variable, depending on distribution of involvement of the lower cranial nerves. The presenting features may be diplopia, difficulty swallowing, dysarthria and facial sensory loss.

Others

Amelioration of hiccups by sleep, vague accompanying symptoms and inconsistencies in the history are suggestive of hysterical hiccups. Uraemia may be responsible for hiccups. Be aware of medication, post-operative and toxic-metabolic causes.

EXAMINATION

A substantial number of causes of intractable hiccups are associated with pyrexia. High swinging fevers are suggestive of collections of pus, such as empyema and subphrenic abscesses.

An abdominal examination should be performed. Areas of tenderness may suggest appendicitis or cholecystitis as a predisposing cause for a subphrenic abscess. More specifically, an abdominal abscess may point to the skin surface, or present with tenderness over the lower chest wall.

Respiratory examination may reveal tracheal deviation with a large empyema or pleural effusion from carcinoma. Areas of percussion dullness correspond to consolidation, effusion and empyema. A large diaphragmatic hernia may elevate the diaphragm sufficiently to produce clinical signs suggestive of an effusion. Localised coarse crepitations may be auscultated, corresponding to areas of consolidation by pneumonia. Vocal resonance is increased with consolidation but attenuated with effusion and empyema.

A neurological examination is performed to identify the presence of and define the anatomical territory of any deficit. Specialised tests should be performed for meningitis. This will include Kernig's sign (pain on extension of the knee from a flexed hip and knee position) and Brudzinski's sign (flexion of the neck produces flexion of the hip and knee).

GENERAL INVESTIGATIONS

In the absence of features in the history to guide specific investigations, the following general investigations should be performed.

- **FBC**
  WCC ↑ with infection, malignancy.
- **ESR**
  ↑ infection, malignancy.
- **Glucose**
  Diabetes, infection.
- **U&Es**
  ↑ urea, ↑ creatinine with renal failure.
- **CXR**
  Peripheral shadow or cavitation, hilar mass, collapse of a lobe may suggest carcinoma. Consolidation is seen with pneumonia. Fluid with a meniscus may be due to empyema, effusion from malignancy or as a result of a subphrenic abscess. Elevation of a hemidiaphragm may be due to phrenic nerve palsy from carcinomatous infiltration or apparent elevation due to the presence of a diaphragmatic hernia.

SPECIFIC INVESTIGATIONS

- **Upper GI endoscopy and biopsy**
  Oesophageal carcinoma.

- ■ **Bronchoscopy and mediastinoscopy**
  Biopsy for bronchial carcinoma.

- ■ **CT thorax with contrast**
  Biopsy for bronchial carcinoma, and empyema characterisation.

- ■ **Drug and alcohol screen**
  To exclude miscellaneous causes.

- ■ **US abdomen**
  Subphrenic abscess; aspiration and drainage may also be performed.

- ■ **CT/MRI head**
  Infarction and tumour may be appreciated as low-density areas. Mass effects may be produced by tumour or bleeding causing midline shifts. Intracranial bleeding may be identified as a high-density area. Cortical swelling may be seen with encephalitis.

- ■ **EEG**
  Encephalitis – periodic complex formation and slowing of the background rhythm.

- ■ **Lumbar puncture**
  Meningitis. Encephalitis – high lymphocyte count as the majority are due to viral aetiology.

- • **If hiccups are persistent, chronic, or are associated with weight loss, a full investigation is required to exclude malignancy.**

HIRSUTISM

Hirsutism is the presence of male-pattern (androgen dependent) hair growth in women. This is not the same as virilism, which, in addition to hirsutism, is associated with the development of male secondary sexual characteristics in women. Whilst hypertrichosis refers to the excessive growth of hair occuring in either sex (i.e. androgen independent).

CAUSES

PHYSIOLOGICAL

- Senility
- Familial (varies with ethnicity)

PATHOLOGICAL

DRUGS

- Ciclosporin
- Antiepileptic drugs, e.g. phenytoin
- Corticosteroids
- Progestogens
- Testosterone (including anabolic steroids)
- Minoxidil

PITUITARY

- Prolactinoma
- Cushing's disease
- Acromegaly

OVARIAN

- Polycystic ovarian syndrome
- Menopause
- IN hyperthecosis
- Androgen-producing ovarian tumour

ADRENAL

- Congenital adrenal hyperplasia
- Cushing's syndrome
- Androgen-producing adrenal tumours

OTHER

- Anorexia nervosa

HISTORY

General

The onset and duration of hirsutism are useful features in the history to help determine the aetiology. Onset in childhood is suggestive of congenital adrenal hyperplasia, whereas sudden onset of hirsutism in adult females needs consideration of androgen-producing tumours of the ovaries or adrenal glands. Enquiries should be undertaken as to whether any relatives have similar problems as the aetiology may be familial. Be aware of family cancer syndromes, such as BRCA gene mutation, which is associated with familial ovarian carcinoma. Excessive androgens may result in virilisation, producing symptoms such as acne, deepening of the voice, increased muscle mass and clitoromegaly.

Menstrual history

A detailed history regarding the onset and regularity of the menstrual cycle should be taken, as amenorrhoea is a feature of polycystic ovarian syndrome, congenital adrenal hyperplasia and prolactinomas. In addition, galactorrhoea may also be an accompanying feature of prolactinomas. Hyperthecosis refers to hyperplasia of the ovarian theca interna leading to increased androgen production.

Drug history

A drug history may identify the use of progestogen-containing hormone replacement therapy or oral contraceptive pills. Hirsutism may also result as a side-effect of anabolic steroid use by body builders; phenytoin for epilepsy; minoxidil for hypertension and ciclosporin as an immunosuppressive agent in organ transplantation.

Associated symptoms

Weight gain may result from Cushing's syndrome, but is also a common complaint with polycystic ovarian syndrome. Symptoms such as headaches, vomiting and visual field loss are suggestive of a pituitary adenoma, which can result in acromegaly, Cushing's disease or hyperprolactinaemia (prolactinoma). Infertility may result from hyperprolactinaemia and polycystic ovarian syndrome.

EXAMINATION

An assessment should be made regarding the pattern of hair distribution. The Ferriman-Gallwey scoring system allows clinicians to quantify the severity of hirsutism. With a degree of normal variation, the distribution of hair growth with hirsutism is on the face, chin, chest and extremities. Careful inspection for virilism may identify increased shoulder-girdle muscle mass and enlargement of the clitoris. Truncal obesity is a feature of Cushing's syndrome, and generalised obesity occurs with polycystic ovarian syndrome. This may also be accompanied by acanthosis nigricans.

Inspection is then continued to identify co-existing endocrine disease. Features of acromegaly are thick greasy skin, prominent supraorbital ridging, broad nose, prognathism, macroglossia, poor jaw occlusion, wide interdental separation, enlarged hands and feet. Features of Cushing's syndrome are moon-like facies, truncal obesity, buffalo hump, skin bruising, striae and proximal muscle weakness. Hypertension, diabetes and visual field defects (bitemporal hemianopia) are associated with both Cushing's disease and acromegaly. In addition, visual field defects may also result from a prolactinoma, whilst hypertension is also associated with congenital adrenal hyperplasia.

Following this, an abdominal and pelvic examination should be performed to exclude a mass, which may be suggestive of a large adrenal or ovarian tumour.

GENERAL INVESTIGATIONS

- Urine dipstick
  The presence of glucose may be due to diabetes, which is a feature of Cushing's syndrome and acromegaly. In addition, polycystic ovarian disease is also associated with insulin resistance.

- U&Es
  ↓ potassium with congenital adrenal hyperplasia.

- Serum glucose
  Diabetes with Cushing's syndrome, acromegaly and polycystic ovarian disease.

- Serum testosterone and DHEA
  A marked increase in both suggests an excess of androgens from a neoplastic origin and warrants detailed investigation.

- FSH/LH
  Polycystic ovarian disease.

SPECIFIC INVESTIGATIONS

- 24-Hour free urinary cortisol
  ↑ with Cushing's syndrome.

- Low-dose dexamethasone suppression test
  Failure of suppression occurs with Cushing's syndrome.

- Oral glucose tolerance test with serial growth hormone estimations
  Failure of suppression or increasing growth hormone concentrations occur with acromegaly.

- IGF-1
  ↑ with acromegaly.

- Plasma prolactin
  ↑ with prolactinomas.

- Plasma 17-hydroxyprogesterone
  ↑ with congenital adrenal hyperplasia.

- **CA125**
  ↑ with ovarian carcinoma.
- **US abdomen and pelvis**
  Polycystic ovaries, ovarian carcinoma.
- **CT abdomen and pelvis**
  Adrenal carcinoma, ovarian carcinoma.
- **CT/MRI head**
  Pituitary tumour.

- Rapid onset and/or severe hirsutism may provide a clue to underlying serious pathology, e.g. androgen-producing tumours of the ovaries or adrenal glands.
- Pituitary tumours may present with hirsutism and associated visual field defects.
- Consider further investigations for women with a raised testosterone and/or 17-hydroxyprogesterone.

HYPERTENSION

Hypertension is the persistent elevation of blood pressure. An individual is classified as hypertensive when there is a sustained rise in blood pressure to more than 140/90 mmHg. Most patients have essential hypertension with contributory factors such as aging, obesity, alcohol and salt intake. An underlying cause is identified in less than 10% of patients. The causes of secondary hypertension are considered below.

Figure 34 MRA renal arteries. The patient presented with poorly-controlled hypertension. Subsequent examination revealed a bruit inferior to the left costal margin. MRA revealed a tight stenosis close to the origin of the left renal artery (arrow). The stenosis was successfully treated with angioplasty and stenting.

CAUSES

RENAL

- Renal parenchymal diseases, e.g. glomerulonephritis
- Diabetic nephropathy
- Renal artery stenosis (Fig. 34)
- Chronic pyelonephritis
- Polycystic kidney disease
- Connective tissue disease (especially systemic sclerosis)

ENDOCRINE

- Adrenal
  - Cushing's syndrome
  - Primary hyperaldosteronism (Conn's Syndrome)
  - Phaeochromocytoma
- Acromegaly

DRUGS

- Oestrogen-containing oral contraceptives
- Corticosteroids
- SNRIs – venlafaxine, sibutramine
- Non steroidal anti-inflammatories – Ibuprofen, diclofenac, celecoxib
- Sympathomimetics – amphetamines, ephedrine

CARDIOVASCULAR

- Coarctation of the aorta

OTHER

- Pregnancy (pre-eclampsia and eclampsia)

HISTORY

Hypertension itself is usually asymptomatic. Hypertensive emergencies (SBP>180 and/or DBP>120 with acute target organ damage) may present with headache, visual changes, chest pain, left ventricular failure, nausea or seizures. Additionally, patients with secondary hypertension may complain of symptoms from the underlying disorder.

Patients with chronic pyelonephritis may have experienced recurrent urinary tract infections or have a history of childhood urinary tract infections. Hypertension can also complicate glomerular disease; in particular it is associated with acute nephritic syndrome. Patients with nephritic syndrome may have experienced an acute illness with malaise, haematuria, oliguria and oedema.

With Conn's syndrome, patients may complain of muscle weakness and fatigue due to hypokalaemia and polyuria from impaired urine-concentrating ability. Paroxysms of headache, sweating, and palpitations with flushing may be experienced by patients with phaeochromocytoma. Classically, these patients have attacks of hypertension; however, in the majority, the hypertension is sustained.

Weight gain, acne, abdominal striae, muscle weakness, and depression may be some of the symptoms experienced by patients with Cushing's syndrome. With acromegaly, patients may complain of headaches, galactorrhoea, deepening of the voice, muscle weakness and joint pains.

A complete drug history will identify offending drugs that may precipitate hypertension.

SECTION A

EXAMINATION

Inspection

On inspection, patients with acromegaly may have thick skin and large hands, feet and tongue. Prominent supraorbital ridging with a large nose and protruding jaw accompanied by interdental separation may be noted on close inspection of the face and teeth. Confrontational testing of the visual fields may reveal bitemporal hemianopia, which may also be present with Cushing's syndrome owing to compression of the optic chiasma by a pituitary adenoma. Additional features of Cushing's disease include truncal obesity, acne, moon-like faces, bruising, striae, kyphosis and proximal muscle weakness.

Palpation and auscultation

In coarctation of the aorta, radiofemoral delay may be appreciated with simultaneous palpation of the radial and femoral arteries; bruits may be auscultated across collateral blood vessels along the axilla, chest wall and scapula. A systolic bruit may also be auscultated over the fourth left posterior intercostal space. Wide discrepancy of measured blood pressure may exist between the arm and leg.

Palpation of the abdomen may reveal bilateral ballotable masses due to enlarged polycystic kidneys, and bruits may be auscultated over stenosed renal arteries.

GENERAL INVESTIGATIONS

- **Urinalysis**
  Dipstick may indicate the presence of blood and protein. Urine microscopy is necessary to confirm the presence of red blood cells and also casts.

- **U&Es**
  Levels of serum potassium may be reduced with Conn's syndrome due to hyperaldosteronism. High levels of creatinine and urea are found with renal failure.

- **Blood glucose**
  Atherosclerosis, renal vascular disease and nephropathy may be associated with diabetes. All of these may contribute to hypertension. Moreover conditions such as Cushing's syndrome, acromegaly and phaeochromocytoma are associated with hyperglycaemia.

- **Serum lipids**
  Serum lipid estimation is used to screen for risk factors for atherosclerosis, and therapy may be initiated for the prevention of cerebrovascular and ischaemic heart disease.

- **ECG**
  A 12-lead ECG is recommended for all patients to provide a baseline and screen for left ventricular hypertrophy, which may result as a complication of hypertension.

SPECIFIC INVESTIGATIONS

- **Autoantibodies**
  Anti-GBM and ANCA may be positive with glomerulonephritis.
  ANA for connective tissue diseases.

- **Plasma catecholamines**
  Elevated in phaeochromocytoma.

- **Urinary catecholamines, metanephrines**
  Elevated in phaeochromocytoma.

- **24-hour urinary free cortisol**
  Excess cortisol in Cushing's syndrome.

- **Low-dose dexamethasone suppression test**
  Failure of suppression of cortisol occurs in Cushing's syndrome.

- **Oral glucose tolerance test**
  Failure of suppression of serum growth hormone occurs in
  acromegaly.

- **Plasma renin and aldosterone**
  Hypersecretion of aldosterone in the presence of low plasma renin
  levels confirms autonomous secretion in Conn's syndrome.

- **Pregnancy test**
  Hypertension occurring with pre-eclampsia and eclampsia.

- **US abdomen**
  Polycystic kidneys. Duplex Doppler can screen for renal artery
  stenosis.

- **Renal biopsy**
  Renal causes of hypertension.

- **MRI – renal and adrenal**
  Renal artery stenosis and adrenal hyperplasia/adenoma.

- **Cardiac echo/MRI**
  Coarctation of the aorta.

- **Hypertensive emergencies must be investigated and treated urgently due to the poor prognosis.**

- **Improvement in cardiovascular outcomes has been clearly shown when hypertension is adequately controlled.**

INTESTINAL OBSTRUCTION

Mechanical obstruction of the bowel may be simple (one-point obstruction) or closed loop (obstruction at two points enclosing a segment of bowel). If the bowel is viable, the obstruction is termed non-strangulating. If the arterial blood supply is compromised, strangulating obstruction occurs with subsequent infarction of the bowel. Intestinal obstruction is a common surgical emergency.

Figure 35 Small bowel obstruction. Distended loops of small bowel are visible in the central abdomen. These are identifiable as small bowel as the valvulae conniventes (arrows) cross the entire lumen of the bowel.

CAUSES

SMALL BOWEL

IN THE LUMEN
- Gallstone ileus ⚠
- Food bolus (after pylorus-destroying or bypass surgery)

IN THE WALL
- Crohn's disease
- Atresia ⚠
- TB ● *(common in areas of the world where TB is endemic)*
- Tumour, e.g. lymphoma, carcinoma

OUTSIDE THE WALL
- Hernia
- Adhesions ⚠

- Volvulus ⚠
- Intussusception ⚠

LARGE BOWEL

IN THE LUMEN
- Faeces

IN THE WALL
- Carcinoma
- Diverticular disease
- Crohn's disease
- Hirschsprung's disease

OUTSIDE THE WALL
- Volvulus ⚠
- Hernia
- Adhesions ⚠

ADYNAMIC OBSTRUCTION/PARALYTIC ILEUS/PSEUDO-OBSTRUCTION
- Peritonitis ⚠
- Postoperative
- Hypokalaemia
- Spinal and pelvic fractures
- Drugs, e.g. ganglion blockers, anticholinergics
- Immobilisation

HISTORY

Small bowel

Central abdominal colicky pain. Vomiting – food, bile, faeculent, depending upon the level of obstruction. Distension – degree depends on level of obstruction. There may be very little distension with proximal small bowel obstruction. It may be gross with distal small bowel obstruction. The patient may report constipation. There may be a history of abdominal surgery to suggest adhesive obstruction. The patient may be aware of a hernia.

Large bowel

Central (right colon to two-thirds of the way along the transverse colon) or lower abdominal colicky pain (remainder of the colon). Constipation. Vomiting is a late feature with large bowel obstruction. Abdominal distension. There may be a previous history of change in bowel habit and bleeding PR to suggest carcinoma. A long history of constipation (years) and abdominal distension suggest Hirschsprung's disease. Development of a constant severe pain suggests infarction.

Adynamic obstruction

Carefully check the drug history. Patients on anticoagulants may have retroperitoneal haemorrhage. Precipitating cause may be obvious, e.g. recent surgery or spinal fracture. The abdominal distension may be painless but uncomfortable. Vomiting, constipation. The elderly immobilised in bed are especially vulnerable.

EXAMINATION

Small bowel

Observe for scars. Exclude obstructed incisional hernia. Check hernial orifices. It is easy to miss a small femoral hernia in an obese patient. Distended tympanitic abdomen usually non-tender. High-pitched tinkling obstructed bowel sounds. Pyrexia, tachycardia and localised tenderness suggest impending infarction. A palpable mass in the right iliac fossa may suggest Crohn's disease or caecal carcinoma (obstructing the ileocaecal valve and causing small bowel obstruction). Carry out a digital rectal examination.

Large bowel

Distended tympanitic abdomen, which may be very tense. Obstructed bowel sounds. Rectum may be empty on examination PR unless obstruction is due to faecal impaction. A mass may be palpable to suggest an obstructing carcinoma. A palpable, tense, tender caecum suggests closed loop obstruction with a competent ileocaecal valve. Caecal perforation may be imminent.

Adynamic obstruction

Abdominal distension. Tense tympanitic abdomen. Absent bowel sounds. Evidence of previous surgery, trauma, retroperitoneal haemorrhage and peritonitis, fractures.

GENERAL INVESTIGATIONS

- Hb, FBC, CRP
  Hb ↓ malignancy. WCC ↑ infection, infarcted bowel.
- U&Es calcium, phosphate
  Dehydration. Electrolyte imbalances leading to paralytic ileus /pseudo-obstruction.
- Clotting screen
  May be abnormal with retroperitoneal haemorrhage, especially if patient on anticoagulants.
- Venous blood gas
  Lactate – indication of infarcted bowel.
- AXR, e.g. Fig. 35
  Small bowel: central abdomen. Lines (i.e. valvulae conniventes) close together and cross the lumen. >3 cm in diameter suggests obstruction.

Large bowel: Periphery of abdomen. Lines (i.e. haustra) do not cross entire lumen. >9 cm in caecal diameter or >6 cm elsewhere indicates obstruction. Sigmoid volvulus – distended loop of bowel will appear like a coffee bean.

Other: Gas in the biliary tree may indicate gallstone ileus.

SPECIFIC INVESTIGATIONS

■ Sigmoidoscopy
Tumour at rectosigmoid. Sigmoid volvulus may be decompressed by careful insertion of sigmoidoscope. Biopsy – carcinoma, absence of ganglion cells in Hirschsprung's disease.

■ CT: abdomen and pelvis
Identify any impingement. Retroperitoneal haemorrhage. Retroperitoneal tumour.

■ Barium enema
Limited barium enema may show 'apple core' lesion of carcinoma. 'Bird's beak' sign of sigmoid volvulus. Intussusception.

■ Small bowel enema follow through study
Crohn's disease/stricture. TB of the terminal ileum. Small bowel carcinoma.

- Urgent surgical exploration should be considered in:
  - Haemodynamically compromised pyrexial patients with neutrophil leucocytosis as bowel infarction/necrosis may lead to perforation.
  - In large bowel obstruction, a tense, tender palpable caecum is a sign of closed loop obstruction, with a risk of impending caecal perforation. This may be supported radiologically with a caecum measuring >9 cm.
- It can be difficult to distinguish between pseudo-obstruction and large bowel obstruction. Gaseous distension all the way along the large bowel, including rectum, suggests pseudo-obstruction. A sharp 'cut-off' of the gas shadow in the colon suggests obstruction.

JAUNDICE

Jaundice is yellow discoloration of the tissues, noticed especially in the skin and sclera (Figs 27 and 36), due to accumulation of bilirubin. Jaundice may be prehepatic (due to haemolysis), hepatic (due to intrinsic liver disease) or cholestatic (due to either intrahepatic cholestasis or post-hepatic biliary tract obstruction).

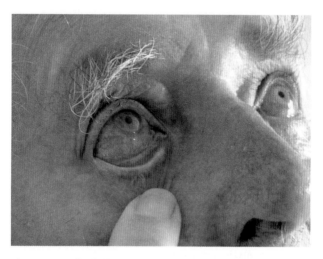

Figure 36 Jaundiced sclera in a patient with hepatitis. Mild jaundice is evident in the sclera. There is no obvious jaundice in the skin. Jaundice in the sclera is usually clinically apparent before progression to the skin.

CAUSES

PREHEPATIC (UNCONJUGATED HYPERBILIRUBINAEMIA)

CONGENITAL DEFECTS
- Gilbert's disease
- Crigler–Najjar syndrome

HAEMOLYSIS
Congenital red cell defects
- Hereditary spherocytosis
- Sickle cell disease
- G6PD deficiency
- Thalassaemia

Acquired

- Malaria ● (common where malaria is endemic)
- Incompatible blood transfusion
- Autoimmune
- Haemolytic disease of the newborn
- Absorbing large haematoma
- Hypersplenism

HEPATIC

ACUTE HEPATOCELLULAR DISEASE ⚠

- Viral hepatitis
  - Hepatitis A, B, C
  - EBV
  - CMV
- Drugs, e.g. paracetamol, halothane
- Other infections
  - Leptospirosis
- Toxins, e.g. carbon tetrachloride
- Autoimmune

CHRONIC HEPATOCELLULAR DISEASE

- Chronic viral hepatitis
- Chronic autoimmune hepatitis
- End-stage liver disease
  - Alcohol
  - Non-alcoholic steatohepatitis related cirrhosis
  - Haemochromatosis
  - Wilson's disease

CHOLESTATIC

INTRAHEPATIC

- Drugs, e.g. chlorpromazine
- Parenteral nutrition
- Viral hepatitis
- Primary biliary cirrhosis
- Pregnancy ⚠

EXTRAHEPATIC (OBSTRUCTIVE)

In the lumen

- Gallstones
- Infestation
  - Clonorchiasis (liver fluke)
  - Schistosomiasis

In the wall

- Stricture, e.g. inflammatory, postoperative
- Cholangitis ⚠
- Congenital biliary atresia
- Cholangiocarcinoma
- Sclerosing cholangitis
- Choledochal cyst

Outside the wall

- Carcinoma of the head of the pancreas
- Carcinoma of the ampulla of Vater
- Malignant nodes in the porta hepatis
- Chronic pancreatitis
- Mirizzi syndrome

HISTORY

General

Fever, malaise, weight loss, dark urine, pale stools, itching.

Newborn

Biliary atresia presents as deepening jaundice within 2–3 days of birth. Liver failure develops over 3–6 months. Physiological jaundice is common and is due to immaturity of liver function. It usually settles within the first week of life.

Prehepatic

Ask about family history, racial origin, drugs, haematuria, history of anaemia. Gilbert's disease is inherited as an autosomal dominant. There is a failure of uptake of unconjugated bilirubin by the hepatocyte. Crigler–Najjar syndrome is a failure of conjugation within the hepatocyte.

Hepatocellular

Occupation. Travel. Alcohol. Sexual activity. Drugs (tablets, injections, anaesthetic agents, drug abuse). Exposure to industrial solvents. Previous episodes of jaundice. Infection. Influenza-like symptoms. Rashes. Joint pains.

Cholestatic

Drugs, e.g. chlorpromazine. Travel abroad. Severe upper abdominal pain preceding jaundice (biliary colic followed by impaction of stone in common bile duct). Insidious onset of painless jaundice (malignancy). Dark urine, pale stools, itching.

EXAMINATION

Prehepatic (haemolytic)

Often the jaundice is not intense, with only a mild lemon tinge.
Anaemia. Splenomegaly.

Hepatic

Tender liver in hepatitis. Signs of liver failure: spider naevi, palmar
erythema, leuconychia, clubbing, gynaecomastia, ascites, Dupuytren's
contracture, caput medusae, liver flap. Haematemesis may have
occurred from bleeding oesophageal varices.

Cholestatic

Hepatomegaly – usually smooth liver with 'sharp' edge. Palpable gall
bladder (Courvoisier's law – in the presence of obstructive jaundice
if the gall bladder is palpable, the cause is unlikely to be due to
gallstones). Epigastric mass, e.g. carcinoma of the pancreas. Other
abdominal masses, e.g. carcinoma of the stomach and carcinoma of
the colon with secondary deposits in the porta hepatis. Recent surgical
scars. Scratch marks on abdomen from itching.

GENERAL INVESTIGATIONS

- FBC, CRP/ESR, blood film
  Hb ↓ malignancy, haemolysis. WCC ↑ infection, e.g. hepatitis,
  cholangitis. CRP/ESR ↑ infection, malignancy. Blood film – red cell
  defects, malaria.

- Reticulocyte count
  Haemolysis.

- U&Es
  Deranged renal function with hepatorenal syndrome.

- LFTs
  See the table below.

Urine and blood biochemistry in jaundice.			
Biochemical parameter	**Prehepatic**	**Hepatic**	**Cholestatic**
Blood			
Bilirubin			
Unconjugated	↑	N/↑	N
Conjugated	N	N/↑	↑
Alkaline phosphatase	N	N/↑	↑↑
Transaminases	N	↑	N/↑
Urine			
Bilirubin	0	↑	↑
Urobilinogen	N/↑	↑	↓↓/0

N, normal; 0, no bilirubin present in urine.

- Clotting screen
  PT ↑.

- Viral antibodies
  Hepatitis A, hepatitis B, hepatitis C, CMV, EBV.

- US
  Gallstones. Dilated biliary tree. Level of obstruction (may not show cause of obstruction). Hepatic secondaries. Cirrhosis.

- ERCP
  Periampullary carcinoma. Stones in common bile duct. Tumour of common bile duct. Stricture of common bile duct. Biopsy. Brush cytology. Stenting.

- PTC
  Undertaken if ERCP fails.

- MRCP
  Bile duct anomalies. Stones.

- CT
  Carcinoma of the head of the pancreas – assess spread and local resectability. Liver secondaries.

- Liver biopsy
  Hepatocellular disease. Carcinoma.

SPECIFIC INVESTIGATIONS

- Serum copper
  Reduced in Wilson's disease.

- Serum ceruloplasmin
  Reduced in Wilson's disease.

- Serum α_1-antitrypsin
  α_1-Antitrypsin deficiency. Serum iron and TIBC.
  Iron raised in haemochromatosis. TIBC saturation > 70%.

- Leptospirosis complement fixation test
  Leptospirosis.

- Blood culture
  Septicaemia. Leptospirosis.

- Lumbar puncture
  Leptospirosis.

- Painless progressive jaundice suggests carcinoma of the pancreas, especially in the presence of a palpable gall bladder (Courvoisier's law).

- Ask about foreign travel contact, drug abuse contact and sexual history in patients with sudden onset of jaundice and fever.

JAW PAIN AND SWELLINGS

Pain or swelling of the jaw results most commonly from dental conditions. In the upper jaw, pain may also result from infection of the paranasal sinuses which is considered under Facial swellings (p. 129).

Figure 37 A large dental cyst in the mandible. *The cyst arose from tooth-forming epithelial remnants in the apical area of the lower left 2nd premolar tooth, which was extracted several months beforehand due to chronic periapical infection.*

CAUSES

TRAUMATIC

INFECTIVE
- Dental abscess
- Tonsilitis
- Mumps (increasing incidence in UK)
- Pericoronitis
- Acute osteomyelitis
- Actinomycosis

TEMPOROMANDIBULAR JOINT
- Temporomandibular joint disorder
- Rheumatoid arthritis

- Osteoarthritis
- Dislocation

CYSTIC

- Dental cysts (Fig. 37)
- Dentigerous cysts

NEOPLASTIC

BENIGN
- Giant cell granuloma

LOCALLY INVASIVE
- Ameloblastoma
- Odontogenic tumours

MALIGNANT
- Osteogenic sarcoma
- Burkitt's lymphoma ● *(endemic in equatorial Africa)*
- Secondary deposits
- Paget's disease

OTHER

- Referred pain (e.g. myocardial ischaemia)
- Giant cell (temporal) arteritis
- Post-herpetic neuralgia
- Osteonecrosis of the mandible (steroid therapy, bisphosphonates for osteoporosis, radiotherapy)
- Systemic conditions (RA, lupus, syphilis)

HISTORY

Traumatic

History of trauma, e.g. fights, road traffic accidents.

Infective

Dental abscess presents with a dull ache in the jaw, becoming throbbing and severe. There is often accompanying malaise and loss of appetite. Acute osteomyelitis of the mandible is rare. It may follow dental infection or tooth extraction. There may be a history of fractures, irradiation, leukaemia, diabetes, malnutrition, alcoholism or immunosuppression. There is a severe, throbbing, deep-seated pain. The patient has difficulty opening the mouth and swallowing due to muscle oedema. Actinomycosis presents with swelling of the jaw with persistent low-grade infection and can lead to abscesses over time.

Temporomandibular joint

Temporomandibular joint pain results from grinding and clenching the teeth but is linked with stress, OA and jaw misalignment. Pain arises in the region of the temporomandibular joint or ear, which may be associated with a clicking noise and is aggravated by wide opening of the mouth, as with yawning and chewing. Rheumatoid arthritis of the temporomandibular joint is rare. Osteoarthritis usually causes pain, swelling and limitation of jaw movement. Temporomandibular joint dislocation may be recurrent, habitual or isolated. The condyle is displaced forwards and upwards into the temporal fossa. The patient presents with an open mouth, which he or she cannot close, and pain due to muscle spasm.

Cystic

Cysts often present as asymptomatic lucencies on radiographs. Otherwise, they present as painless swellings, which may reach a large size. If the cyst becomes infected, the patient presents with pain, swelling and discharge. Occasionally pathological fractures occur. A dental cyst is attached to the root of a normally erupted but decayed tooth, and the swelling grows slowly. Dentigerous cysts are associated with an unerupted tooth.

Neoplastic

The patient presents with a jaw swelling which grows steadily and often painlessly. Giant cell granuloma may erode through bone to produce a soft-tissue purplish swelling on the gum. Ameloblastomas are rare, usually occur around the age of 30–50 years and are symptomless until the swelling becomes obtrusive. Osteogenic sarcoma of the jaw is extremely rare. Initially it is painless but becomes painful as it grows. The patient may complain of paraesthesia due to involvement of the mental nerve. Burkitt's tumour is associated with EBV. It is a malignant tumour of B lymphocytes. It is endemic in certain parts of Africa and New Guinea. Most commonly it affects children below the age of 12 years. The child presents with a progressive painless swelling of the jaw. Secondary deposits in the jaw are uncommon but may arise from lung, breast, thyroid, prostate or kidney.

Others

With post-herpetic neuralgia, there is usually a history of herpes zoster in the distribution of the trigeminal nerve. The pain tends to be distributed in a division of the trigeminal nerve. Referred pain to the jaw is common with angina; the patient usually complains of associated chest pain and radiation of the pain down the left arm. With giant cell arteritis, there will be pain in the jaw on chewing (jaw claudication). In addition, there will be other symptoms of temporal arteritis, e.g. headache precipitated by touch and tenderness in the temporal area. With osteonecrosis of the jaw, ask about steroid and bisphosphonate therapy for osteoporosis and past history of radiotherapy.

EXAMINATION

Traumatic

Check for bite marks, bruising, swelling, crepitus, tenderness. Bloodstained saliva. Broken teeth. Step deformities in occlusion.

Infective

With dental abscesses, there is reddening of the mucosa with a firm, hot, acutely tender, boggy swelling. The dental abscess may point on the outer side of the jaw. There may be associated dental caries and gingivitis. Cervical lymphadenopathy is usually present. With acute osteomyelitis, there is usually difficulty in opening the mouth and swallowing due to muscle oedema. There is a tender, red, painful swelling overlying the mandible. In actinomycosis, there may be multiple discharging sinuses, usually near the angle of the jaw, on which characteristic 'sulphur granules' may be seen discharging.

Temporomandibular joint

Diagnosis of temporomandibular joint disorder is usually made from the history. There is usually trismus and spasm around the joint. In rheumatoid arthritis, there may be tenderness and swelling over the joint. In osteoarthritis, there may be swelling over the joint and limitation of movement. In temporomandibular joint dislocation, the condyles are palpable anterior to the articular eminence. The mouth is gagged open.

Cystic

Often the only abnormality on examination is a swelling in the bones. Sometimes the bone is so thin that it crackles when touched, like a broken eggshell. With dentigerous cysts, the tooth remains unerupted and therefore a tooth will be missing when the teeth are counted.

Neoplastic

Often the only abnormality is a bony swelling, which grows steadily, initially without pain. In osteogenic sarcoma check for loose teeth and paraesthesia. With burkitt's lymphoma, there is progressive painless swelling. The eye may be displaced and the mouth partly occluded by the swelling. Secondary deposits often present as painful lesions within the bone. Check for a previous history of malignancy and check the lungs, breast, prostate, kidney and thyroid to identify the primary site.

Other

The diagnosis of post-herpetic neuralgia is usually made on the history, as well as referred pain from myocardial ischaemia.

General Investigations

- FBC, ESR
  Hb ↓ malignancy. WCC ↑ infection, leukaemia, acute osteomyelitis.

- ■ **LFTs**
  Alcoholism (acute osteomyelitis).
- ■ **Blood glucose**
  Diabetes (acute osteomyelitis).
- ■ **Swab**
  C&S. Dental infection. Actinomycosis.
- ■ **Temporomandibular joint X-rays**
  Dislocation. Osteoarthritis. Rheumatoid arthritis.
- ■ **Skull X-rays with special views**
  Fractures, cysts, tumours.
- ■ **CXR**
  Secondary deposits.

SPECIAL INVESTIGATIONS

- ■ **Blood cultures**
  Osteomyelitis.
- ■ **ECG**
  Myocardial ischaemia.
- ■ **EBV serology**
  Burkitt's lymphoma.
- ■ **CT/MRI**
  Rule out malignancy.
- ■ **Biopsy**
  Benign versus malignant lesions.

- • **Painless, progressive swelling of the jaw may suggest malignancy and requires urgent dental referral.**

JOINT DISORDERS

Disorders of joints are common problems. They may be acute, as in gout or rheumatic fever, or chronic, as in osteoarthritis. Some acute disorders go on to become chronic, e.g. rheumatoid arthritis. The first part of this section deals with general causes of arthropathy and the second part deals with specific joint disorders.

Figure 38 Osteoarthritis of the right hip joint. The joint space is diminished and there is sclerosis of the surrounding bone. On the left side, the patient has had an arthroplasty (hip replacement).

CAUSES

CONGENITAL

- Achondroplasia (dwarfism)
- Ehlers–Danlos syndrome
- Marfan's syndrome
- Osteogenesis imperfecta

ACQUIRED

INFECTIVE
- Septic arthritis ⚠
- Viral
- TB ● *(very common in the developing world and on the increase in developed countries)*
- Rheumatic fever ● *(very common in developing countries)*
- Endocarditis
- Brucellosis
- Typhoid ● *(very common in developing countries)*

INFLAMMATORY
- Rheumatoid arthritis
- Polymyalgia rheumatica
- Psoriatic arthritis
- Henoch–Schönlein disease
- Reactive arthritis (Reiter's disease)
- Ankylosing spondylitis
- Connective tissue disease

DEGENERATIVE
- Osteoarthritis (Fig. 38)

ENTEROPATHIC
- Acute gastrointestinal infections (e.g. hepatitis B/C)
- Inflammatory bowel disease

ENDOCRINE
- Acromegaly

METABOLIC
- Gout
- Pseudogout
- Haemochromatosis

NEUROPATHIC
- Charcot's joints

HAEMATOLOGICAL
- Haemophilia
- Leukaemia
- Sickle cell disease

DRUGS
- Anticoagulants
- Steroids

NEOPLASTIC

- Hypertrophic pulmonary osteoarthropathy ⚠

OTHER

- Avascular necrosis of bone
- Sarcoidosis
- Behçet's disease ● *(more common in certain Mediterranean countries)*

HISTORY

Congenital

Premature osteoarthritis may occur in achondroplasia. In Ehlers–Danlos syndrome, a genetic disorder of connective tissue, patients display hypermobile joints and hyperextensible skin. They may present with joint subluxation, dislocation and swelling due to effusions. In Marfan's syndrome, generalised joint laxity occurs with patients presenting with joint pain and swelling due to effusions. In osteogenesis imperfecta, bony fracture is common.

Acquired

Infective

Septic arthritis usually presents as a monoarthritis with a red, swollen, painful, immobile joint. Spread has usually occurred by the haematogenous route but may occur from adjacent osteomyelitis. Organisms responsible include *Staphylococcus aureus streptococci*, gonococcus, *Brucella* and *Salmonella* spp. With TB, the patient usually presents subacutely with swelling and stiffness of the joint. It is not as erythematous or warm as with acute septic arthritis. Viral arthritis may occur with rubella, mumps, hepatitis and certain enteroviruses. Rheumatic fever usually follows a streptococcal infection, e.g. scarlet fever or tonsillitis. There is a history of migratory polyarthritis, together with erythematous skin lesions and subcutaneous nodules.

Inflammatory

Rheumatoid arthritis often presents in multiple joints involvement, with swollen, painful, stiff hands and feet. Eventually characteristic hand deformities with swelling of the metacarpophalangeal joints, swan-neck and boutonnière deformities and ulnar deviation occur. The patient may complain of extra-articular manifestations, i.e. rheumatoid nodules, pulmonary disease and eye changes. Psoriatic arthritis can occur in patients with psoriasis. Reactive/Reiter's disease may present when a history of gastrointestinal or genitourinary infection is present with associated urethritis and conjunctivitis. Ankylosing spondylitis most commonly affects young males and initially presents with morning stiffness in the lower spine. The sacroiliac joints are invariably involved. Arthritis may occur in SLE. Other manifestations may be present, e.g. cutaneous, pulmonary or renal. Polymyalgia rheumatica presents with morning stiffness with a mild polyarthritis. Henoch–Schönlein purpura presents with a purpuric rash, often over the buttocks and extensor surfaces. There may be associated nephritis and abdominal pain. Pain, swelling and stiffness in the joints, usually the ankles and knees, are transient.

Degenerative

Osteoarthritis usually occurs after the age of 50, unless it is secondary to previous joint pathology or injury. The patient complains of pain on movement, worse at the end of the day, together with stiffness and instability of joints. Bony swelling may be present.

Enteropathic

Check for a history of Crohn's disease or ulcerative colitis. There may also be a history of gastric bypass surgery. The spine or the peripheral joints may be affected.

Endocrine

Acromegaly will lead to arthralgia. The patient will usually complain of other symptoms, namely, enlarged hands and feet (increase in shoe size) and deepening of the voice.

Metabolic

Gout usually presents with severe pain, redness and swelling in the first metatarsophalangeal joint; however, any joint may be affected. There may be a history of polycythaemia, leukaemia or medication with cytotoxic or immunosuppressive drugs.

Neuropathic

The patient usually complains of painless, swollen joints, which are unstable. There may be a history of diabetes, tabes dorsalis (syphilis), syringomyelia or leprosy.

Haematological

Bleeding into joints (haemarthrosis) occurs in haemophilia. A family history will be apparent. Eventually severe arthropathy occurs. Pain in bones and joints may occur in both childhood and adult leukaemia along with fever, fatigue and recurrent infections. In sickle cell disease, painful crises may occur in bones and joints. Avascular necrosis of bone may occur.

Drugs

Anticoagulants may cause bleeds into joints, whilst steroids may lead to septic arthritis or avascular necrosis of bone, with subsequent secondary degenerative disease.

Neoplastic

Rarely, a patient will present with direct infiltration of a joint with malignant disease. However, hypertrophic pulmonary osteoarthropathy is more common, occurring usually in association with bronchial/ovarian carcinoma, but it may occur in association with congenital heart disease.

Other

Avascular necrosis of bone may lead to secondary arthritis. The most common sites are the head of the femur, proximal tibia, proximal scaphoid, talus and lunate. Check for a history of steroid use. Arthralgia may occur in sarcoidosis presenting with fever, malaise, lymphadenopathy and erythema nodosum. Behçet's disease may present with arthritis but usually there are eye signs, mouth ulcers and genital ulcers.

EXAMINATION

Congenital

In Ehlers–Danlos syndrome, there will be hypermobile joints and hyperextensible skin. There may be evidence of dislocation or subluxation of joints. In Marfan's syndrome, the patient will be tall with long extremities, long fingers (arachnodactyly), high-arched palate, lens dislocation and aortic incompetence. Diagnosis of osteogenesis imperfecta will present as stunted growth due to repeated fractures with deformities. The patient has blue sclerae and often hypotonia.

Acquired

Infective

With infective arthritis there is usually a red, painful, swollen, tender joint with limited movement. The patient will be pyrexial and a single joint is usually involved. With viral infections, there may be signs of childhood illness, e.g. mumps (swollen salivary glands), rubella (rash), hepatitis (jaundice). With rheumatic fever, there will be murmurs, migratory polyarthritis, subcutaneous nodules, erythema marginatum and occasionally chorea (Sydenham's).

Inflammatory

With rheumatoid arthritis, there will be swelling of the metacarpophalangeal, PIP and wrist joints. Swan-neck and boutonnière deformities will be apparent, as will ulnar deviation. There may be subluxation at the wrist. Tendon ruptures may occur. Large joint involvement is common and atlantoaxial subluxation with myelopathy may develop. General signs include anaemia, nodulosis and eye signs. With psoriatic arthritis psoriasis of the skin is usually present. With reactive/Reiter's disease, there may be urethritis, conjunctivitis, keratoderma blenorrhagica, circinate balanitis, plantar fasciitis and Achilles tendonitis. With ankylosing spondylitis, there may be minimal signs initially, the first sign usually being a reduced range of movement of the lumbar spine, but eventually there will be involvement of the sacroiliac joints, together with a loss of the lumbar lordosis and a fixed kyphotic spine. SLE may present with malaise, arthralgia, myalgia, a butterfly rash on the face, Raynaud's phenomenon, splenomegaly, pleurisy, pleural effusion, pericarditis. Polymyalgia rheumatica is associated with tender muscles and mild polyarthritis, and there may be associated temporal arteritis.

Degenerative

Osteoarthritis usually involves the distal interphalangeal joints (Heberden's nodes), the metacarpophalangeal joint of the thumb, the first metatarsophalangeal joint, the cervical spine, the lumbar spine, the hips and knees. There will be joint tenderness and limitation of movement.

Enteropathic

There is normally spondyloarthritis with sacroiliitis. Large joint monoarthropathy is common, although many peripheral joints may be involved.

Endocrine

With acromegaly, there will be large hands and feet, a macroglossia, prognathism, arthralgia, kyphosis, deep voice and heart failure. There may be signs of the pituitary tumour (i.e. bilateral hemianopia) due to local pressure on the optic chiasma.

Metabolic

There is an acutely painful, red, swollen joint with gout. The first metatarsophalangeal joint is most often involved but any joint may be affected. There may be evidence of gouty tophi, e.g. pinna, tendons, joints. With haemochromatosis, in addition to arthropathy, there may be evidence of hepatomegaly, cirrhosis, diabetes, cardiomyopathy and skin pigmentation.

Neuropathic

Deformed, painless joints with subluxation may occur. There is usually limited warmth or tenderness in relation to the joint. Abnormal movement may occur. If the condition is due to syphilis (tabes dorsalis), there may be Argyll Robertson pupils.

Haematological

With haemophiliacs, the patient will present with an acute, painful, immobile joint following a bleed. Eventually, there will be deformed joints. Joints may be involved in leukaemia and acute sickle cell crises.

Drugs

Steroids may cause avascular necrosis, especially of the hips. There will be pain and limitation of movement. Osteoarthritis develops eventually. Patients on anticoagulants may have acute haemarthroses.

Neoplastic

Hypertrophic pulmonary osteoarthropathy usually occurs in association with bronchial/ovarian carcinoma. The ends of long bones are affected by symmetrical but irregular widespread thickening. Clubbing usually occurs. Pain from local tumours may progress to a pathological fracture.

Other

With avascular necrosis of bone, there is usually severe pain, tenderness and limitation of movement leading to osteoarthritis. With sarcoidosis, there is usually fever, lymphadenopathy, hepatosplenomegaly, erythema nodosum, eye signs, cardiac signs and CNS involvement.

GENERAL INVESTIGATIONS

- **FBC, ESR**
  Hb ↓ anaemia of chronic disease, e.g. rheumatoid arthritis, SLE. WCC ↑ infective causes, leukaemia. ESR ↑ chronic infection, rheumatoid arthritis, ankylosing spondylitis, rheumatic fever.

- **CRP**
  ↑ infective and inflammatory causes.

- **U&Es**
  Renal involvement, e.g. SLE.

- **LFTs**
  Hepatic involvement, e.g. haemochromatosis.

- **Serum uric acid**
  Gout.

- **Rheumatoid factor, anti-CCP antibodies**
  Rheumatoid arthritis.

- **PSA**
  Prostatic carcinoma.

- **Joint X-ray**
  Osteoarthritis – loss of joint space, subchondral sclerosis and cyst, osteophytes. Rheumatoid arthritis – soft-tissue thickening, juxta-articular osteopenia, loss of joint space, erosion of bone, subluxations. Avascular necrosis – avascular bone is more dense than adjacent bone. Gout – soft-tissue swelling initially, then 'punched-out' lesions in juxta-articular bone. Ankylosing spondylitis – syndesmophytes, bamboo spine, obliteration of sacroiliac joints.

- **CXR**
  Bronchial carcinoma.

SPECIFIC INVESTIGATIONS

- **Blood culture**
  Septic arthritis – *Staphylococcus aureus, Brucella, Salmonella, Streptococci.*

- **Antibody screen**
  ANA positive. Anti-double-stranded DNA ↑ SLE.

- **Brucella serology**
  Brucellosis.

- Viral titres
  Viral infections.
- Hepatitis screen
  Hepatitis B-associated arthralgia.
- Sickling test
  Sickle cell disease.
- Coagulation screen
  Anticoagulant therapy. Haemophilia.
- Mantoux test/ELISpot assay
  TB.
- Skeletal survey
  Tumours are usually visible only when more than 50% of bone mineral is lost. Acromegaly – pituitary fossa, hand and skull changes.
- Bone scan
  Metastatic disease. Primary bone tumours. Paget's disease. Inflammatory bone lesions. Osteoarthritis. Rheumatoid arthritis. Bone fractures.
- MRI
  Soft-tissue injuries. Meniscal injuries. Ligamentous injuries. Early rheumatoid arthritis.
- Joint aspirate
  Microscopy and culture and sensitivity in septic arthritis. Crystals in gout.
- Synovial biopsy
  Arthritis in rare cases.

INDIVIDUAL JOINTS

The following section covers individual joints. The conditions described under the individual joints (below) will refer to those conditions that normally affect, or cause pain in, the region of the particular joint.

SHOULDER

CAUSES

CONGENITAL

- Klippel–Feil syndrome

ACQUIRED

TRAUMATIC

- Dislocation
- Fracture of the neck of the humerus

- Fracture of the clavicle
- Fracture of the scapula

DEGENERATIVE

- Supraspinatus tendinosis
- Impingement syndromes
- Rotator cuff tears
- Frozen shoulder (adhesive capsulitis)
- Osteoarthritis
  - Acromioclavicular
  - Glenohumeral

INFLAMMATORY

- Rheumatoid arthritis
- Crystal disease (gout, pseudogout)

INFECTIVE

- Septic arthritis
- TB arthritis

NEOPLASTIC

- Metastases in the upper end of the humerus/ribs/neck

REFERRED PAIN

- Cervical spondylosis
- Diaphragmatic irritation
- Pancoast's tumour

NEUROLOGICAL

- Winged scapula

HISTORY

Congenital

In Klippel–Feil syndrome, the neck is short and there are anomalies of the cervical vertebrae; the scapula is placed superiorly.

Acquired

Traumatic

With dislocation of the shoulder, there is usually a history of a fall on the outstretched hand. Recurrent dislocation may occur. The patient presents in pain supporting the arm, which is abducted. Anterior dislocation is the most common, but posterior dislocation is often missed and can occur after trauma such as fits or electric shocks. Clavicular fracture is usually caused by a fall on the outstretched hand or point of the shoulder. Scapular fractures are usually high-energy injuries often due to RTAs.

Degenerative

Supraspinatus tendinosis results from degeneration, inflammation or calcification of the tendon. There may be sudden pain or there may be just a painful arc at the initiation of movement. With impingement syndromes, the rotator cuff becomes compressed under the acromion or acromioclavicular joint, resulting in pain on abducting the arm. Rotator cuff tears often occur in older patients and probably relate to degeneration of the cuff. The patient is unable to initiate abduction of the arm but passive movement is normal. Frozen shoulder (adhesive capsulitis) usually affects the middle-aged and there may be a history of minor injury. There is pain and limitation of both active and passive movement of the shoulder. It may occur in the elderly following immobilisation of the arm, e.g. following a Colles' fracture or stroke. It is more common in diabetics. Osteoarthritis of the acromioclavicular joint presents as pain associated with overhead movement and a high painful arc (>140°). Osteoarthritis of the glenohumeral joint may be idiopathic, or follow avascular necrosis or radionecrosis following radiotherapy for carcinoma of the breast. The patient complains of pain on shoulder movement and night pain.

Inflammatory

Rheumatoid arthritis is more common than osteoarthritis in the shoulder joint. There is usually a history of rheumatoid arthritis elsewhere.

Infective

The patient presents with a painful, red, swollen joint with limited movement. TB of the shoulder is extremely rare in the UK. There are systemic symptoms of malaise and fever and there is usually wasting of the muscle around the shoulder joint.

Neoplastic

Secondary deposits may occur in the upper end of the humerus, giving rise to pain. Pathological fractures may occur. Check for a history of carcinoma of the bronchus, breast, thyroid, prostate or kidney.

Referred pain

This is an extremely common cause of shoulder pain. Cervical spondylosis often results in referred pain to the upper part of the shoulder. Check for a history of neck pain with limitation of movement of the neck. Irritation of the diaphragm may refer pain to the dermatome C4 at the shoulder tip. This may be due to peritonitis below the diaphragm or pleurisy if above. A history of chest problems should be sought if Pancoast's tumour is suspected, especially if Horner's syndrome is present.

Neurological

Winged scapula may cause difficulty with shoulder movements. Check for recent surgery to the neck or axilla, e.g. axillary clearance in breast carcinoma, which may damage the long thoracic nerve. Carrying heavy loads on the shoulders over a prolonged period may also be responsible.

EXAMINATION

Congenital

Klippel–Feil syndrome. The patient will present with a short neck and a highly placed scapula.

Acquired

Traumatic

With dislocation of the shoulder, the patient supports the arm. The normal contour of the shoulder is lost. Check for axillary nerve damage (anaesthesia over the 'badge' area). With acromioclavicular dislocation, there will be a palpable lump at the site of dislocation. With fracture of the surgical neck of the humerus, there will be pain and tenderness, and inability to abduct the arm due to pain. With fractures of the clavicle, the patient supports the weight of the arm with the other hand. The site of the break is usually palpable.

Degenerative

There will be limitation of movement. Check for a painful arc. Check for the ability to initiate abduction (supraspinatus tendon tears). With frozen shoulder and osteoarthritis, there is limitation of active and passive movements. With osteoarthritis of the acromioclavicular joint, there is usually obvious prominence of the joint, with localised tenderness and a high painful arc. Check for mastectomy scars or signs of radiotherapy.

Inflammatory

With rheumatoid arthritis. There may be fever, malaise and heat in the joint. Features of gout may be evident such as the presence of tophi.

Infective

There will be a red, hot, swollen, tender joint with a focus of infection elsewhere in the body.

Neoplastic

There may be a pathological fracture with pain, local tenderness and limitation of movement.

Referred pain

Check for movements of the cervical spine. Carry out a full neurological examination. With referred pain from the diaphragm, examine the abdomen for tenderness, guarding and rigidity. Examine the chest for signs of pneumonia, pleurisy or tumour.

Neurological

Check for scars in the neck or axilla. Note the winging of the scapula when the patient pushes the hand against a wall with the arm forward, flexed to 90° (protraction of the scapula).

GENERAL INVESTIGATIONS

- **FBC, ESR**
  Hb ↓ anaemia of chronic disease, e.g. rheumatoid arthritis.
  WCC ↑ infection. ESR and CRP ↑ infection/inflammatory disease.
- **X-ray**
  X-rays in two planes (AP and lateral). Arthritis. Dislocation.
  Fracture. Secondary deposits.

SPECIFIC INVESTIGATIONS

- **Blood culture**
  Septic arthritis.
- **Mantoux test/ELISpot assay**
  TB.
- **Bone scan**
  Secondary deposits.
- **Aspiration**
  Gram stain. C&S. Septic arthritis. Characteristic crystals in gout and
  pseudogout.
- **Arthroscopy**
  Cause of arthritis.
- **CT/MRI**
  Impingement syndromes. Rotator cuff tears.

ELBOW

CAUSES

TRAUMATIC

- Supracondylar fracture of the humerus
- Dislocation of the elbow
- Pulled elbow
- Fracture of the radial head
- Fractured olecranon
- Fractured epicondyle/condyle
- Myositis ossificans

DEGENERATIVE

- Osteoarthritis
- Osteochondritis dissecans

INFLAMMATORY

- Rheumatoid arthritis

NEUROLOGICAL

- Nerve entrapment, e.g. ulnar, posterior interosseous and median

OTHER

- Olecranon bursitis
- Tennis elbow
- Golfer's elbow
- Cubitus varus/valgus

HISTORY

Traumatic

Supracondylar fracture is chiefly a fracture of childhood. There is a history of a fall on the outstretched hand followed by pain and swelling around the elbow. Dislocation of the elbow may occur in children or adults. The symptoms are similar to those of supracondylar fracture. Pulled elbow occurs in children aged 2–6 years. The radial head slips out of the annular ligament. The child may have been 'swinging' with the parents holding the hands. Fractures of the olecranon may result as a fall on the point of the elbow or by sudden contraction of the triceps. Condylar and epicondylar fractures are rare but easily missed. With myositis ossificans, there will be a history of a supracondylar fracture or dislocation of the elbow. A calcified haematoma forms in front of the joint. Movement of the joint, especially flexion, is affected. It may follow physiotherapy with passive stretching of the joints after trauma or after surgery.

Degenerative

Osteoarthritis of the elbow may occur in heavy manual workers or following fractures involving the joint. Osteochondritis dissecans may cause elbow pain and restrict movement because of a loose body in the joint.

Inflammatory

Rheumatoid arthritis may affect the elbow joint. If there is gross disorganisation of the joint with deformity, the ulnar nerve may be involved and there may be symptoms of ulnar nerve palsy. Gout may also affect the elbow joint.

Neurological

Various nerve entrapment syndromes can occur around the elbow. Symptoms may present in the distribution of ulnar, median or posterior interosseous nerves.

Other

Olecranon bursitis results in painful or painless swelling over the olecranon. It is common in carpet layers and students. The bursa may become infected with a red, tender, hot swelling. Tennis elbow is common between the ages of 30 and 50 years. It presents with pain on the lateral side of the elbow. It affects tennis players and anyone whose job involves extending and twisting the forearm. The pain is often worse on gripping. Golfer's elbow is similar to tennis elbow but affects the medial epicondyle. The patient complains of pain and tenderness over the medial epicondyle and also of pain on hyperextending the fingers and wrists. Cubitus valgus/varus may follow fractures around the elbow in childhood. Cubitus valgus may progressively stretch the ulnar nerve, slowly developing ulnar nerve palsy.

EXAMINATION

Traumatic

With supracondylar fractures, there will be swelling around the elbow joint and limitation of movement. The olecranon, medial epicondyle and lateral epicondyle preserve their normal relationship with one another in an equilateral triangle. With posterior dislocation at the elbow, the triangular relationship referred to above is lost. It is important to check the distal circulation and to assess for median and radial nerve palsies. With a fracture of the olecranon, there is swelling and tenderness directly over the olecranon. With damage to the medial epicondyle, it is important to test the integrity of the ulnar nerve. With myositis ossificans, a calcified mass occurs in front of the elbow joint and there will be limitation of flexion. With radial head fractures, the patient will be focally tender over the radial head and there will be lack of full extension.

Degenerative

With osteoarthritis. There may be bony swelling of the joint with loss of movement and crepitus. With osteochondritis dissecans, there may be restriction in movement, crepitus and locking of the joint due to a loose body.

Inflammatory

In longstanding arthritis, there will be a swollen, disrupted joint with deformity. Check the integrity of the ulnar nerve. Tophi may be present in gout.

Neurological

Examine carefully in the distribution of the median, ulnar and radial nerve.

Other

With olecranon bursitis, there will be a swelling over the olecranon. This is fluid-filled and exhibits fluctuation and transilluminates. With infection it may become red and tender. With tennis elbow, there is tenderness over the lateral epicondyle. Pronating the forearm while extending the elbow exacerbates the pain. With golfer's elbow, there is tenderness over the medial epicondyle. With cubitus valgus/varus, the deformity is usually obvious. Check the integrity of the ulnar nerve.

GENERAL INVESTIGATIONS

- **FBC, ESR**
  Hb ↓ anaemia of chronic disease, e.g. rheumatoid arthritis.
  WCC ↑ septic arthritis. ESR and CRP ↑ in infection/inflammatory disease.
- **Rheumatoid factor/anti-CCP antibodies**
  Rheumatoid arthritis.
- **X-ray**
  Fractures around the elbow. Fracture of the radial head – anterior fat pad sign ('sail' sign). Dislocation of the elbow. Osteoarthritis. Rheumatoid arthritis. Osteochondritis dissecans with loose body. Myositis ossificans.

SPECIFIC INVESTIGATIONS

- **US**
  Olecranon bursitis (diagnosis should be obvious on clinical examination).
- **MRI**
  Will detect abnormalities of all structures, e.g. synovitis in rheumatoid arthritis ligament disruption in tennis and golfer's elbow.
- **Aspiration**
  Gram stain. C&S – infection. Crystals – gout.

WRIST

CAUSES

TRAUMATIC

- Distal radial fracture, e.g. Colles', Smith's
- Scaphoid fracture
- Dislocations
- Carpal dislocations

DEGENERATIVE

- Osteoarthritis

INFLAMMATORY

- Rheumatoid arthritis

OTHER

- Ganglion
- Tenosynovitis
  - de Quervain's
  - Extensor tenosynovitis
- Carpal tunnel syndrome
- Avascular necrosis of the lunate (Kienböck's disease)

HISTORY

Traumatic

The patient with a Colles' fracture is usually an elderly osteoporotic woman. There is a history of a fall on the outstretched hand (extended wrist). The patient presents with pain and deformity. A Smith's fracture is the reverse of a Colles' (fall onto flexed wrist). Again there is pain and deformity. Dislocations of the carpus are rare, the most common being dislocation of the lunate. This is usually due to a fall on the dorsiflexed hand. Fracture of the scaphoid results from a fall on the outstretched hand or a blow to the palm of the hand. The patient presents with a painful, swollen wrist.

Degenerative

Osteoarthritis of the wrist is uncommon and usually a sequel to injury, e.g. a fracture of the scaphoid. The patient complains of pain and stiffness in the wrist.

Inflammatory

The wrist is commonly affected in rheumatoid arthritis. In the early stages, there will be swelling, heat, pain and stiffness.

Other

A ganglion is a painless lump, usually on the dorsum of the wrist. de Quervain's tenosynovitis usually occurs in the middle-aged. It involves the abductor pollicis longus and extensor pollicis brevis. The patient complains of pain on movement of the wrist and a weakness of the grip. Extensor 'tenosynovitis crepitans' follows excess activity and may affect all or only one of the extensor tendons. The patient usually complains of pain and tenderness over the dorsum of the wrist occurring with activity. With carpal tunnel syndrome there is often a history of pregnancy, rheumatoid arthritis, hypothyroidism, osteoarthritis, anterior dislocation of the lunate or an arteriovenous fistula created for dialysis. The diagnosis is often a clinical one. Middle-aged women are most affected with carpal tunnel syndrome. There is pain in the distribution of the median nerve in the hand, worse in bed at night. It is relieved by hanging the hand out of bed and shaking the hand. The patient often complains of clumsiness with fine movements due to median nerve involvement. With avascular necrosis of the lunate, there may be a history of trauma with aching and stiffness.

EXAMINATION

Traumatic

With a Colles' fracture, there is a classical 'dinner fork' deformity. The distal fragment is displaced backwards and radially. With Smith's fracture, there is forward angulation of the distal fragment. Pain, limitation of movement and swelling occur. With dislocation, there is a swollen wrist. Scaphoid fractures result in swelling around the wrist, with localised tenderness in the anatomical snuff box. Test the median nerve.

Degenerative

With osteoarthritis. There may be limited painful movement with crepitus.

Inflammatory

With rheumatoid arthritis, there may be gross swelling with increased local heat, pain and stiffness. Ultimately, ulnar deviation occurs and there may be palmar subluxation with significantly reduced movement.

Other

A ganglion is a well-defined cystic non-tender lump which transilluminates. With tenosynovitis, there is usually localised tenderness and occasionally swelling. There may be wasting of the thenar eminence and sensory abnormalities in the distribution of the median nerve. Tinel's sign (percussion over the median nerve in the carpal tunnel causes paraesthesia in the median nerve distribution) and Phalen's sign (paraesthesia following prolonged wrist flexion) may be positive. With AVN there will be localised tenderness and limited dorsiflexion.

GENERAL INVESTIGATIONS

- **FBC, ESR**
  Hb ↓ anaemia of chronic disease, e.g. rheumatoid arthritis.
  WCC ↑ infection. ESR and CRP ↑ infection/inflammatory disease.
- **Rheumatoid factor/anti-CCP antibodies**
  Rheumatoid arthritis.
- **X-ray**
  Fractures. Dislocation. Scaphoid views for suspected scaphoid fractures. Increased density of bone in avascular necrosis. Osteoarthritis. Rheumatoid arthritis.

SPECIFIC INVESTIGATIONS

- **Blood culture**
  Septic arthritis.
- **Aspiration**
  Infection – Gram stain, C&S. Crystals in gout.

- ■ Nerve conduction studies
  Carpal tunnel syndrome.
- ■ Bone scan
  Fracture or avascular necrosis.
- ■ MRI
  Fracture or avascular necrosis.

HIP

CAUSES

CONGENITAL

- Developmental dysplasia of the hip

ACQUIRED

TRAUMATIC

- Fractured neck of femur
- Fracture of the pubic ramus
- Dislocation of the hip
- Acetabular fracture

INFECTIVE

- Acute septic arthritis
- TB ● *(common in developing countries)*

INFLAMMATORY

- Rheumatoid arthritis
- Reactive/Reiter's syndrome
- Ankylosing spondylitis

DEGENERATIVE

- Osteoarthritis (Fig. 38)
  - ● Primary
  - ● Secondary
- Avascular necrosis

NEOPLASTIC

- Metastases
- Leukaemia (in childhood)

OTHER

- Transient synovitis
- Perthes' disease (childhood)
- Slipped upper femoral epiphysis (childhood)
- Transient osteoporosis of the hip

HISTORY

Congenital

DDH is usually picked up on routine examination of the neonate with Ortolani's/Barlow's test and confirmed by US scan. If the diagnosis is missed on routine testing, the child may present with a limp and waddling gait (Trendelenburg gait). There is an increased risk of DDH if one parent has a history of the disease and it is commoner with breech delivery, primigravidas and female infants. Consider checking for other congenital anomalies.

Acquired

Traumatic

Fracture of the neck of the femur usually occurs in an elderly frail patient. The trauma may be minor, e.g. tripping over the carpet. The patient presents with pain in the hip, especially with movement, and weight-bearing is often impossible. Dislocation of the hip, which is usually posterior, is associated with other severe injuries. It often occurs with road traffic accidents, the knee striking the dashboard. Pelvic fractures (usually pubic rami) are usually a result of a fall in the elderly. The patient feels deep-seated pain in the region of the hip. Walking is painful. Acetabular fractures usually result from direct violence, e.g. a fall on the side, or indirect, such as a fall on the feet or from impact of the knee on a car dashboard.

Infective

The infection is usually blood-borne. It may occur in children where the metaphysis is intracapsular, as in the hip. Check for a history of steroid medication or other immunosuppression. With TB, there is usually a history of contact. The patient presents with malaise, weight loss and night sweats.

Inflammatory

Reactive/Reiter's disease presents with a history of genitourinary or gastrointestinal infection, urethritis and conjunctivitis. There may be a history of sexual contact or dysentery. Rheumatoid arthritis usually presents with a symmetrical small joint polyarthritis; however, the hip may be involved.

Degenerative

Osteoarthritis presents with pain and stiffness and the patient often has difficulty walking. Secondary osteoarthritis may follow a history of fractures, Perthes' disease, slipped upper femoral epiphysis, avascular necrosis, haemophilia. Avascular necrosis of the head of the femur may occur following intracapsular fractures of the neck of the femur. It may also occur in patients on steroid therapy.

Neoplastic

The upper end of the femur near the neck is a common site for metastases. Hip pain in children may be due to leukaemia.

Other

Transient synovitis gives rise to an irritable hip with a limp, pain and restriction of movement. Perthes' usually occurs with a maximum incidence around 7–8 years. There is pain in the hip and a limp. The pain may be referred to the knee joint. Slipped upper femoral epiphysis usually presents between 11 and 16 years. It occurs more commonly in boys. There is usually pain in the hip and a limp and it may present with referred pain to the knee. Transient osteoporosis of the hip may occur during pregnancy and is a self-limiting condition.

EXAMINATION

Congenital

Ortolani's test is carried out after birth. The hips and knees are flexed to a right angle and the thighs are abducted. There is a 'clunk' as the head of the femur slips into the joint over the acetabulum (Ortolani's test). In Barlow's test, the surgeon holds the upper femur between the middle finger on the great trochanter and the thumb in the groin and levers the femoral head in and out of the acetabulum, readily demonstrating dislocation.

Acquired

Traumatic

The patient with a fractured neck of femur classically shows shortening, adduction and external rotation of the leg. If the fracture is undisplaced, limb alignment may be normal; however, movements are painful. With posterior dislocation, the thigh is flexed, adducted and internally rotated. Check for sciatic nerve injury. There may be associated injury to femur or patella. With isolated fractures of the pubic ramus, there may be little to find on examination, although a second fracture/joint injury is common at the back of the pelvic ring.

Infective

Acute pyogenic arthritis presents with a hot, tender, painful, swollen hip. All movements are painful. There is spasm in the surrounding muscles. The patient usually has a high fever. TB presents with local tenderness, swelling and effusion. There is muscle wasting and spasm.

Inflammatory

With rheumatoid arthritis, other joints are usually involved and the patient may describe constitutional symptoms. The hip is often held in flexion and movements are painful. Ankylosing spondylitis usually presents with a stiff spine with a limited range of movement, although the hips may also be stiff.

Degenerative

Osteoarthritis usually presents with a limp. The leg lies externally rotated and appears shortened because of fixed adduction. There is usually a degree of fixed flexion. Restriction in movement occurs: abduction, extension and internal rotation loss occurring early and being most restricted. There is apparent shortening. Avascular necrosis results in distortion of joint shape with stiffness, limitation of movement and ultimately secondary osteoarthritis.

Neoplastic

Check for localised pain over the hip joint. Check for any tumour of breast, bronchus, thyroid, prostate or kidney. In children with leukaemic infiltration, there may be other signs, e.g. spontaneous bruising, lymphadenopathy, splenomegaly.

Other

Transient synovitis presents with a limp and limitation of movement at the joint. Perthes' disease presents with a limp and a decreased range of joint movement whilst with slipped upper femoral epiphysis the leg lies in external rotation and passive internal rotation is diminished. Limitation of movement due to pain is usually present in transient osteoporosis of the hip.

GENERAL INVESTIGATIONS

- **FBC, ESR**
  Hb ↓ anaemia of chronic disease, e.g. rheumatoid arthritis.
  WCC ↑ infection. ESR and CRP ↑ in infection/inflammatory disease.
- **Hip X-ray**
  AP and lateral. Fractures, osteoarthritis, rheumatoid arthritis, dislocation, Perthes' disease, slipped upper femoral epiphysis, TB, avascular necrosis, transient osteoporosis.

SPECIFIC INVESTIGATIONS

- **Blood culture**
  Septic arthritis.
- **Aspiration**
  Infection – Gram stain, C&S. Crystals in gout.
- **US**
  Developmental dysplasia of the hip.
- **Bone scan**
  Avascular necrosis. Fracture.
- **MRI**
  Fractures, osteoarthritis, rheumatoid arthritis, dislocation, Perthes' disease, slipped upper femoral epiphysis, TB, avascular necrosis, transient osteoporosis.

KNEE

CAUSES

TRAUMATIC

BONES
- Patellar fractures
- Supracondylar fractures of the femur
- Tibial fractures

LIGAMENTS
- Medial and lateral collateral ligament damage
- Cruciate ligament damage
- Rupture of quadriceps tendon
- Rupture of the patellar tendon

MENISCI
- Meniscal tears

INFECTIVE
- Septic arthritis

INFLAMMATORY
- Rheumatoid arthritis
- Reactive/Reiter's syndrome
- Ankylosing spondylitis

DEGENERATIVE
- Osteoarthritis

METABOLIC
- Gout
- Pseudogout

NEUROPATHIC
- Charcot's joint

NEOPLASTIC
- Osteogenic sarcoma

OTHER
- Bursitis
  - Pre-patellar bursitis (housemaid's knee)
  - Infra-patellar bursitis (clergyman's knee)
  - Semi-membranosus bursitis

- Baker's cyst
- Disorders of alignment
  - Genu varum (bow legs)
  - Genu valgum (knock knee)
- Patellofemoral instability
- Referred pain from the hip/back
- Osteochondritis dissecans
- Osgood–Schlatter's disease (osteochondritis of the tibial tuberosity)
- Chondromalacia patellae

HISTORY

Traumatic

With fractures around the knee joint, there will usually be an obvious history of trauma. Fractures of the patella may arise because of violent contraction of quadriceps or because of direct blows to the patella. With ligamentous tears, there is often a history of damage during sport, e.g. footballers. The patient will present with a painful, swollen knee joint. Posterior cruciate ligament injury is usually due to a force drawing the tibia backwards on the femur with the knee flexed, e.g. in a car accident when the upper tibia strikes the dashboard. Meniscal tears often occur in sportsmen when the knee is twisted while it is flexed. The patient presents with a swollen knee with pain and tenderness on the side on which the meniscus is torn. The knee may be 'locked', i.e. lacks the last 10°–15° of extension.

Infective

May occur in children and adults on steroids or who are immunosuppressed. The patient presents with a hot, painful, tender joint with malaise and fever. The patient is reluctant to move the joint.

Inflammatory

In rheumatoid arthritis, the patient complains of pain, swelling and stiffness together with constitutional upset. Reactive/Reiter's syndrome may present with swelling and discomfort in the knee.

Degenerative

Osteoarthritis is common in the knee. The patient may be overweight and elderly. There is pain on movement, stiffness and deformity. There may be a history of previous joint pathology, e.g. septic arthritis, meniscal tear, meniscal surgery or osteochondritis dissecans.

Metabolic

Gout may present with pain and swelling of the knee. Pseudogout (pyrophosphate deposition disease) may also present in the knee joint. The condition is associated with chondrocalcinosis, i.e. there is calcification visible in hyaline and fibrocartilage.

Neuropathic

The patient presents with a painless joint, which is grossly deformed and hypermobile. There may be a history of diabetes, syphilis or leprosy.

Neoplastic

The lower end of the femur and the upper end of the tibia are common sites of osteogenic sarcoma. The patient is usually male and under the age of 30 years. There is pain, swelling and deformity around the knee.

Other

Bursitis

Bursitis presents with swelling, either in front of or behind the knee. The swelling may be painless. Patients who work on their knees leaning forwards, e.g. carpet fitters, may get prepatellar bursitis (housemaid's knee). Infrapatellar bursitis occurs in those who sit back on their heels (e.g. vicars praying, hence the name clergyman's knee). A bursa may become infected, in which case the patient will present with a tender, red, hot swelling.

Baker's cyst

Baker's cyst presents in the midline of the popliteal fossa. The patient will notice a lump and reduced flexion of the knee. There may also be pain associated with concurrent osteoarthritis of the joint.

Disorders of alignment

With genu varum, the patient presents with bow legs. In children, this is usually associated with a disorder of growth, often with a bony injury to the area of epiphyses. In adults, there may be a history of rickets, Paget's disease, rheumatoid or osteoarthritis. In genu valgum (knock knee), the patient is often a child who has flat feet. In adults, there may be a history of rheumatoid arthritis.

Patellofemoral instability

Dislocation of the patella may occur. In the acute form, there may be a history of a blow to one side of the knee. Recurrent dislocation is usually associated with flattening of the lateral condyle, a high-riding patella (patella alta) or genu valgum.

Referred pain

It is very common for pain to be referred from the hip or the back to the knee. Always enquire about hip and back symptoms.

Osteochondritis dissecans

This occurs most commonly in the second decade of life. A segment of bone undergoes avascular necrosis, separates and forms a loose body in the joint. The patient complains of pain, swelling and intermittent 'locking' of the joint.

Osgood–Schlatter's disease

The patient is usually a boy aged between 10 and 14 years. There is a history of physical activity, e.g. football. Pain and swelling occur, accurately located to the area of the tibial tuberosity.

Chondromalacia patellae

The patient presents with localised pain in front of the knee. It is most common in females in the 15–35 years age group. There may be a history of injury. There is usually some swelling, and pain occurs, especially when climbing stairs. The knee tends to give way.

EXAMINATION

Traumatic

Fractures will usually be obvious. There will be pain, tenderness, deformity and crepitus. With supracondylar fractures, it is important to check the distal circulation. With ligamentous injuries, test for joint stability, effusion and tenderness over the affected ligament. Testing for active straight-leg raising will exclude injury to the extensor mechanism (rupture of quadriceps, rupture of patellar tendon, patellar fracture). Valgus and varus strain testing may be necessary to diagnose ligamentous injury. Test for anterior and posterior drawer signs and carry out Lachman's test. With meniscal injuries, there is tenderness, swelling and effusion in the acute phase. In the chronic phase, there will be wasted quadriceps, effusion, tenderness over the meniscus in the joint line. McMurray's test will be positive with medial meniscus injury, although it is rarely carried out these days.

Infective

The patient will be febrile, with a hot, red, tender, painful, swollen joint. There will be spasm in the surrounding muscles and often no active or passive movement will be possible.

Inflammatory

With rheumatoid arthritis, there will be fever, pain and swelling with decreased range of movement and synovial thickening. There will often be signs of rheumatoid arthritis in other joints.

Degenerative

With osteoarthritis, there will be swelling due to osteophytes, and possibly thickened synovium or effusion. There will be wasting of quadriceps, reduced mobility of the joint and gait is invariably disturbed. Alignment may be distorted if only one side of the joint is affected.

Metabolic

With gout, the joint is red, hot and swollen and there is limitation of movement. A similar appearance occurs in pseudogout.

Neuropathic

The joint will be grossly swollen and deformed. Test for abnormality of dorsal column sensation (joint position sense).

Other

Bursitis – soft, fluctuant swelling in front of the patella (prepatellar bursitis) or below the patella (infrapatellar bursitis). Semi-membranosus bursitis presents as a cystic swelling on the medial aspect of the popliteal fossa. If the bursa becomes infected, then the swelling becomes hot, red and tender. With osteochondritis dissecans, there will be joint swelling due to effusion, and intermittent locking of the joint. Genu valgum and genu varum will be apparent on examination. Patellofemoral instability may result from acute or chronic dislocation. With acute dislocation, the patella is visibly displaced laterally with the knee flexed. There will be localised tenderness and swelling. With chronic dislocation, the knee locks in semiflexion. Spontaneous reduction often occurs. Always remember to examine the hip joint and spine as pain may be referred. Baker's cyst is a soft, diffuse swelling in the popliteal fossa. Pain occurs if the cyst ruptures and can mimic a DVT.

GENERAL INVESTIGATIONS

- **FBC, ESR**
  Hb ↓ anaemia of chronic disease, e.g. rheumatoid arthritis.
  WCC ↑ infection, e.g. pyogenic arthritis. ESR and CRP ↑ infection/inflammatory disease.

- **Rheumatoid factor/anti-CCP antibodies**
  Rheumatoid arthritis.

- **Serum uric acid**
  Gout.

- **Knee X-ray (AP, lateral, tunnel and skyline views)**
  Fractures. Osteoarthritis. Rheumatoid arthritis. Loose bodies. Osteogenic sarcoma. X-ray stressing the joints may be necessary to diagnose ligamentous injuries.

- **CXR**
  Secondary deposits in osteogenic sarcoma.

SPECIFIC INVESTIGATIONS

- **Blood culture**
  Septic arthritis.

- **Joint aspiration**
  Gram stain and culture and sensitivity – infection. Microscopy shows crystals in gout and pseudogout.

- **Isotope scan**
  Tumour. Infections.

- MRI
  All pathology, but especially good for meniscal and other cartilage injuries. Ligamentous injuries. Avascular necrosis. Synovitis.
- Arthroscopy
  Loose bodies. Effusion. Meniscal injuries.
- Synovial biopsy
  Confirmation of diagnosis.

ANKLE

CAUSES

TRAUMATIC

- Sprains (lateral ligaments)
- Fractures around the ankle
- Rupture of the Achilles tendon

INFECTIVE

- Septic arthritis
- TB

INFLAMMATORY

- Rheumatoid arthritis

DEGENERATIVE

- Osteoarthritis

OTHERS

- Tenosynovitis
- Footballer's ankle
- Tarsal tunnel syndrome
- Osteochondritis of the talus

HISTORY

Traumatic

History of recent injury. Sprains usually affect the lateral ligament. With fractures, there will be swelling, deformity, bruising and crepitus around the ankle. With tibiofibular diastasis, there may be a high fibular fracture. Rupture of the Achilles tendon often occurs during sport particularly in middle-aged men. Patients feel as though they have been kicked in the back of the heel.

Infective

Septic arthritis will result in a red, hot, tender joint with pain on walking.

Inflammatory

Rheumatoid arthritis is the commonest cause of chronic pain and swelling at the ankle joint. Fever and malaise may also be present.

Degenerative

Primary osteoarthritis of the ankle is rare. Osteoarthritis is often a sequel to an imperfectly reduced fracture or avascular necrosis of the talus.

Others

Tenosynovitis may occur in the tendons behind either the lateral or medial malleolus. Pain is present on either side of the ankle, particularly during inversion or eversion. Footballer's ankle, as the name implies, occurs in those who play football. The patient presents with poorly localised pain in front of the ankle. Osteochondritis of the talus is rare. It occurs in teenagers and young men. There is often severe pain in the ankle. In tarsal tunnel syndrome, the tibial nerve may be compressed as it passes beneath the flexor retinaculum, giving rise to paraesthesia and a burning pain in the medial aspect of the sole of the foot and toes.

EXAMINATION

Traumatic

In fractures, there will be deformity, a palpable swelling, tenderness and crepitus. With ruptures of the Achilles tendon, there is usually an obvious gap in the Achilles tendon, and a weakness of plantar flexion of the foot against resistance. Apply the Thomson squeeze test. Normally, when the calf is squeezed, the foot plantar flexes. This does not occur with rupture of the Achilles tendon.

Infective

In septic arthritis, there will be a hot, tender, swollen, painful ankle. With TB, the ankle will be swollen, with wasting of calf muscles.

Inflammatory

Rheumatoid arthritis seldom affects the ankle only. It presents with a swollen, tender ankle but there will be signs of arthritis elsewhere.

Degenerative

In osteoarthritis, there is swelling, with a decreased range of movements of the ankle with crepitus.

Others

With tenosynovitis, there is a puffy swelling and tenderness along the tendons. There may be pain on forced eversion (peroneus longus) and inversion (tibialis posterior). With footballer's ankle, there is tearing of the anterior capsule of the joint with subsequent calcification. Examination often reveals restriction in dorsiflexion. With osteochondritis of the talus, there is ankle swelling and tenderness. Loose bodies may present in the joint.

GENERAL INVESTIGATIONS

■ FBC, ESR
Hb ↓ anaemia of chronic disease, e.g. rheumatoid arthritis.
WCC ↑ infection, e.g. pyogenic arthritis. ESR and CRP ↑ infection/inflammatory disease.

■ Ankle X-ray
Fractures. Stress X-rays may be required to delineate the type of fracture. Always include the upper fibula in the X-ray, as in diastasis of the joint there may be a fracture of the upper part of the shaft of the fibula. Rheumatoid arthritis. Osteoarthritis. Osteochondritis of the talus. Calcification of the anterior part of the capsule in footballer's ankle.

SPECIFIC INVESTIGATIONS

■ Blood culture
Septic arthritis.

■ Joint aspiration
Gram stain and C&S in infection. Crystals in the fluid in gout.

■ Bone scan
Infections. Acute arthritis.

■ MRI
Osteochondritis of the talus. Fractures. Synovitis. Avascular necrosis. Tenosynovitis.

* Septic arthritis is an emergency. Immediate assessment and management is required in order to avert long-term joint damage.

* New onset inflammatory arthritis dictates rapid referral to a specialist, as early intervention has been shown to markedly improve prognosis.

KIDNEY SWELLINGS

Kidney swellings are common. They may present silently or may be associated with haematuria, urinary tract infections and pyrexia.

Figure 39 Abdominal CT scan. *A large renal cell carcinoma (hypernephroma) of the right kidney can be seen (arrow).*

CAUSES

CONGENITAL
- Polycystic kidney

ACQUIRED

INFECTIVE
- Perinephric abscess ▲
- TB ● *(common where TB is endemic)*

OBSTRUCTIVE
- Hydronephrosis
- Pyonephrosis

DEGENERATIVE
- Solitary cyst

NEOPLASTIC ▲
- Hypernephroma (Fig. 39)
- Nephroblastoma

HISTORY

Congenital

There will often be a family history with adult polycystic kidney disease; however, it does not usually present until the third or fourth decade, when the patient may present with an abdominal mass, haematuria, loin pain (infection or bleeding into a cyst) or chronic renal failure. Hypertension may be a presenting symptom. Rarely, hydronephrosis may present at birth. Hydronephrosis in infants may be a cause of failure to thrive.

Acquired

There may be a history of TB. The patient may present with haematuria, dysuria or pyuria. With perinephric abscess, there may be a history of diabetes. Nephroblastoma presents with an abdominal mass, pain, haematuria, pyrexia and weight loss within the first three years of life.

EXAMINATION

A mass may be palpated in either the right or the left loin. This moves with respiration and is palpable bimanually and ballotable. Generally, a kidney swelling is dull to percussion, but there may be a strip of resonance across the swelling due to the gas-filled overlying transverse colon. A solitary cyst may be large, tense and smooth. Polycystic kidneys may be very large and extend down to the groin. They are smooth and embossed with many cysts. They may be tender if the cysts are infected or tense following bleeding. Hydronephrotic kidneys may be very large, smooth and tense. Perinephric abscesses may be associated with redness, swelling and oedema in the loin. Hypernephromas are usually firm, irregular, nodular, and may be fixed. A nephroblastoma presents with a large mass in the loin and abdomen.

GENERAL INVESTIGATIONS

- **FBC, CRP, ESR**
  Hb ↑ (hypernephroma may be associated with polycythaemia).
  Hb ↓ blood loss due to haematuria. WCC ↑ pyonephrosis, perinephric abscess. ESR ↑ hypernephroma, nephroblastoma, TB, infection.

- **U&Es**
  Urea and creatinine raised if bilateral disease.

- **Blood glucose**
  Perinephric abscess in diabetes.

- **Urinalysis and urine culture**
  Blood, pus cells, organisms.

- **CT kidney, ureter and bladder (CT KUB)**
  Hydronephrosis due to renal or ureteric stones. Renal outline.

- **CXR**
  Metastases – hypernephroma (cannonball metastases), nephroblastoma. TB.
- **US**
  Cystic versus solid. Biopsy.

SPECIFIC INVESTIGATIONS

- **Intravenous pyelogram (IVP) or intraveneous urogram (IVU)**
  Hydronephrosis. Distortion of calyces (hypernephroma).
- **CT abdomen**
  Solid versus cystic. Spread of tumour. Biopsy.
- **Cystoscopy**
  Bladder tumour obstructing ureters. TB. Bladder outlet obstruction.
- **Antegrade/Retrograde pyelography**
  Identify site of obstruction.
- **MRI**
  Renal parenchymal lesions. Vascular lesions.

- Painless, frank haematuria in association with an abdominal mass is an ominous sign and indicates malignancy.
- If polycystic kidney is a possible diagnosis, others in the family may be affected or there may be a past history of deaths in the family from chronic renal failure.

LEG PAIN

This section deals with causes of pain arising from local lesions within the leg, or referred into the leg. Pain in the leg is a common complaint and the majority of cases are of vascular or orthopaedic origin. Joint problems are dealt with in the section on Joint disorders (p. 247).

Figure 40 MRA femoral vessels. *A block in the left (superficial) femoral artery in the adductor canal (arrow) can be seen. The distal artery fills via numerous collaterals. The patient presented with intermittent claudication in the left calf.*

CAUSES

TRAUMATIC

- Fractures
- Dislocations ▲
- Crush injuries ▲

INFLAMMATORY

- Rheumatoid arthritis
- Reiter's disease
- Ankylosing spondylitis

INFECTIVE

- Cellulitis
- Septic arthritis ▲

- Osteomyelitis ⚠
- Myositis

DEGENERATIVE

- Osteoarthritis
- Meniscal lesions
- Baker's cyst

VASCULAR

- Intermittent claudication
- Varicose vein
- Deep vein thrombosis ⚠
- Acute arterial occlusion ⚠

NEUROLOGICAL

- Sciatica
- Peripheral neuropathy
- Neurogenic claudication

METABOLIC

- Gout/pseudogout

NEOPLASTIC

- Secondary deposits
- Osteogenic sarcoma

OTHER

- Cramp
- Strenuous exercise
- Polymyalgia rheumatica

HISTORY

Traumatic

Obvious history of trauma.

Inflammatory

History of joint swelling, stiffness, limitation of movement. Pain on walking. There may be an obvious history of rheumatoid arthritis with signs elsewhere, e.g. the hands. Reiter's disease – conjunctivitis, urethritis. Ankylosing spondylitis – stiffness of the spine, especially in the morning; hip and knee involvement.

Infective

Cellulitis may arise from puncture wounds, e.g. insect bites or in a lymphoedematous leg. The patient presents with pain, redness, tenderness, malaise and fever. Myositis may occur in association with collagen diseases, e.g. scleroderma, dermatomyositis. Osteomyelitis is rare but more common in childhood. History of immunosuppression or diabetes. Recent history of infection elsewhere. Pain aggravated by movement. Swelling and redness of the affected area. Septic arthritis presents with a red, hot, tender, painful joint. More common in children. In adults, enquire about a history of steroid therapy or diabetes.

Degenerative

Osteoarthritis presents with pain, stiffness and deformity. The pain is often worse on starting walking and then improves. Baker's cyst presents with a lump behind the knee. The patient may complain of pain and swelling of the calf if the cyst ruptures. With meniscal lesions, there is usually a history of twisting the knee, e.g. playing football. The knee may lock.

Vascular

Deep vein thrombosis presents with painful swelling of the leg. There may be a history of the contraceptive pill, prolonged immobilisation, recent surgery, malignancy. Acute arterial occlusion results in sudden onset of severe pain in the affected limb. The patient is unable to move the leg and complains that the leg feels cold. With intermittent claudication, there is pain on walking, which is relieved by rest. It may affect the calf, thigh or buttock. Rest pain in the foot may occur with advanced arterial disease. The pain is often worse in bed at night and the patient obtains relief by hanging the foot out of bed. Varicose vein disease may be evident if pain is reported whilst standing, most prominent at the end of the day.

Neurological

Pain down the back of the leg (sciatica) often made worse by coughing, movement or straining. The patient may also complain of backache with painful spasm in the back muscles. There are restricted movements of the spine. Neurogenic claudication results from central spinal canal stenosis. Symptoms improve with flexion, as this increases the diameter of the canal. Therefore, patients find it easier to cycle than walk and easier to walk upstairs than downstairs. With neurogenic claudication, the claudication distance becomes progressively shorter with each bout of pain during one walk but not with vascular claudication. It also takes the pain of neurogenic claudication longer to settle than the pain of vascular claudication. The two forms of claudication may co-exist, making diagnosis difficult.

Metabolic

Gout/pseudogout presents as acute severe pain with redness and swelling of a joint. There may be a history of previous episodes.

Neoplastic

Osteogenic sarcoma usually presents in men between 20 and 40 years old. There is usually swelling around the knee, with the commonest sites of the tumour being the lower femur or upper tibia. The patient often complains of bone pain, swelling or cough due to lung secondaries. Pain or pathological fractures may be due to secondary deposits. These may occur from the breast, lung, thyroid, prostate or kidney. Check for symptoms related to these or previous surgery for malignancy.

Other

Polymyalgia rheumatica usually occurs in elderly women. There is aching, morning stiffness in proximal muscles and often associated arthritis. Cramp is painful muscle spasm. The patient often complains of severe pain in the legs, especially at night or after exercise. It may occur with salt depletion, myopathy or muscle ischaemia. It is common in chronic renal failure.

EXAMINATION

Traumatic

Pain, loss of function, tenderness, deformity, crepitus, abnormal mobility. Check for associated nerve and vascular injuries.

Inflammatory

Pain in joints, swelling, tenderness, loss of movement, fixed deformities, disturbances of gait. Signs of rheumatoid arthritis elsewhere. Reiter's disease – conjunctivitis, urethritis. Ankylosing spondylitis – stiffness of the spine, reduced thoracic excursion, fixed kyphotic spine, hyperextended neck.

Infective

In acute cellulitis, there is redness and tenderness over the affected area. Inguinal lymphadenopathy may be present. With acute osteomyelitis, there is tenderness and heat over the site of infection. With myositis, there is tenderness and wasting of the muscles. There may be other signs of collagen diseases, e.g. polyarteritis nodosa, SLE, scleroderma or dermatomyositis. In septic arthritis, there is a hot, tender, painful, swollen joint and all movements are painful. Surrounding muscle spasm is present.

Degenerative

In osteoarthritis, there is deformity, synovial thickening, bony enlargement due to osteophytes, effusion, loss of movement and fixed deformities. Baker's cyst presents as a swelling in the popliteal fossa. If it has ruptured there is pain and swelling of the calf. Meniscal lesions present with swelling of the knee and tenderness over the joint line in the early phase. Later, there may be a continued effusion with wasted quadriceps and a positive McMurray sign.

Vascular

Deep vein thrombosis presents with pain, tenderness, swelling and heat, usually over the calf. There is ankle oedema. With iliofemoral thrombosis, there may be phlegmasia alba dolens (white leg) or phlegmasia cerulea dolens (painful blue leg). Acute ischaemia presents with the six Ps: pain, pallor, pulselessness, perishingly cold, paraesthesia and paralysis. Check for atrial fibrillation. With intermittent claudication, examine for absent pulses. Perform Buerger's test. Varicose vein disease may be evidence by the presence of prominent superficial veins.

Neoplastic

There is usually a hot, tender swelling around the knee joint in either the lower femur or upper tibia. Examine the chest for lung metastases. With secondary deposits, check the lung, breast, thyroid, prostate and kidney.

Neurological

Lordosis, limited straight leg raising, restricted back movements. Reduced reflexes in the lower limb. Areas of absent sensation.

Metabolic

With gout/pseudogout, there will be a tender, red, swollen joint with limitation of movement. Check for gouty tophi elsewhere.

Other

Polymyalgia rheumatica presents with tenderness over muscles and arthritis. Occasionally there is associated giant cell arteritis.

Examine the temporal artery for tenderness. With cramp, there may be signs of chronic renal failure.

GENERAL INVESTIGATIONS

- **FBC, ESR, CRP**
  Hb ↓ anaemia of chronic disease, e.g. rheumatoid arthritis, collagen disease. WCC & CRP ↑ infection, e.g. osteomyelitis, septic arthritis. ESR ↑ inflammation, e.g. rheumatoid arthritis, malignancy, polymyalgia rheumatica.

- **U&Es**
  Chronic renal failure may lead to peripheral oedema.

- **LFTs**
  Alkaline phosphatase ↑ in liver secondaries.

- **Blood glucose**
  Diabetes – neuropathy, peripheral vascular disease.

- **Local X-rays**
  Fractures. Osteoarthritis. Rheumatoid arthritis. Chronic osteomyelitis. Tumours.
  Disc lesions. Osteophytes. Narrowing of joint spaces. Lordosis. Secondary deposits in osteogenic sarcoma.

SPECIFIC INVESTIGATIONS

- **Rheumatoid factor antinuclear antibodies (ANA), antineutrophil cytoplasmic antibodies (ANCA)**
  Rheumatoid arthritis.

- **Serum uric acid calcium, phosphate**
  Gout/Pseudogout.

- **CT**
  Local lesion. Spine, e.g. disc lesion, tumour, neurogenic claudication – narrowing of canal.

- **MRI**
  Spine, disc lesion, tumour.

- **Duplex Doppler**
  DVT. Arterial disease. Varicose vein.

- **Arteriography**
  Vascular disease (Fig. 40). CT angiography or catheter angiogram if acute occlusion is suspected. MR angiography for critical limb ischaemia.

- **Magnetic resonance venogram**
  Complex DVT. Varicose vein.

- **Nerve conduction studies**
  Nerve lesions, peripheral neuropathy.

- Always carefully examine the pulses. Vascular disease in the lower limbs is a common condition.
- Acute ischaemia presents with the five Ps (see above). Treatment is urgent.
- Vague swelling and thickening around the knee joint in 20–40-year-olds may be due to osteogenic sarcoma. Refer for X-ray.

LEG SWELLINGS

Swelling of the lower limb may be unilateral or bilateral. Bilateral swellings are usually due to medical conditions such as cardiac, renal or hepatic failure. Unilateral swellings are commonly due to trauma, venous disease or lymphatic disease.

Figure 41 Phlegmasia cerulea dolens. *The painful, swollen, blue leg results from a massive ilio-femoral venous thrombosis. It may lead to venous gangrene unless the resulting high tissue pressure is relieved by thrombectomy. In this patient, blood-filled blisters and gangrene of the toes have already developed. This is a relatively rare presentation of deep vein thrombosis.*

CAUSES

LOCAL

ACUTE SWELLING
- Trauma
- Deep venous thrombosis (DVT) (Fig. 41)

- Cellulitis
- Rheumatoid arthritis
- Allergy

CHRONIC SWELLING
- Venous
  - Varicose veins
  - Obstruction to venous return, e.g. pregnancy, pelvic tumours, inferior vena cava (IVC) obstruction, post-phlebitic limb
- Lymphoedema
- Congenital malformations, e.g. arteriovenous fistulae
- Paralysis (failure of muscle pump)

GENERAL
- Congestive cardiac failure
- Hypoproteinaemia, e.g. liver failure, nephrotic syndrome, malnutrition
- Renal failure
- Fluid overload
- Myxoedema

HISTORY

Bilateral leg swelling is usually due to systemic conditions, e.g. cardiac failure, while unilateral leg swelling is more often due to local causes, e.g. DVT and cellulitis. Pain will be associated with trauma, DVT, infection or complications of varicose veins. Other causes of swelling of the lower limb may be painless, although the limb may be uncomfortable if the oedema becomes tense. Evidence of the following should be sought in the medical history: trauma to the limb, recent pregnancy (DVT), abdominal or pelvic malignancy, previous surgery or radiotherapy to lymph nodes, thyroid disease, congestive cardiac failure, renal failure, liver failure, malnutrition, poliomyelitis in childhood and nerve lesions. With primary lymphoedema, the leg may have been swollen since birth or oedema may have developed at puberty (lymphoedema praecox) or in the third decade (lymphoedema tarda).

EXAMINATION

The presence of fracture, contusion or haematoma should be obvious. With cellulitis, the limb will be red, swollen, hot and tender. A puncture wound may be visible. DVT may be suspected if the limb is tender and swollen, particularly the calf, with a positive Homans' sign, i.e. pain in the calf on dorsiflexion of the foot. Tenderness may be present over the femoral vein with femoral vein thrombosis.

The limb may be pale and swollen to the groin (phlegmasia alba dolens) or tense and purplish and extremely painful (phlegmasia cerulea dolens) with iliofemoral thrombosis. Bilateral swelling with dilated collateral veins on the abdominal wall suggests IVC thrombosis. Swelling and tenderness over the joints may suggest rheumatoid arthritis. Lymphoedema pits in the early stages, but in the later stage, it becomes nonpitting, when the skin and subcutaneous tissue become thick and eventually hyperkeratotic and warty. Previous scars in the groin, a mass of malignant nodes or signs of previous radiotherapy suggest lymphoedema as a possible cause.

In the presence of an arteriovenous fistula, there will be dilated veins that do not collapse on elevation of the limb. The limb will be warmer than the opposite limb; palpation will reveal a thrill and auscultation will reveal a continuous machinery bruit.

Localised swelling of the limb may be due to a tumour. There may also be associated distal swelling due to venous or lymphatic obstruction.

Swelling due to neurological damage, e.g. nerve lesions or poliomyelitis, will result in wasting, which should be apparent. Examination of the abdomen may reveal hepatomegaly or an abdominal mass, which could obstruct the venous outflow. It is appropriate to carry out a rectal examination for a pelvic tumour, which may be causing back pressure on the venous and lymphatic system or may have resulted in a 'frozen' pelvis.

GENERAL INVESTIGATIONS

- **FBC, ESR**
  A large haematoma associated with trauma or fracture may result in a low Hb. WCC ↑ will suggest infection. Haematoma may be associated with a reduced platelet count.

- **Urinalysis**
  Proteinuria may suggest a renal cause.

- **U&Es and creatinine**
  Raised urea and creatinine will be associated with renal failure.

- **LFTs**
  May indicate impaired liver function with associated hypoalbuminaemia.

- **Blood glucose**
  Cellulitis or other infections of the leg may be associated with diabetes.

- **CXR**
  Findings suggestive of cardiac failure are cardiomegaly, pulmonary oedema and pleural effusions. Pulmonary oedema may be associated with fluid overload associated with renal failure. Secondary deposits may be seen in association with sarcoma of the limb.

- **Limb X-ray**
  May show fracture, tumour or gas in the tissues associated with gas gangrene.

SECTION A

SPECIFIC INVESTIGATIONS

- **Clotting screen**
  There may be abnormal clotting associated with coagulopathy, resulting in spontaneous haematoma.

- **TFTs**
  Myxoedema

- **US**
  Haematoma or soft-tissue sarcoma.

- **CT**
  Haematoma or tumour.

- **MRI**
  Soft-tissue sarcoma.

- **US or CT pelvis**
  May show an abdominal or pelvic mass causing extrinsic pressure on the veins.

- **Duplex Doppler**
  Will show DVT or arteriovenous fistula.

- **Venography**
  Will confirm DVT.

- **Arteriography**
  Will confirm the presence of an arteriovenous fistula.

- **Lymphangiography**
  May demonstrate the cause of lymphoedema, e.g. hypoplasia or obstruction.

- **Lymph node biopsy**
  Infection or tumour.

- Patients with unexplained DVT may have underlying malignancy. Take a full systematic history.

- In the young patient with unilateral oedema of slow onset, always consider lymphoedema. Lymphoedema does not pit.

LEG ULCERS

An ulcer is a discontinuity of an epithelial surface. Leg ulcers are common and the site of an ulcer on the leg may provide a clue to its aetiology.

Figure 42 Venous ulcer. The ulcer is in a characteristic position on the distal medial aspect of the lower limb.

CAUSES

INFECTIVE

- Syphilis
- TB ● *(common where TB is endemic)*

NEOPLASTIC

- Squamous cell carcinoma ⚠
- Malignant melanoma ⚠
- Basal cell carcinoma

VASCULAR

- Venous ulcers (Fig. 42)
- Arterial (ischaemic) ulcers
- Arteriovenous fistulae

NEUROPATHIC

- Diabetes
- Leprosy
- Tabes dorsalis (syphilis)

AUTOIMMUNE/VASCULITIC

- Rheumatoid arthritis
- SLE

HAEMATOLOGICAL

- Sickle cell anaemia
- Polycythaemia rubra vera
- Thrombotic thrombocytopenic purpura

OTHER

- Dermatitis artefacta (self-inflicted)
- Pyoderma gangrenosum

HISTORY

A history of trauma may be apparent. In self-inflicted injury, it may not. Pain suggests trauma, ischaemia or infection. Lack of pain suggests a neuropathic cause, e.g. diabetes mellitus or tabes dorsalis. A history of varicose veins or DVT suggests a venous ulcer. A prior history of intermittent claudication suggests ischaemic ulcers, as does a history of atrial fibrillation or subacute bacterial endocarditis (embolic). The presence of a longstanding venous ulcer with recent change in the shape of the ulcer suggests development of a squamous cell carcinoma (Marjolin's ulcer).

A history of rheumatoid arthritis or collagen disease may suggest a vasculitic lesion. A pigmented ulcerating lesion arising at the site of a previous mole or de novo may suggest a malignant melanoma, especially if there is a history of prolonged exposure to the sun or sunburn. A history of any haematological conditions should be sought. Pyoderma gangrenosum may occur in association with Crohn's disease or ulcerative colitis.

EXAMINATION

Site

The site of an ulcer may give a clue to the aetiology. Venous stasis ulcers usually occur on the medial aspect of the lower third of the leg, usually over the medial malleolus. Arterial ulcers occur over the metatarsal heads, tips of the toes, lateral aspect of the head of the fifth metatarsal, around the heel, in between the toes and on the tips of the toes. Diabetic ischaemic ulcers occur at the same sites. Diabetic neuropathic ulcers usually occur at pressure points, e.g. under the heel, under the heads of the first and fifth metatarsals and under the toes. They are often associated with callosities.

Edge

Classically, five types are described. A sloping edge suggests a healing ulcer, e.g. venous stasis ulcer. A punched-out edge suggests an ischaemic ulcer or a syphilitic gummatous ulcer (rare). An undermined edge suggests a tuberculous ulcer (rare). A rolled edge is characteristic of a rodent ulcer, while an everted edge is suggestive of a malignant ulcer, e.g. squamous cell carcinoma.

Base

This may contain slough or granulation tissue. Ischaemic ulcers may contain no granulation tissue but have black necrotic tissue, or tendon or bone visible in the base. Syphilitic ulcers have a classical appearance of slough in the base, which resembles a wash leather.

Surrounding tissues

Is the surrounding skin pink and healthy with normal innervation? Are there black satellite lesions associated with malignant melanoma?

Examine the regional lymph nodes for sites of secondary infection or metastases. Examine for varicose veins, changes following DVT or the absence of pulses and the presence of bruits. Examine the whole patient, e.g. signs of rheumatoid arthritis.

Remember that, although the initial lesion may have been caused by trauma, other abnormalities may be present to prevent healing, e.g. poor circulation, malnutrition or steroid therapy. Ulcers over the shin in elderly women with thin skin may have been due to minor trauma. However, the fact that the skin there is poorly supported on the periosteum of the underlying bone means that they may be extremely slow to heal. Ulcers occurring in inflammatory bowel disease may be due to pyoderma gangrenosum. The ulcers may be multiple and may have started as pustules.

GENERAL INVESTIGATIONS

- FBC, ESR, CRP
  Hb ↓ suggests haematological disease. WCC & CRP ↑ infection. ESR & CRP ↑ collagen diseases (vasculitis), syphilis, TB.

- U&Es
  Renal involvement may suggest autoimmune disease.

- Blood glucose
  Diabetes mellitus.

- Swab of ulcer
  C&S.

- Doppler assessment
  Assess pulse for arterial disease.

SPECIFIC INVESTIGATIONS

- **Duplex ultrasound**
  Venous/arterial disease.

- **MR venogram**
  Assess varicose veins, including venous patency.

- **MR/CT angiography**
  Assess arterial tree.

- **VDRL**
  Syphilis.

- **Rheumatoid factor**
  Rheumatoid arthritis.

- **Antibody screen**
  E.g. ANCA (SLE).

- **Biopsy**
  Incision biopsy for possible squamous cell carcinoma or diagnosis
  of the cause of an obscure ulcer. Excision biopsy is required for
  suspected malignant melanoma.

- **Always carefully describe the ulcer in the notes,
  especially the edge. Rolled everted edges suggest
  malignancy.**

- **Deep ulcers punched out with tendon or periosteum in
  the base suggest an arterial aetiology.**

- **Painful ulcers usually have an arterial aetiology.**

LIP LESIONS

Lip lesions are common. They may be extremely painful and interfere with speech and feeding. There is often a social stigma attached for the patient that leads to embarrassment. In the elderly, carcinoma is a common cause of a lump on the lip, especially in those with outdoor occupations and non-healing ulcers.

Figure 43 A squamous cell carcinoma on the lower lip. The patient, a man of 60, had smoked a pipe for most of his life. He presented with a short history of a non-healing ulcer of the lip, which proved to be a well-differentiated squamous cell carcinoma on biopsy.

CAUSES

CONGENITAL

- Cleft lip

ACQUIRED

FLAT LESIONS

- Junctional naevus
- Telangiectasia (hereditary haemorrhagic telangiectasia)
- Peutz–Jeghers syndrome
- Lichen planus

RAISED LESIONS

- Mucous retention cysts
- Warts
- Pyogenic granuloma
- Squamous cell carcinoma (Fig. 43) ⚠
- Malignant melanoma ⚠
- Syphilitic chancre
- Vascular malformations

EROSIONS

- Herpes simplex (Type 1 or Type 2)
- Impetigo
- Pemphigus

SWELLING

- Trauma, e.g. burns, bites, assault
- Angioedema
- Drug reactions
- Crohn's disease

CHEILITIS

- Infection (e.g. candidiasis)
- Contact dermatitis (e.g. lipstick, pen-sucking)
- Lip biting (especially in children)

HISTORY

Congenital

Cleft lip occurs due to failure of fusion of the nasal and maxillary processes which form the upper lip and the maxilla. The only abnormality may be a slight indentation in the outer part of the middle third of the upper lip. However, it may extend to the anterior nares and therefore involve the cleft palate. Abnormal phonation occurs.

Acquired

Flat lesions

Junctional naevi develop at or before puberty. Ensure that there has been no change in a junctional naevus to suggest development of malignant melanoma. There will usually be a family history (autosomal dominant). These pigmented lip lesions do not become malignant. There may be associated history of bowel problems, e.g. bleeding or intussusception. In hereditary telangiectasia, the patient may also have noticed lesions in the mouth and on the skin, especially the fingertips. In Peutz–Jeghers syndrome, pigmentation will be on the gums as well as the lips. Lichen planus can occur on the lips in isolation, but this is rare, and there is often mucosal involvement. This often occurs in the elderly.

Raised lesions

Mucous retention cysts may occur at any age. The patient complains of a lump on the inner aspect of the lip, which interferes with eating. With warts, pyogenic granuloma and squamous cell carcinoma, the patient's only complaint is usually of a lump on the lip. With carcinoma, there may be a history of leucoplakia or pipe smoking. Classically, it used to relate to clay-pipe smoking. There may also be a history of exposure to sunlight, and carcinoma is common in outdoor workers, e.g. sailors, farmers, fishermen and fair-skinned people in sunny climates. Ulcerating and bleeding of the lesion are often the presenting complaints. Syphilitic lesions are now extremely rare but a primary chancre may present on the lip. They are highly contagious. A gummatous lesion on the lip is extremely rare. Malignant melanoma may present as a black, ulcerating or raised lesion at the site of a junctional naevus. Vascular malformations can be present from birth involving blood vessels. They are usually benign.

Erosions

The commonest are herpes simplex lesions, which are painful ulcers that itch. They are common in immunocompromised patients. Impetigo is common around the mouth and face of children but may affect any age. Pemphigus is a blistering disorder, which affects the mucosa and skin.

Swelling

Swelling of the lips may be due to a variety of causes. Trauma is probably the most common, usually following assault, but may arise as a result of burns (hot fluids), sun rays or angioedema, which is rare, and may affect the tongue. Drug reactions may also cause oedema along with urticaria. They usually affect the whole face rather than just the lips. Crohn's disease may also cause swelling of the lips.

Cheilitis

This usually refers to inflammation of the lips and may occur at the angles of the mouth, i.e. angular cheilitis or angular stomatitis. Contact dermatitis may be apparent from either lipstick or pen-sucking. A history of lip-biting should be sought, especially in children. *Candida* may cause cheilitis in the immunocompromised, infants, those with dentures and those with iron-deficiency anaemia.

EXAMINATION

Congenital

Cleft lip is obvious at birth. Cleft palate is discovered on routine inspection soon after birth or may be discovered when difficulties occur with feeding. Beware missing a submucous cleft in which the palate initially appears intact. Later presentation may occur with speech and hearing difficulties.

Acquired

Flat lesions

Junctional naevi are flat, pigmented lesions. In hereditary telangiectasia, telangiectasia may also be present in the mouth, on the palate and on the skin, especially the fingertips. The lesions of Peutz–Jeghers syndrome are also flat lesions but, in addition to occurring on the lips, occur also on the gums. Lichen planus may occur on the lips with lip erosion and crusting. It more commonly appears on the gingivae, tongue and oral mucosa.

Raised lesions

Mucous retention cysts tend to occur on the inner aspects of the lips. They are generally pale pink with a grey glairy appearance when the cyst contents show through the stretched overlying mucosa. They are usually smooth, well localised and rarely become larger than 2 cm in diameter. A warty lesion is usually obvious, with a rough hyperkeratotic surface. Warts may be pedunculated. A pyogenic granuloma is a firm, small, cherry-red nodule consisting of hyperplastic granulation tissue. A squamous cell carcinoma is usually a hard centrally ulcerated lesion with a raised everted edge. The regional lymph nodes may be palpable due to metastases. Malignant melanoma may arise *de novo* or in a pre-existing junctional naevus. The lesion is usually raised, pigmented, occasionally friable and bleeds easily. In syphilitic lesions, the initial lesion is elevated, flat, hard and painless. Eventually, however, ulceration may occur, to give a slightly painful ulcer which crusts over. The regional lymph nodes become enlarged and tender, usually 7–10 days after the appearance of the chancre.

Erosions

Herpetic lesions begin as a patch of painful, itchy erythema. Vesicles form subsequently, which dry up and crust over after 4–5 days, with the crust eventually separating, leaving tiny scars. Impetigo causes golden-coloured crusts. In pemphigus, blisters erode quickly and become painful erosions on the mucous membrane and skin.

Swellings and cheilitis

These are usually diagnosed from a thorough history. They usually cause entire reddening and inflammation of the lips.

GENERAL INVESTIGATIONS

- ■ FBC, ESR
  Hb ↓ iron-deficiency anaemia (associated with cheilitis). WCC ↑ infection. WCC ↓ immunosuppression. ESR ↑ Crohn's disease, syphilis, malignancy.

- ■ Swab
  C&S. Dark-ground illumination of fluid from syphilitic chancre (spirochaetes visible).

SPECIFIC INVESTIGATIONS

- **B12/Folate Level**
  B12/folate deficiency.

- **VDRL**
  Syphilis.

- **Biopsy**
  Benign versus malignant. Pyogenic granuloma. Squamous cell carcinoma. Malignant melanoma (excision biopsy). Crohn's disease.

- **FNAC**
  May be diagnostic when local lymph node enlargement is associated with lip lesion.

- **Gastroscopy/Colonoscopy**
  Peutz–Jeghers syndrome. Mucosal lesions.

- Lip lesions associated with fever may suggest infection and warrant further review.

- Non-healing ulcers on the lips in the elderly are likely to be malignant. Biopsy is indicated.

- Recurrent herpetic lesions suggest an immunosuppressed state. Further investigation is necessary.

LYMPHADENOPATHY

Lymphadenopathy is a common presenting condition. It may be localised or generalised. The causes are multiple but a careful history and clinical examination will often simplify the diagnosis. Lymphadenopathy, especially cervical, is extremely common in children who are otherwise healthy. Painful tender nodes are usually associated with infection. Firm or hard, painless nodes are commonly the seat of malignancy. Only the more common causes, which the student would be expected to know, are described in this section.

CAUSES

PRIMARY INFECTION

VIRAL
- Infectious mononucleosis
- HIV
- CMV
- Rubella
- Measles

BACTERIAL
- TB ● *(common in parts of the world where TB is endemic)*
- Syphilis
- Brucellosis
- Cat scratch disease
- Septicaemia

PROTOZOAL
- Toxoplasmosis

PARASITIC
- Filariasis ● *(common in tropical regions of Asia, Africa)*

SECONDARY INFECTION
- E.g. tonsillitis with cervical lymphadenitis, abscess with regional lymphadenitis

PRIMARY MALIGNANCY
- Acute lymphoblastic leukaemia
- Chronic lymphatic leukaemia
- Hodgkin's disease
- Non-Hodgkin's lymphoma
- Myeloproliferative disorders

SECONDARY MALIGNANCY

- Metastases from local malignancy
- Metastases from distant malignancy

OTHERS

- Sarcoidosis
- SLE
- Rheumatoid arthritis

HISTORY

Infection

Local infections will be usually obvious, e.g. dental abscess with cervical lymphadenopathy. With generalised lymphadenopathy, there may be a history of malaise, lethargy and fever. Check for exposure to TB, which may be a cause of lymphadenopathy in the immunocompromised patient. Check for visits abroad. Check if there are animals in the household, e.g. cats (cat scratch fever) or dogs (toxoplasmosis). In the case of cat scratch fever, the scratches are often healed before the patient presents. Note any history of local trauma.

Primary malignancy

There will normally be a history of malaise, fever or night sweats. The patient may have noticed lumps at several sites. Spontaneous bruising and bleeding associated with thrombocytopenia may also be present.

Secondary malignancy

The primary may be obvious or may be very small and have not been noticed by the patient (e.g. a malignant melanoma in an inaccessible site). There may be a history of malignancy that has been treated several years previously with metastases presenting late (e.g. axillary lymphadenopathy or cervical lymphadenopathy occurring several years after an apparently curative operation for carcinoma of the breast). Occasionally the lymph node swelling is distant from the primary, e.g. cervical lymphadenopathy (left supraclavicular fossa) from testicular cancer; Virchow's node in gastric cancer.

Other conditions

Sarcoidosis causes bilateral hilar lymphadenopathy but may present with lymphadenopathy at other sites. Check for a history of SLE or rheumatoid arthritis.

EXAMINATION

Examine the enlarged lymph nodes. Are they painful and tender, suggesting infection, or are they firm and painless, suggesting malignancy? Check the sites draining to these nodes for a site of infection or primary malignancy. Check for linear scratches suggestive of cat scratch disease. Examine for bruising. Examine all other sites of potential lymphadenopathy: cervical, axillary, inguinal, popliteal and epitrochlear nodes. Check for splenomegaly and hepatomegaly. Carry out a full general examination.

GENERAL INVESTIGATIONS

- **FBC, CRP/ESR**
  Hb ↓ blood dyscrasias. Platelets ↓ dyscrasias. WCC ↑ infection, leukaemia. CRP/ESR ↑ tumour, infection. Blood film. Leukaemia.

- **LFTs**
  Malignant infiltration of the liver.

- **Clotting screen**
  Blood dyscrasias.

- **Viral titres**
  Viral infections, e.g. EBV, HIV.

- **CXR**
  Hilar glands in sarcoidosis. TB. Secondary deposits.

- **Mantoux test**
  TB.

- **Swab**
  Local infection. C&S.

SPECIFIC INVESTIGATIONS

- **Antibody screen**
  SLE, rheumatoid arthritis.

- **Blood film**
  Filariasis.

- **Blood cultures**
  Septicaemia.

- **VDRL**
  Syphilis.

- **Serum angiotensin-converting enzyme (ACE)**
  Sarcoidosis. Positive in 50–80% of patients with active sarcoidosis.

- **Toxoplasma screen**
  Toxoplasmosis.

- **PCR**
  Filariasis.

- **OGD**
  Virchow's node with gastrointestinal malignancy.

- **CT**
  Nodal distribution. Staging of Hodgkin's disease.

- **FNAC of lymph node**
  Malignancy versus other conditions.

- **Biopsy**
  Lymph node, e.g. Hodgkin's disease, secondary deposit. Biopsy of local lesion, e.g. infective versus malignant.

- An enlarged left supraclavicular lymph node in a patient with weight loss suggests gastrointestinal malignancy.

- Persistent generalised lymphadenopathy with night sweats suggests lymphoma or AIDS.

- Persistent cervical lymphadenopathy in the older patient suggests malignancy and, in the absence of an obvious cause, an ENT assessment is required.

- A solitary left supraclavicular node in a young male should prompt examination of the testes.

MELAENA

Melaena is the passage of altered blood per rectum (PR). A melaena stool is black and tarry and has a characteristic smell. The blood is degraded by hydrochloric acid and intestinal enzymes high in the gastrointestinal tract. Melaena is unlikely to occur if bleeding comes from lower than the jejunum, although occasionally melaena may result from a bleeding Meckel's diverticulum.

CAUSES

SWALLOWED BLOOD
- Epistaxis
- Haemoptysis ⚠

OESOPHAGUS
- Oesophageal varices ⚠
- Oesophageal carcinoma

STOMACH
- Peptic ulceration
- Acute gastric erosions
- Mallory–Weiss syndrome
- Carcinoma
- Leiomyoma (gastrointestinal stromal tumour – GIST)
- Hereditary haemorrhagic telangiectasia

DUODENUM
- Peptic ulceration
- Duodenal diverticulae
- Aortoduodenal fistulae ⚠
- Invasive pancreatic tumours
- Haemobilia

SMALL INTESTINE
- Leiomyoma (gastrointestinal stromal tumour – GIST)
- Meckel's diverticulum

BLEEDING DISORDERS
- Liver disease-associated
- Thrombocytopenia
- Haemophilia

DRUGS

- Anticoagulants
- Aspirin
- NSAIDs
- Steroids

OTHERS

- Uraemia
- Connective tissue disorders

OTHER CAUSES OF DARK STOOLS

- Iron therapy
- Bismuth preparations
- Liquorice
- Charcoal biscuits

HISTORY

Swallowed blood

Check for a recent history of epistaxis haematemsis, or haemoptysis.

Oesophagus

There may be a history of excess alcohol consumption or a history of other liver disease to suggest oesophageal varices. Check for retrosternal burning pain and heartburn, which would suggest oesophagitis/carcinoma. Check for a history of dysphagia. The bleeding associated with varices is often torrential.

Stomach

History of epigastric pain to suggest peptic ulceration. There may be a history of steroid or NSAID medication. Mallory–Weiss syndrome usually occurs in the younger patient who has had a large meal with much alcohol and has a forceful vomit. The first vomit contains food, the second contains blood. Acute gastric erosions may occur with stressful illnesses, e.g. major surgery, acute pancreatitis, burns (Curling's ulcer) and head injuries (Cushing's ulcer). It is unusual to get a large bleed with a carcinoma. Anaemia is a common presentation, and there may be 'coffee ground' vomit. Leiomyoma causes a moderate haematemesis. There is usually no preceding history. There will also be no preceding history with vascular malformations. Hereditary haemorrhagic telangiectasia is rare. The patient may present with a history of the condition, or it may be apparent from the telangiectasia around the lips and oral cavity.

Duodenum

Melaena tends to be a more common symptom than haematemesis with duodenal lesions. There may be a history of chronic duodenal ulceration, although often presentation may be acute with little background history. Bleeding from invasive pancreatic tumours is rare. The patient will present with malaise, lethargy, weight loss and vomiting. Haemobilia is rare. Aortoduodenal fistula is rare and usually follows repair of an aneurysm with subsequent infection of the graft. There is massive haematemesis and malaise.

Small intestine

Leiomyomas are rare but may bleed, resulting in melaena. Bleeding from a Meckel's diverticulum, if it occurs fast enough, usually causes dark-red bleeding rather than characteristic melaena.

Other causes of dark stools

Take a full dietary and drug history.

EXAMINATION

Depending upon the severity of the bleed, there may be shock. The patient will be cold, clammy, with peripheral vasoconstriction; there will be a tachycardia and hypotension.

Swallowed blood

Check for blood around the nose. Examine the chest for a possible cause of haemoptysis.

Oesophagus

There may be little to find on examination except clinical signs of anaemia and weight loss, unless the cause is oesophageal varices, in which case there may be jaundice, abdominal distension due to ascites, spider naevi, liver palms, clubbing, gynaecomastia, testicular atrophy, caput medusae, splenomegaly or hepatomegaly.

Stomach

There may be little to find on examination. There may be an epigastric mass with a carcinoma, or a palpable left supraclavicular node (Virchow's nodes). There may be epigastric tenderness. With hereditary haemorrhagic telangiectasia, there may be telangiectasia on the lips and mucous membrane of the mouth.

Duodenum

Again, there may be little to find on examination other than epigastric tenderness. In the rare case where duodenal bleeding comes from an invasive pancreatic carcinoma, there may be a palpable mass in the region of the pancreas.

Small intestine

Often, there is little to find. Leiomyomas may be palpable.

Bleeding disorders

There may be sites of bruising or bleeding from other orifices.

GENERAL INVESTIGATIONS

- **FBC, ESR**
  Hb ↓ anaemia due to chronic bleeding, e.g. from carcinoma.
  ESR ↑ connective tissue disease.
- **U&Es**
  Urea and creatinine will be raised in uraemia. Urea may be raised
  due to absorption of blood from the bowel.
- **LFTs**
  Liver failure, oesophageal varices, haemobilia.
- **Clotting screen**
  Liver disease. Bleeding diatheses. Anticoagulants.

SPECIFIC INVESTIGATIONS

- **Gastro-oesophageal duodenoscopy**
  Will demonstrate most lesions, e.g. varices, oesophagitis, peptic
  ulcer, gastric erosions, Mallory–Weiss tear, carcinoma and rarer
  causes of bleeding. Biopsy may be carried out where necessary.
- **Small bowel follow-through**
  Leiomyoma. Meckel's diverticulum.
- **Angiography**
  Vascular malformations. Also may diagnose rarer distal duodenal
  causes, e.g. aortoduodenal fistulae.
- **Technetium scan**
  Meckel's diverticulum containing gastric mucosa.
- **Labelled red cell scan**
  Rare small bowel causes of bleeding.

- Melaena is altered blood PR. It is black and tarry and
  has a characteristic smell. Take care to distinguish it
  from rectal bleeding, which is either bright red or dark
  red and free from odour.

MOUTH ULCERS

Mouth ulceration is common but it is important to be able to distinguish between simple benign ulcers (e.g. traumatic or aphthous) and those that are malignant. Tongue disorders are dealt with on p. 431.

Figure 44 Aphthous ulcers. These commonly occur in isolation, but they may be an indication of an underlying intestinal disease such as coeliac disease or inflammatory bowel disease.

CAUSES

- Traumatic
- Aphthous (Fig. 44)

INFLAMMATORY

- Inflammatory bowel disease

INFECTIVE

BACTERIAL

- Acute ulcerative gingivitis (Vincent's angina)
- Syphilis
- TB

VIRAL

- Herpes simplex
- Herpes zoster

- Hand, foot and mouth
- HIV

FUNGAL
- Candidiasis

NEOPLASTIC
- Squamous cell carcinoma ⚠
- Haematological disorders
- Agranulocytosis

HAEMATOLOGICAL DISORDERS
- Anaemia
- Leukaemia
- Agranulocytosis

SKIN DISEASE-ASSOCIATED
- Lichen planus
- Pemphigus
- Pemphigoid
- Erythema multiforme

CONNECTIVE TISSUE DISEASE
- Folate/B12 deficiency
- SLE

OTHER
- Drugs
- Radiotherapy
- Behçet's syndrome
- Reiter's disease

HISTORY

Traumatic

Diagnosis is usually obvious, such as ill-fitting dentures or sharp teeth with ulcers healing when the precipitating cause is removed.

Aphthous

Patient presents with small, painful ulcers, usually inside the cheeks or lips. They heal in about one week but others may occur while the initial ulcers are healing. A number of patients will have a history of gastrointestinal disease, e.g. coeliac disease or Crohn's disease. They may also arise in patients who are immunocompromised.

Inflammatory

Crohn's disease may affect the oral cavity. The patient may complain of painful ulcers, swelling of the lips or gum swelling.

Infective

Acute ulcerative stomatitis presents with swollen gums with small ulcers, which may spread to the buccal mucosa. The patient will complain of bleeding gums, together with constitutional upset with fever and malaise. Syphilis is now rarely seen but chancres, snail-track ulcers and gummas may occur within the mouth. *Candida* is common in the oral cavity. There may be a history of chronic disease diabetes or immunosuppressive therapy. Herpes simplex presents as painful vesicles, which ulcerate. The patient may be immunocompromised. Herpes zoster may occur on the palate in the distribution of the maxillary division of the trigeminal nerve. There will be severe pain and ulceration. A history of TB will include symptoms of a cough, night sweats and weight loss. HIV is rare but can present as ulcers, leukoplakia and Kaposi's sarcoma in advanced stages. Hand, foot and mouth is highly contagious and is often associated with fever. malaise and ulcers appearing on the tongue or mouth.

Neoplastic

Squamous cell carcinomas occur as non-healing ulcers with hard edges, which bleed. They tend to occur in the older patient. There may be a history of leucoplakia or the six Ss: syphilis, smoking, sharp tooth, spirits, spices, sepsis.

Haematological disorders

Agranulocytosis may be due to drugs or bone marrow infiltration. Take a careful drug history. The ulceration may be due to bacterial infection consequent to low WCC. Anaemia and leukaemia may also present with mouth ulcers.

Skin disease-associated

These include lichen planus, pemphigus pemphigoid, erythema multiforme and dermatitis herpetiformis. The reader is referred to a textbook of dermatology for the characteristics of these conditions.

Connective tissue disease

Oral ulceration may be associated with SLE. The patient may present with other vague features of this disease, e.g. skin lesions, joint pains or renal failure.

Other

Although Behçet's disease may present with mouth ulcers, the patient may also complain of arthritis, eye disease, scrotal or labial ulcers. With Reiter's disease, the patient will also complain of urethritis, conjunctivitis and arthritis. There is usually a history of sexual contact. Medication history and recent radiotherapy will often be verbalised by the patient.

EXAMINATION

Traumatic

There will be ulceration related to ill-fitting dentures or sharp teeth.

Aphthous

Small, white, circular, deep, painful ulcers with surrounding erythema. Consider signs and symptoms of gastrointestinal disease.

Inflammatory

With Crohn's disease, there may be lip swelling, nodular thickening of the buccal mucosa, diffuse granular gingival swelling or painful linea oral ulcers.

Infective

Ulcerating gingivitis presents with red, swollen, bleeding gums covered with yellowish ulcers. The ulcers may also be seen on the buccal mucosa and occasionally on the tonsils. There is usually associated tender lymphadenopathy. Herpes simplex presents with small 2-mm vesicles, which ulcerate and coalesce and produce erosions with surrounding erythema. Herpes zoster shows small ulcers surrounded with erythema in the distribution of the maxillary nerve on the palate. There will usually be skin lesions in the distribution of the nerve. Candidiasis appears as red patches on the buccal mucosa, which are covered with white patches of desquamated epithelium mixed with fungus.

Neoplastic

There will be an ulcer with hard, everted edges that bleeds on touching. Cervical lymphadenopathy may be present.

Haematological disorders

These present with bleeding gums, ulceration and skin lesions.

Other

Behçet's disease presents with painful ulcers. Other features may be apparent on examination, e.g. arthritis, keratitis, iritis, scrotal or labial ulcers. With Reiter's syndrome, there will be urethritis, conjunctivitis and arthritis, as well as mouth ulcers.

GENERAL INVESTIGATIONS

- **FBC, ESR**
  Hb ↓ malignancy, chronic disease. WCC ↑ infection, leukaemia. ESR ↑ malignancy, connective tissue disease, chronic infection, e.g. syphilis.

- **U&Es**
  Renal disease – SLE.

- **Ferritin**
  Iron-deficiency anaemia.
- **Folate/B12**
  Folate/B12 deficiency.
- **Swab**
  C&S. Infections – *Borrelia vincentii* candidiasis.
- **Antibody screen**
  SLE – ANA positive. Anti-double-stranded DNA ↑.
- **Serum IgA-TtG**
  Coeliac disease.
- **VDRL**
  Syphilis.
- **Viral serology**
  Herpes simplex. Herpes zoster. HIV. EBV.
- **Biopsy**
  Squamous cell carcinoma. Crohn's disease.

- A solitary persistent ulcer that feels hard to the touch is potentially malignant. Urgent referral is required.
- Mouth ulcers may be associated with inflammatory bowel disease so consider systemic illness.
- Mouth ulcers may further be associated with vitamin and iron deficiency. Check for associated glossitis and angular cheilitis.

MUSCLE WEAKNESS AND WASTING

Muscle weakness and wasting may be caused by a variety of conditions both systemic and those confined to the muscles only.

CAUSES

LOCALISED

- Peripheral nerve lesions
  - Peripheral nerve compression
  - Motor neuropathy
  - Peripheral nerve transection
- Disuse atrophy
- Anterior horn cell lesions
  - Previous poliomyelitis ● *(common in developing countries)*

GENERALISED

NUTRITIONAL DEFICIENCY
- Vitamin D deficiency

SYSTEMIC DISEASE
- Malignancy
- Cardiac and/or respiratory cachexia
- Thyrotoxicosis
- Sarcoidosis
- Guillain–Barré syndrome
- Cushing's disease
- Addison's disease

MUSCLE AND MOTOR END PLATE DISORDERS
- Myasthenia gravis
- Muscular dystrophies
- Motor neurone disease
- Myotonic dystrophy
- Polymyositis/dermatomyositis/inclusion body myositis

DRUGS AND TOXINS
- Alcohol
- Statins
- Steroids
- Ciclosporin

HISTORY

Onset

Muscle weakness and wasting in childhood is often due to congenital disease such as inherited muscular dystrophies (e.g. Duchenne's muscular dystrophy), a diagnosis further supported by a positive family history of a first-degree relative with similar problems. With myotonic dystrophy, first symptoms occur around the age of 15–30 years, while with motor neurone disease, the peak age of onset is in the 50s.

Site

The distribution of muscle wasting may characterise the disease. Atrophy may be confined to the motor supply of a single nerve, such as the thenar eminence with the median nerve affected by carpal tunnel syndrome. It may also occur with a group of muscles such as the leg, with polio. The distribution may be generalised in conditions such as motor neurone disease. Distal weakness ascending to involve proximal muscles is characteristic of Guillain–Barré syndrome.

Precipitating factors

Precipitating factors such as trauma may result in transection of a peripheral nerve such as the ulnar nerve, commonly at the wrist.

Past medical history

The presence of carcinoma or chronic cardiorespiratory disease may give rise to peripheral muscle wasting from cachexia. Previous infection with polio is significant because, in a minority of affected individuals, degeneration of anterior horn cells with subsequent paralysis and muscle wasting occurs (post-polio syndrome). Disuse atrophy can be localised or generalised. Conditions that result in immobility such as a long-bone fracture will cause disuse atrophy of the surrounding muscles; this is commonly seen upon removal of plaster casts. Localised disuse atrophy may also result from joint pains such as quadriceps wasting with painful knee disorders. Prolonged immobility will result in generalised muscle wasting.

Associated symptoms

Most of the causes are associated with weakness of the affected muscles. Diplopia, ptosis and fatiguability are associated features suggestive of myasthenia gravis. Motor neurone disease may present with progressive weakness and wasting of the hand or leg accompanied with dysarthria and dysphasia. Cushing's disease may be associated with weight gain, hair growth, acne, abdominal striae, muscle weakness, back pain and depression.

EXAMINATION

Inspection will identify the areas of muscle wasting. Central obesity with limb wasting occurs with Cushing's disease. Generalised uniform muscle wasting should lead to a careful examination of the organ systems for malignancy and organ failure. Muscle tenderness may occur with polymyositis.

Characteristic features of myotonic dystrophy are frontal balding, ptosis, temporal and facial muscle wasting. Cataracts may be seen with inspection of the eyes. Ptosis may also be a feature of myasthenia gravis; this is accompanied by diplopia, facial weakness and a weak nasal voice. Muscle wasting with fasciculations occurs with motor neurone disease, no sensory loss is experienced and mixed upper and lower motor neurone signs may be present.

Assessment of tone, reflexes and pattern of weakness will determine whether it is an upper or lower motor neurone lesion. Delayed relaxation of muscle contraction occurs with myotonic dystrophy and proximal muscle weakness occurs with Cushing's disease. With localised muscle wasting, examination of each muscle will allow you to determine whether the lesion arises from a single nerve or a nerve root. Weakness, areflexia and sensory loss are seen with Guillain–Barré syndrome.

The joint surrounded by wasted muscles should be examined for deformity or pain that may restrict movement. Measurements of circumference can be obtained to assess asymmetrical muscle wasting of the limbs.

Proximal muscle weakness may be more evident than distal weakness in many of the conditions listed. Specific assessment for this, such as rising from a low chair or from a squatting position, is required.

GENERAL INVESTIGATIONS

- FBC
  Anaemia with nutritional disorders and chronic disease.
- ESR and CRP
  ↑ with malignancy, polymyositis.
- U&Es
  ↑ urea and ↑ creatinine with renal failure.
- Glucose
  ↑ with diabetes.
- LFTs
  ↓ Albumin with malnutrition.
- Creatine phosphokinase
  ↑ with myopathies.
- TFTs
  ↓ TSH ↑ T_4 with thyrotoxicosis.
- EMG
  Allows assessment for denervation of muscle, myopathies and myotonic dystrophy, motor neurone disease.
- Nerve conduction studies
  Radiculopathies, peripheral neuropathy, peripheral nerve compression, motor neurone disease.

SPECIFIC INVESTIGATIONS

- **Tensilon test**
  Injection of edrophonium reverses symptoms of myasthenia gravis.
- **MRI**
  May reveal areas of abnormal muscle in myositis.
- **Lumbar puncture**
  Elevated protein in Guillain–Barré syndrome.
- **Muscle biopsy**
  Diagnosis of muscle dystrophies and the various myositides.

- A patient presenting with rapid-onset muscle weakness requires an urgent full assessment, as respiratory muscle involvement may lead to respiratory failure.

NAIL ABNORMALITIES

Nail abnormalities are common and can give invaluable clues to underlying systemic illness. Clubbing is dealt with in a separate section (p. 56).

Figure 45 Psoriasis with onychodystrophy of toenails. *(Courtesy of Dr G Wright and the EULAR Image Database.)*

CAUSES

CONGENITAL

- Epidermolysis bullosa
- Anonychia congenita

ACQUIRED

INFECTIONS

- Fungal infection (onychomycosis)
- Paronychia

TRAUMATIC

- Nail biting
- Nailbed trauma

SYSTEMIC ILLNESS

- Severe systemic illness (Beau's lines)
- Iron deficiency anaemia (koilonychia)
- Chronic liver disease (leuconychia)
- Diabetes mellitus (leuconychia)
- Psoriatic arthritis (onycholysis)
- Plummer–Vinson syndrome (koilonychia)

DERMATOLOGICAL

- Psoriasis (Fig. 45)
- Eczema

OTHER

- Onychogryphosis
- Raynaud's syndrome
- Hypo/hyperthyroidism
- Autoimmune disease
- Yellow nail syndrome
- Malignancy (melanoma/SCC)

HISTORY

Congenital

A history of severe skin disease from birth will be apparent with epidermolysis bullosa. Equally anonychia is obvious from missing nails.

Acquired

Infections

A history of discoloration of the nail will be present with chronic fungal infections. This is seen with increasing age and patients with diabetes. Paronychia leads to pain, swelling and tenderness in the area of the nailfold and can lead to cellulitis.

Traumatic

A history of severe or recurrent damage to the nail may be present. Enquiry as to whether the patient is a nail-biter is important.

Systemic illness

The patient must be asked about severe illness trauma or infection of any description, as this may have led to trophic nail changes with transverse ridges (Beau's lines), which may occur up to three months following the insult. Symptoms of joint pain, stiffness and swelling will be present with psoriatic arthritis. In iron deficiency anaemia, patients often describe lethargy, shortness of breath and/or chest pain on minimal exertion. Frank blood loss (haematemesis, melaena) will usually be disclosed by the patient. Plummer–Vinson syndrome occurs in middle-aged women. This is an iron deficiency anaemia associated with koilonychia, a smooth tongue and dysphagia. A history for the possible causes of chronic liver disease should be sought such as alcohol abuse or hepatitis. Symptoms of polyuria, polydipsia and lethargy commonly suggest diabetes mellitus.

Dermatological

The scaly rash of psoriasis is classically found on the extensor areas of the knees, elbows and scalp; however, lesions may be described in the external meatus, umbilicus, glans penis and natal cleft. An eczematous rash may be present diffusely and is often itchy.

Other

Onychogryphosis is a 'ram's horn' deformity of the nail. It usually affects the great toenail. The nail thickens and curls over as it grows. Common in the elderly, it may follow trauma to the nail in the younger patient. The nail is greatly deformed and difficult to cut. In autoimmune disease, the patient may describe hair loss in alopecia areata and sclerodactyly in systemic sclerosis. In classic Raynaud's phenomenon, the fingers turn white, blue, then red upon exposure to cold environments. In yellow nail syndrome, the nails are typically slow growing with yellow discoloration. It is associated with lymphoedema, pleural effusions and in some cases, bronchiectasis and chronic sinusitis. In thyroid disease there will be systemic symptoms including bowel, hair and weight changes. For malignancy this is rare but can occur as a lontigudinal line in the nail for melanoma whilst in SCC a pigmented lesion may be seen.

EXAMINATION

Congenital

Severe skin disease will be apparent with epidermolysis bullosa.

Acquired

Infections

A discolored, thick and possibly malformed nail will be seen with chronic fungal infections. A swollen, red, tender nailfold will be present with paronychia.

Traumatic

A malformed nail will be seen. Severe nail-biters will have nails bitten back to the nailbed.

Systemic illness

Swollen deformed joints may be seen with psoriatic arthritis. Further nail changes in psoriasis include onycholysis loss of nail and subungal hyperkeratosis. Check for associated psoriatic plaques. If the patient suffered from severe systemic illness, this may have resolved; however, trophic nail changes may be seen following this. In iron deficiency anaemia, pallor, angular cheilitis and spoon-shaped nails (koilonychia) may be present. Features of chronic liver disease might be present along with leuconychia. Leuconychia may also be seen with diabetes and chronic kidney disease.

Dermatological

Scaly, silvery plaques of psoriasis will be seen, which may be localised or diffuse. Eczema may also be present either as localised or diffuse lesions.

Other

A grossly deformed, usually great toenail, will be seen with onychogryphosis. The nail thickens and curls over as it grows. Distal finger atrophic changes may be seen following longstanding Raynaud's phenomenon. In yellow nail syndrome, the nails are typically slow growing with yellow discoloration. Lymphoedema usually affects the lower limb. Examine the chest for signs of bronchiectasis and pleural effusions. Abdominal examination may reveal ascites. In malignancy, the signs may be subtle with melanoma (longitudinal line) and SCC, a keratotic hyperpigmented lesion also causing onycholysis.

GENERAL INVESTIGATIONS

The diagnosis of most nail abnormalities is made on clinical examination alone.

- FBC
  ↓ Hb, ↓ MCV, ↓ MCHC.
- Blood film
  Microcytic RBCs in iron deficiency.
- Serum iron and TIBC
  ↓ serum iron, ↑ TIBC with iron deficiency.
- Serum ferritin
  ↓ iron deficiency anaemia.
- Blood glucose
  Diabetes.
- LFTs
  Cirrhosis.
- Urinalysis
  Diabetes.

SPECIFIC INVESTIGATIONS

- Nail clippings
  Fungal infections.
- Biopsy
  Malignancy.
- Skin biopsy
  Psoriasis, eczema.
- Hand X-rays
  Psoriatic arthritis.

- CXR
  Chest abnormalities with yellow nail syndrome, e.g. bronchiectasis, pleural effusion.
- Vasculitis screen (e.g. ANA)
  Systemic sclerosis.

- Always examine the nails. It may be necessary to ask patients to remove nail varnish.
- It may be difficult to differentiate between psoriatic nail dystrophy and fungal infections. Always confirm the diagnosis with nail clippings before starting a patient on a lengthy course of anti-fungal treatment requiring blood monitoring.
- Malignancy, although rare, is an important differential to consider, especially in the absence of trauma or systemic symptoms.

NASAL DISCHARGE

Nasal discharges are common. The most frequent causes are the common cold and allergic rhinitis, however persistent bloodstained nasal discharge is a serious symptom requiring urgent investigation.

CAUSES

CONGENITAL

- Choanal atresia
- Cystic fibrosis

ACQUIRED

INFECTIVE

- Common cold (coryza)
- Chronic rhinitis
- Sinusitis (acute or chronic)
- Adenoiditis (large adenoids)
- Viral infections
- Bacterial infections (e.g. whooping cough)
- Fungal infections
- Chronic infections (e.g. syphilis)
- AIDS ● *(common in certain developing countries)*

ALLERGIC

- Allergic rhinitis

INFLAMMATORY

- Nasal polyps
- Decongestant spray overuse
- Non-eosinophilic vasomotor rhinitis
- Eosinophilic vasomotor rhinitis

NEOPLASTIC

- Carcinoma
  - Nasopharynx ● *(common in South east Asia)*
  - Sinuses
- Lymphoma (malignant granuloma)

GRANULOMATOUS DISEASE

- Granulomatosis with Polyangiitis (GPA – formerly Wegener's granulomatosis)
- Eosinophilic Granulomatosis with Polyangiitis (EGPA – formerly Churg-Strauss syndrome)

TRAUMATIC

- Foreign body
- Crying
- Fracture of the anterior or middle fossa
- Irritant gases, e.g. chlorine, tobacco smoke

DEGENERATIVE

- Senile rhinorrhoea

MISCELLANEOUS

- Pregnancy
- Cluster headache

HISTORY

Congenital

Choanal atresia is rare and linked with other congenital abnormalities. Bilateral choanal atresia is a life-threatening condition in newborn infants. Unilateral atresia may not be picked up until 5–10 years of age, when it becomes apparent that one nostril is blocked and there is a thick mucus discharge. Cystic fibrosis is an autosomal recessive condition resulting in increased viscosity, leading to recurrent chest infections, failure to thrive as well as nasal polyps.

Acquired

Infective

The most frequent cause is the common cold. There is a mucoid nasal discharge, which settles rapidly once the cold has settled. With chronic rhinitis, there may be a chronic purulent discharge that is often thick and mucoid. With sinusitis, there may be pain or discomfort over the maxillary sinuses or a headache with pain over the frontal sinuses. With large adenoids, there may be a complaint of mouth breathing, recurrent pharyngeal infections, snoring and recurrent ear infections. Bacterial infections can also occur, for example whooping cough, leading to a paroxysmal cough, inspiratory whoop and apneic episodes. Fungal infections of the nose are rare, occurring in immunosuppressed patients, with *Candida albicans* and *Aspergillus* spp. being the most common organisms. Chronic infective lesions include syphilis. Secondary syphilis can affect the nose and cause a catarrhal rhinitis. AIDS may be associated with a watery nasal discharge, but check for HIV risk factors.

Allergic

Allergic rhinitis

There may be a history of infantile eczema, allergic asthma, nasal or conjunctival allergy. It may be seasonal with an allergy to pollen or perennial with exposure to animal dander (cats) or house-dust mites. The patient complains of watery rhinorrhoea, sneezing attacks, nasal obstruction, conjunctival irritation and lacrimation. There is usually a family history.

Inflammatory

Nasal polyps

These occur in non-allergic eosinophilic vasomotor rhinitis. The patient will complain of nasal obstruction and discharge.

Decongestant spray overuse

This phenomenon relates to the overuse of medication, resulting in a rebound in symptoms often worse than the initial presenting symptoms.

Non-eosinophilic vasomotor rhinitis

The patient presents with watery nasal discharge, nasal obstruction and sneezing attacks. This condition may be associated with: (1) certain antihypertensive drugs, particularly ganglion blockers and vasodilators; (2) hormonal disturbances; (3) congestive cardiac failure; (4) anxiety states; (5) occupational irritants, e.g. ammonia, smoke.

Eosinophillic vasomotor rhinitis

Eosinophilic vasomotor rhinitis presents with a watery nasal discharge and sneezing. The condition is associated with nasal polyps, aspirin sensitivity and asthma called Samter's triad.

Neoplastic

Nasopharyngeal carcinoma

Nasopharyngeal carcinoma is rare in Europe but is common in South east Asia. The patient presents with nasal obstruction and bloodstained discharge. Unilateral otitis media may occur from eustachian tube blockage. Nerve palsies may occur due to invasion of the base of the skull. The patient may complain only of a swelling in the neck due to lymphadenopathy, with lymphatic spread occurring at an early stage. With this disease, unilateral deafness, cervical lymphadenopathy and cranial nerve palsies are often diagnostic.

Carcinoma of the maxillary sinus

This is often diagnosed late. Early presenting symptoms include bloodstained nasal discharge and unilateral nasal obstruction. Later, swelling of the cheek occurs, with ulceration of the palate. Epiphora may occur due to invasion of the nasolacrimal duct. Erosion into the orbit results in proptosis and diplopia. Pain may be referred to the ear.

Malignant granuloma

Malignant granuloma (now thought to be lymphomatous) presents with slowly progressive ulceration, starting in the region of the nose. The chronic inflammatory reaction causes a nasal discharge.

Granulomatous disease

GPA and EGPA affect the nose and are associated with disease of the kidneys, lungs and respiratory tract. The patient may present with either lung signs or renal failure and can be challenging to diagnose formally.

Traumatic

The commonest trauma causing a nasal discharge is a foreign body. The patient is usually a child aged between 1 and 5 years. The child is usually miserable with a smelly, bloodstained nasal discharge.

In adults, rhinoliths may occur, resulting in unilateral obstruction and discharge. There is usually a large concretion blocking the nose, which may have a foreign body at the centre, with calcium and magnesium laid down around it. Crying is another example where excess tears are drained into the nasal cavity, resulting in increased congestion. Following fracture of the anterior fossa, sustained during head injury, the patient may complain of a clear nasal discharge (CSF rhinorrhoea) or a bloodstained nasal discharge. Irritant gases, e.g. chlorine, which may be industrial or in excess in swimming pools, may cause irritation of the nasal mucosa, with discharge.

Degenerative

Senile rhinorrhoea occurs in the elderly. It is thought to be due to failure of vasomotor control.

Miscellaneous

Pregnancy has been associated with increased congestion. Cluster headache can present as nasal stuffiness, lacrimation and lid swelling.

EXAMINATION

Choanal atresia

Pass a probe or catheter into the nasal cavity. It will not pass. Posterior rhinoscopy under general anaesthetic will confirm the diagnosis.

Infective

With a common cold, there will be oedematous nasal mucosa with clear mucus in the nose. With chronic rhinitis, there will be thick mucus or a purulent nasal discharge. With enlarged adenoids, mirror examination will reveal the diagnosis. Consider a full systemic examination in chronic infections.

Allergic

Allergic rhinitis reveals an oedematous nasal mucosa with clear mucus in the nose.

Inflammatory

The appearance of eosinophilic vasomotor rhinitis is similar to that of allergic rhinitis, except that nasal polyps may be seen. Nasal polyps are usually pink and smooth or a yellowish-grey and pedunculated. With non-eosinophilic vasomotor rhinitis, excessive secretions will be noted on examination, with engorgement of the inferior turbinates. Often, the signs are not as severe as the symptoms would suggest.

Neoplastic

Examination should include visualisation of the post-nasal space, under general anaesthetic if necessary. A full examination of the cranial nerves must be made (including proptosis and diplopia due to invasion of the orbit). With carcinoma of the maxillary sinus, there may be swelling of the cheek with ulceration of the palate. Epiphora may occur due to invasion of the nasolacrimal duct. Examine the neck for cervical nodes. With malignant granuloma, there is slowly progressive ulceration of the face, starting in the region of the nose.

Granulomatous disease

With GPA or EGPA, necrotic mucosal ulceration occurs. There may be co-existing otitis media, ulceration of the mouth or involvement of the trachea or larynx. There may be lung involvement, eye involvement and renal disease, and therefore a full examination may be needed.

Traumatic

Examination with a nasal speculum will usually reveal the foreign body. With CSF rhinorrhoea, it may be difficult to distinguish bleeding from blood mixed with CSF. Place a drop of the bloodstained discharge on a clean white gauze. If CSF is present, there will be a spreading yellowish ring around the central stain of blood (halo sign). With irritant gases, there will be redness and oedema of the nasal mucosa. There will almost certainly be eye irritation and a skin reaction accompanying it.

Degenerative

With senile rhinorrhoea, there are usually no physical signs apart from the nasal drip.

Miscellaneous

In a cluster headache, look for miosis, ptosis, erythema, lid swelling and general patient unrest.

GENERAL INVESTIGATIONS

- **FBC, ESR and CRP**
  Hb ↓ malignancy, granulomatous disease. WCC ↑ infection, e.g. adenoiditis. ESR and CRP ↑ infection, malignancy, granulomatous disease.
- **Clotting screen**
  Clotting needed for nasal biopsies and history of epistaxis.
- **Swab**
  Culture and sensitivity. Bacterial versus fungal.
- **Skull X-ray**
  Anterior and middle cranial fossa fracture involving ethmoid bone – CSF rhinorrhoea. Carcinoma of the maxillary antrum.
- **Saline nasal flush**
  Dislodge foreign body or obtain tissue to be sent for histopathology.

SPECIFIC INVESTIGATIONS

- Biopsy
  Carcinoma. GPA. Malignant granuloma. Chronic inflammation.
- RAST
  Measures allergen-specific Ig.
- CT and MRI
  Carcinoma and granulomatous disease: diagnosis and assessment of extent of disease.

- Persistent bloodstained nasal discharge or unilateral symptoms is a serious sign and further investigation is required to exclude malignancy.
- Consider referring nasal polyps to ENT for further evaluation.

NECK LUMPS

A lump in the neck is a common problem. It is necessary to be able to distinguish the different causes, which may vary from a simple benign swelling to part of a generalised malignant condition.

Figure 46 Thyroglossal cyst. There is a midline swelling in the neck, which moved on swallowing, and tongue protrusion.

CAUSES

SUPERFICIAL

- Sebaceous cyst
- Lipoma
- Lymph nodes
- Abscess
- Dermoid cyst

DEEP

- Lymph nodes

ANTERIOR TRIANGLE

Move on swallowing
- Thyroid
- Thyroglossal cyst (Fig. 46)

Do not move on swallowing
- Salivary glands
- Branchial cyst
- Carotid body tumour

- Carotid aneurysm ⚠
- Sternomastoid 'tumour'

POSTERIOR TRIANGLE
- Cervical rib
- Subclavian artery aneurysm ⚠
- Pharyngeal pouch
- Cystic hygroma

HISTORY

Symptoms

The diagnosis of superficial swellings of the neck should be obvious. A sebaceous cyst will usually have grown slowly and may have been painful and red if infected. Lipomas tend to grow slowly. An abscess will be obvious from pain and tenderness. Lymphadenopathy may be associated with a recent pyrexial illness, local lesions in the head and neck, generalised infection or generalised malignancy. Swelling during mastication suggests a salivary gland origin. Blackouts or dizziness may suggest a carotid body tumour. A lump in the lower part of the posterior triangle, increasing in size after eating, and gurgling when full, suggests a pharyngeal pouch. The patient may experience bouts of coughing or choking when lying down as the pouch empties itself and aspiration occurs. Neurological or vascular symptoms in the upper limb may be associated with a cervical rib. Sternomastoid tumours are rare and occur in the neonate. Cystic hygromas are rare and occur in infancy.

Past medical history

A history of HIV infection, TB and malignancy is relevant. Breech or forceps delivery may be relevant to the development of a sternomastoid tumour.

EXAMINATION

Decide whether the swelling is superficial or deep. Decide whether it is likely to be due to lymphadenopathy. If the swelling is deep, decide whether it is in the anterior triangle of the neck or the posterior triangle. If it is in the anterior triangle, decide whether it moves on swallowing (thyroid-associated) or not.

Sebaceous cyst

This is usually obvious, being in the skin and having a punctum.

Lipoma

May occur anywhere in the neck but often occurs in the midline posteriorly. Lipomas are soft and lobulated and not fixed to the skin.

Dermoid cyst

These may be congenital or acquired. The congenital ones are most common in the head and neck and occur where skin dermatomes fuse.

They are not unlike sebaceous cysts on examination but lack a punctum. Acquired implantation dermoids usually occur in relation to scars.

Abscess

The diagnosis will usually be obvious. There will be a tender, red, inflamed swelling. They may occur in relation to lymph nodes or salivary glands.

Lymphadenopathy

Depending upon the cause of the condition, lymph nodes will be enlarged and tender; non-tender and firm or rubbery or small, hard and matted together. A check should be made for enlarged lymph nodes elsewhere in the body and for hepatosplenomegaly. Generalised lymphadenopathy and splenomegaly will occur with blood dyscrasias.

Thyroid

Thyroid swellings move on swallowing. Associated lymphadenopathy will suggest malignancy. The thyroid status of the patient should be checked on clinical examination.

Thyroglossal cyst

This is a painless cystic swelling in the midline of the neck that moves on swallowing. It also moves on protrusion of the tongue. It is commonly attached to the body of the hyoid bone. Occasionally, it may become infected, with pain, tenderness and increased swelling.

Salivary gland

Swelling of the submandibular salivary gland is most frequently due to obstruction of the submandibular duct. Swelling will be noted on mastication. A stone may be palpated in the submandibular duct in the floor of the mouth. Swelling of the parotid gland may be due to duct obstruction, although tumour is more common with this gland. Malignant tumours of the parotid gland may be associated with facial nerve palsy.

Branchial cyst

A branchial cyst feels soft and putty-like and abuts from the anterior border of sternocleidomastoid at the junction between its upper and middle thirds.

Carotid body tumour

This feels firm and is located at the bifurcation of the common carotid artery.

Carotid aneurysm

These are extremely rare. False ones may follow surgery or trauma to the neck. A tortuous carotid artery may be mistaken for a carotid aneurysm.

Sternomastoid 'tumour'

This appears only in babies and is a result of birth trauma. There is a swelling in the middle third of the sternomastoid. The head becomes turned to the opposite side and tilted towards the shoulder on the side of the lesion.

Cervical rib

A bony, hard swelling may be palpable in the posterior triangle of the neck.

Subclavian artery aneurysm

Obvious as a pulsatile, expansile swelling in the lower part of the posterior triangle. Often associated with a cervical rib.

Pharyngeal pouch

Presents behind the lower border of sternomastoid in the posterior triangle. It may fill after a meal and empty after lying down. Signs of aspiration pneumonitis may be present.

Cystic hygromas

This is a collection of dilated lymphatics, which presents in infancy. It is soft, lobulated, fluctuant, compressible and brilliantly transilluminable.

GENERAL INVESTIGATIONS

■ **FBC, ESR, CRP**
  Hb ↓ malignancy. WCC ↑ infection and leukaemia. ESR and CRP ↑ infection and malignancy.

■ **TFTs**
  If clinical examination reveals a swelling to be a goitre.

■ **CXR**
  May show TB or primary or secondary tumour. Tracheal deviation may be associated with thyroid swellings. A cervical rib may be seen. Count the ribs. If there are 13, it is likely that there is a cervical rib.

■ **US**
  This may be helpful in almost any lump in the neck. It will also distinguish between solid and cystic swellings, e.g. in the thyroid.

SPECIFIC INVESTIGATIONS

A detailed history and examination may suggest the aetiology of the swelling. Further confirmatory investigations may be required for specific cases.

■ **Paul–Bunnell test**
  For glandular fever.

■ **Toxoplasma screen**
  Toxoplasmosis.

■ **Mantoux test**
  For TB.

■ **Viral titres**
  For any viral infection that may cause cervical lymphadenopathy.

- **FNAC**
  Especially useful for swellings of lymph nodes, thyroid or salivary glands.

- **CT**
  Helpful with the diagnosis of almost any mass but particularly helpful with confirming the diagnosis of carotid body tumours.

- **Duplex Doppler**
  For suspected carotid artery aneurysm or subclavian artery aneurysm.

- **Floor of mouth X-ray**
  Will identify a calculus in the submandibular duct.

- **Sialography**
  Contrast study of salivary duct to locate possible cause and site of obstruction, e.g. stone or stricture.

- **Barium swallow**
  To confirm the presence of a pharyngeal pouch. Never perform an endoscopy if a pouch is suspected, as it may result in perforation of the pouch.

- **OGD**
  To check for a primary oesophageal or gastric carcinoma causing cervical lymphadenopathy.

- **If cervical lymphadenopathy is thought to be due to malignancy, the patient should be referred for an urgent ENT opinion.**

- **Dysphagia in association with a neck swelling is likely to represent serious underlying pathology.**

NECK PAIN

Neck pain is a common presenting complaint. The majority of cases are due to poor posture or cervical spondylosis. If there has been a history of trauma, extreme care must be taken in examination of the neck and any X-rays must be strictly supervised.

CAUSES

CONGENITAL

- Torticollis
- Klippel–Feil syndrome

ACQUIRED

TRAUMATIC
- Fractures
- Dislocations
- Whiplash injury

INFLAMMATORY
- Rheumatoid arthritis

INFECTIVE
- Herpes zoster
- TB ● *(common where TB is endemic)*

DEGENERATIVE
- Cervical spondylosis
- Cervical radiculopathy
- Degenerative cervical myelopathy

NEOPLASTIC
- Secondary deposits

OTHER
- Postural
- Exposure to cold
- Meningitis ⚠
- Subarachnoid haemorrhage ⚠
- Osteomyelitis

HISTORY

Congenital

Torticollis may be congenital and present at birth due to sternomastoid 'tumour'. This is a rare condition often associated with breech delivery.

Klippel–Feil syndrome is also rare and is characterised by developmental abnormalities of the cervical vertebrae and a high-riding scapula involving fusion of two or more spinal bones.

Acquired

Traumatic

History of trauma may be evident and it is important to screen for any neurological sequelae, e.g. arm pain or weakness as well as bladder symptoms. Whiplash injuries occur in road traffic accidents where the car is struck from behind. The neck extends with sudden acceleration and flexes forward with sudden deceleration.

Inflammatory

Rheumatoid arthritis frequently affects the neck, particularly the atlantoaxial joints, which may undergo subluxation (atlanto-axial subluxation). There will usually be a history of rheumatoid arthritis elsewhere. The patient complains of pain in the neck, difficulty in walking.

Infective

TB of the cervical spine is rare in the UK and there is usually a history of TB elsewhere. In herpes zoster, a particular dermatome may be affected by a neuropathic rash or equally result in post-herpetic neuralgia.

Degenerative

Cervical spondylosis (cervical osteoarthritis) is the commonest condition involving the neck. The patient complains of neck pain and stiffness with radiation of pain into the occiput, shoulder or arms. There may be complaints of weakness of grip and wasting of the hand. Cervical radiculopathy may cause neck pain, with referred pain to the arm with weakness. Central disc protrusion may cause loss of coordination as well as bladder problems or even paraplegia. Degenerative cervical myelopathy (DCM) is a progressive condition caused by multiple risk factors, leading to neck pain, loss of sensory and motor function as well as bowel or bladder loss.

Neoplastic

Primary tumours of the cervical vertebrae are extremely rare. Secondary deposits may occur from breast, bronchus, lung, prostate or kidney. The patient may have had surgery for carcinoma of one of these organs. The patient will present with pain and collapse of a vertebra, perhaps with neurological symptoms.

Other

Postural neck pain is common and relates to changes in neck posture, with the patient often complaining of sleeping in an 'awkward' position. The pain is usually across the neck and shoulders. Meningitis may cause a stiff neck with pain, as does subarachnoid haemorrhage. The diagnosis of these will usually be obvious from the history of sudden thunderclap headache that radiates into the neck and causes neck stiffness.

EXAMINATION

Congenital

Torticollis – the head is pulled down to the affected side and often rotated to the opposite side. Klippel–Feil syndrome presents with a short neck, a high-riding scapula with restricted neck movement.

Acquired

Traumatic

Treat the patient as for spinal injury, with stabilisation of the neck. Any X-ray examination should be strictly supervised by an experienced orthopaedic surgeon. With whiplash injuries, there is usually only ligamentous and soft-tissue damage. Localised tenderness may be present. Consider a full neurological examination. Check for pain and paraesthesia in the arms and hands.

Inflammatory

Rheumatoid arthritis will be apparent elsewhere, e.g. hand deformities, ulnar deviation. Carry out a full neurological examination.

Infective

With TB, the patient will be generally unwell with spasm in the neck muscles. There may be evidence of paravertebral abscess. Carry out a full neurological examination. In herpes zoster, a rash may be vesicular, which consists of vesicles that scab over and are often painful.

Degenerative

In spondylosis, there will be reduced neck movements. There will often be weakness of grip, muscle wasting and reduced reflexes. Cervical radiculopathy can result in pain and spasm of the neck muscles. There may be weakness of the arm and reduced reflexes. In DCM, this may present with gait abnormalities, increased tone and muscle weakness. Carry out a full neurological examination in all instances.

Neoplastic

Examine the possible sites of primary tumours, e.g. breast, bronchus, prostate, thyroid, kidney. Carry out a full neurological examination.

Other

With postural neck pain or cold exposure, there is usually little to find on examination. There may be some localised muscular tenderness. With meningitis, the patient is usually ill, with photophobia, headache, stiff neck and a positive Kernig's sign. Subarachnoid haemorrhage is usually diagnosed from the history.

GENERAL INVESTIGATIONS

- ■ FBC, ESR
  Hb ↓ anaemia of chronic disease, e.g. rheumatoid arthritis.
  WCC ↑ infection. ESR ↑ rheumatoid arthritis, TB, malignancy.

- ■ Rheumatoid factor (or anti-CCP)
  Rheumatoid arthritis.

- ■ Cervical spine X-ray
  Fractures (supervised X-rays), cervical spondylosis – narrowing
  of joint spaces, osteophytes. Rheumatoid arthritis – atlantoaxial
  subluxation. Secondary deposits. Congenital anomalies.

SPECIFIC INVESTIGATIONS

- ■ Cervical CT
  Fracture. Disc lesion. TB. Subarachnoid haemorrhage.

- ■ Cervical spine MRI
  Disc lesions – cord compression. Degenerative cervical myelopathy.

- ■ Bone scan
  Secondary deposits. Acute arthritis.

- ■ Lumbar puncture
  Meningitis. Subarachnoid haemorrhage.

- • If there has been a history of trauma, extreme care
  must be exercised in examination of the neck and
  any X-rays must be strictly supervised involving neck
  immobilisation.

- • Neck pain and stiffness may be early signs of meningitis.
  Check carefully for petechiae or palpable purpura.

- • In neck pain, carefully consider red flags (e.g. altered
  mental status, weakness, incontinence, weight loss).

NIPPLE DISCHARGE

This is a common problem and can be embarrassing for the patient, as discharge may leak through and stain clothing. Bloodstained nipple discharge may be due to an underlying carcinoma. We have classified below according to consistency.

CAUSES

SEROUS

- Early pregnancy
- Fibroadenosis
- Medication (e.g. antipsychotics, antidepressants)

MILKY

- Late pregnancy
- Lactation
- Lactorrhoea of the newborn (witch's milk)
- Puberty
- Prolactinoma

COLOURED

YELLOW, BROWN, GREEN
- Fibroadenosis

THICK AND CREAMY
- Mammary duct ectasia

PURULENT

- Retroareolar abscess
- Breast abscess
- TB

BLOODSTAINED

- Intraduct carcinoma
- Intraduct papilloma
- Paget's disease of the nipple
- Jogger's nipple

HISTORY

Pregnancy or lactation will be apparent. Discharge may occur from the nipples of newborn babies of either sex (witch's milk). It is due to the passage of female hormones across the placenta. A serous or milky discharge may occur at puberty. Cyclical mastalgia with a coloured discharge, especially greenish, suggests fibroadenosis. Always consider medication as a possible cause of galactorrhoea (e.g. antipsychotics or antidepressants). A patient in the fifth decade (around menopause) with a history of retroareolar pain and a thick creamy discharge may have duct ectasia. This is also more common in smokers. A bloodstained discharge must be taken seriously and fully investigated. The patient may describe this as frank, red blood or altered blood, which may be darkish brown. It is important to know whether it has come from one duct or several. Does the patient have an underlying lump? Profuse milky discharge associated with amenorrhoea will suggest the possibility of prolactinoma of the anterior pituitary gland. There may also be associated visual changes. Intraductal papilloma is more common in younger women and can cause bloodstained discharge. There is usually no palpable lump. Jogger's nipple is fairly common in male athletes. Jogger's nipple occurs when the nipple and the areola become irritated as the nipple rubs up against damp, rough fabric. Crusting, soreness and even bleeding of the nipple tissue occur.

EXAMINATION

Is the discharge obvious? It may have stained the clothes and the colour of it may be apparent. Is it associated with a painful and lumpy breast to suggest fibroadenosis? Is it possible to express the discharge by manual pressure? Occasionally it is possible, by manual pressure on specific areas of the breast, to express blood from one particular duct. Is there an underlying discrete lump, suggestive of a carcinoma or axillary lymphadenopathy? Is there retroareolar tenderness, lumpiness and nipple retraction, suggestive of duct ectasia? Are there any signs of infection or abscess? Has the nipple been destroyed (i.e. Paget's disease)? If prolactinoma is suspected (galactorrhoea, amenorrhoea, infertility), the visual fields should be checked, as a macroadenoma of the anterior pituitary gland may impinge on the optic chiasma, leading to bitemporal hemianopia. In jogger's nipple, there will be crusting, fissuring and bleeding from nipple tissue.

GENERAL INVESTIGATIONS

- **FBC, ESR**
  WCC ↑ in infection. ESR ↑ in tumour and TB.
- **TSH and Prolactin**
  Rule out endocrine causes (e.g. hypothyroidism or prolactinoma).
- **Swab**
  C&S. Infection, abscess, TB.
- **FNAC**
  Breast carcinoma.
- **Dipstick testing**
  Blood versus other fluid.

SPECIFIC INVESTIGATIONS

- **Mammography**
  Carcinoma, duct ectasia, fibroadenosis.
- **Ductogram**
  Detailed mammogram of ductal system.
- **Ultrasound**
  Carcinoma, duct ectasia.
- **Microdochectomy**
  If bleeding is localised to an individual duct, this is an appropriate surgical investigation. It may demonstrate intraduct papilloma or intraduct carcinoma.
- **CT head**
  Tumour of the pituitary gland (i.e. prolactinoma).

- A bloodstained nipple discharge can be serious. An underlying carcinoma is the most likely diagnosis. Urgent referral to a breast surgeon for full assessment is required.
- Consider pregnancy in the patient with bilateral serous discharge.
- Destruction of the nipple suggests Paget's disease.
- Nipple discharge in a male is always abnormal. Full investigation is required to rule out underlying carcinoma.

OLIGURIA

Oliguria is the passage of less than 400 mL of urine in 24 hours. Anuria is defined as the failure to pass urine (less than 100 mL in 24 hours). Oliguria is an important feature of acute renal failure.

CAUSES

RENAL CIRCULATORY INSUFFICIENCY

- Dehydration, e.g. vomiting, diarrhoea
- Shock, e.g. haemorrhage, burns

RENAL

- Nephrotoxins
- Acute tubular necrosis
- Acute cortical necrosis
- Acute glomerulonephritis
- Acute interstitial nephritis
- Vascular lesions

POST-RENAL (OBSTRUCTIVE)

- Prostatic hypertrophy
- Post-renal calculi
- Pelvic tumours
- Haematoma
- Retroperitoneal fibrosis

OTHERS

- Mismatched transfusion (haemoglobinuria)
- Crush injuries (myoglobinuria)

ANURIA

- Blocked catheter
- Ureteric damage (bilateral)
- Stone in solitary functioning kidney

HISTORY

Pre-renal

There will usually be a recent history of a condition which causes renal hypoperfusion. This may include haemorrhage, burns or dehydration, e.g. from vomiting, diarrhoea or acute pancreatitis.

Renal

In the absence of adequate resuscitation, shock will proceed to cause damage to the tubules, resulting in acute tubular necrosis. Acute cortical necrosis may arise as a result of antepartum haemorrhage, eclampsia or septic abortion. It may also follow insults similar to those that cause acute tubular necrosis. With acute interstitial nephritis, there may be a history of drug ingestion, e.g. antibiotics, NSAIDs or diuretics, or there may be a history of infection. Nephrotoxins may cause acute renal failure and drugs implicated can again include antibiotics such as aminoglycosides, amphotericin or radiographic contrast media. Paraquat, snake bites and mushrooms may also cause acute renal failure. Vascular lesions may also lead to acute renal failure; these include renal vein thrombosis, renal artery stenosis and intravascular coagulation occurring in haemolytic uraemic syndrome.

Post-renal

Often the patient will present with complete anuria. This may occur if there is ureteric damage following surgery or a stone impacted in the ureter of a solitary functioning kidney. The patient may have a history of calculous disease or may have recently suffered an attack of ureteric colic. There may be a history of pelvic tumour or symptoms of prostatic hypertrophy (e.g. difficulty in starting and a poor stream). Retroperitoneal fibrosis often develops insidiously.

Others

Oliguria may follow a mismatched transfusion, due to haemoglobinuria, or crush injuries, due to myoglobinuria. The history will usually be obvious.

Anuria

Before diagnosing anuria, make sure that the patient does not have a palpable bladder (if not catheterised) and is not therefore in acute retention, or, if the patient is catheterised, that the catheter is not blocked. Anuria is more likely to be a symptom of an obstructive lesion rather than one of renal hypoperfusion or an intrinsic renal lesion.

EXAMINATION

General

If the patient has a catheter in situ, make sure that it is not blocked. If the patient does not have a catheter in situ, palpate the lower abdomen for a distended bladder associated with acute retention as well as excluding swellings of the kidneys. Consider performing a rectal examination to exclude prostatic hypertrophy.

Specific

All causes of oliguria are likely to have some common features on examination. The patient will be dyspnoeic due to pulmonary oedema and will either have sacral oedema (if confined to bed) or ankle oedema (if ambulant). There may be confusion, drowsiness, fitting or coma. Hypertension and arrhythmias may be present. The patient will be nauseated, may be vomiting, have hiccups and there may be evidence of gastrointestinal haemorrhage. Spontaneous bruising may eventually occur.

GENERAL INVESTIGATIONS

- **FBC, ESR**
  Hb ↓ anaemia, renal failure, haemorrhage. WCC ↑ infection.
  ESR ↑ some causes of glomerulonephritis.

- **U&Es**
  Urea ↑, creatinine ↑ in renal and post-renal causes. These may rise in renal hypoperfusion if not adequately treated.

- **ECG**
  Arrhythmias. Associated with electrolyte imbalance, e.g. hyperkalaemia.

- **CXR**
  Pulmonary oedema. Cardiomegaly.

- **ABGs**
  Metabolic acidosis.

- **Urine dipstick and MSU**
  Red cells, casts and protein in intrinsic renal disease. Hb-positive but no red blood cells suggest myoglobinuria or haemoglobinuria.

- **Urine electrolytes**
  See table below.

- **Urine osmolality**
  See table below.

Physiological oliguria	
Urine	**Physiological oliguria**
Specific gravity	>1020
Osmolality (mmol/kg)	>500
Sodium (mmol/L)	<15
Urine/serum creatinine	>40
Fractional sodium excretion[a]	<1
Renal failure index[b]	<1

[a]Fractional sodium excretion = (urine sodium × plasma creatinine/plasma sodium × urine creatinine) × 100.
[b]Renal failure index = (urine sodium × plasma creatinine)/urine creatinine.

SPECIFIC INVESTIGATIONS

- **US**
  Obstructive lesion.
- **Cystoscopy with retrograde pyelography**
  Cause of obstruction, possible relief of obstruction.
- **Antegrade pyelography**
  Cause of obstruction. Relief of obstruction.
- **DMSA scan**
  Renal function. Structure and morphology.

- The commonest cause of oliguria is hypovolaemia. Always check the patients hydration status. CVP monitoring may be required.
- Consider catheter blockage before diagnosing oliguria/anuria as well as urinary retention.

PALPITATIONS

Palpitation is an awareness of the heartbeat. Although benign in the vast majority, palpitations are occasionally a manifestation of a life-threatening disorder.

Figure 47 ECG of atrial fibrillation. *The irregularly irregular QRS complexes occur in the setting of a saw-tooth baseline of uncoordinated atrial activity with absent P waves.*

CAUSES

SINUS TACHYCARDIA

- Anxiety/emotional stress
- Caffeine
- Nicotine
- Alcohol
- Infection
- Hyperthyroidism
- Electrolyte disturbances

CARDIAC ARRHYTHMIA

- Premature ventricular contractions (ventricular ectopic beats)*
- Premature atrial contractions (atrial ectopic beats)*
- Atrial fibrillation* (Fig. 47)
- Supraventricular tachycardia (AVRT, AVNRT)
- Ventricular tachycardia (long QT syndrome)

*Indicates causes that tend to present as irregular palpitations.

HISTORY

A variety of symptoms is used to describe palpitations and this includes 'fluttering', 'pounding' and 'skipping a beat'. Symptoms may also be experienced in the neck. Important aspects are frequency, regularity of palpitation (e.g. fast and irregular) and precipitating factors. Asking the patient to tap the rate and rhythm of the palpitation (on a table for example) can be very informative. Arrhythmias associated with irregular palpitations are listed above.

Knowledge of precipitating factors is important. Palpitations can be a normal manifestation of anxiety or panic reactions. However, it is vitally important that organic causes are excluded as it is common for anxiety disorders to co-exist in a patient with supraventricular tachycardia. Exercise is associated with excess catecholamines and also a precipitator of arrhythmia (supraventricular tachycardia, atrial fibrillation and ventricular tachycardia usually originating from the right ventricle). Excessive caffeine, smoking and alcohol intake are also thought to be precipitators.

A history of any underlying heart disorder is important, as arrhythmia is associated with ischaemic heart disease (ventricular arrhythmia), hypertensive heart disease (atrial fibrillation), heart failure (ventricular arrhythmia), heart valve disease.

Early age of onset of arrhythmia (childhood or teenage years) suggests the presence of a congenital abnormality such as a bypass tract that can lead to supraventricular tachycardia.

Additional features

Dizziness (p. 97) or syncope (p. 410) is usually associated with more serious underlying arrhythmia such as ventricular tachycardia and occasionally supraventricular tachycardia. Also ask about chest pain and shortness of breath as these symptoms may warrant urgent management.

EXAMINATION

Examination during an episode of palpitation is very informative, as assessment of the rhythm and rate of the pulse can be determined. Auscultation of the rate at the cardiac apex is more accurate as not all beats are conducted to the pulse (e.g. in atrial fibrillation).

It is important to measure the blood pressure and screen for any evidence of underlying structural heart disease, especially mitral valve prolapse (systolic murmur and a systolic click), as this condition is associated with supraventricular tachycardia and atrial fibrillation.

INITIAL INVESTIGATIONS

12-Lead ECG

All patients should have a resting ECG, although it is unlikely that any arrhythmia can be picked up during this investigation; however, conditions that predispose to arrhythmia may be diagnosed. The presence of an accessory pathway (and hence predisposition to supraventricular arrhythmia) is indicated by a short PR interval (less than 0.12 seconds).

Also, the presence of left ventricular hypertrophy on ECG can indicate underlying structural heart disease (hypertensive heart disease, or hypertrophic obstructive cardiomyopathy). Ischaemic heart disease can be suggested by Q waves, or ST segment/T wave abnormalities.

Occasionally, atrial or ventricular premature contractions (ectopic beats) may be evident and often benign.

SPECIFIC INVESTIGATIONS

- TFT
  Rule out hyperthyroidism
- U&Es
  Electrolyte disturbance
- FBC
  Anaemia

FURTHER INVESTIGATIONS

Further investigations are best reserved for those who are at high risk of arrhythmia: patients with evidence of underlying structural heart disease, family history of arrhythmia, regular palpitations (especially during sleep) and dizziness or syncope associated with palpitations.

Ambulatory ECG monitoring

Continuous ambulatory ECG monitoring is an excellent method to detect and identify arrhythmia. This can include 24-hour tapes, extended loop or implantable loop recorders. Upon further investigation, ventricular and atrial premature contractions (ectopic beats) are the most commonly identified arrhythmia. Sinus rhythm is the usual remaining finding with a serious arrhythmia detected in approximately 7%. Consult ECG textbooks for a detailed discussion of the numerous configurations of each arrhythmia.

- Palpitations are benign in the vast majority of cases.
- Palpitations can occasionally be a manifestation of life-threatening disorders, especially in the presence of associated symptoms including chest pain. Consider emergency admission to hospital.
- Sudden onset of tachycardia in childhood or teenage years associated with breathlessness, dizziness and chest pain suggests supraventricular tachycardia and possible congenital abnormality.

PENILE LESIONS

Penile lesions are common. They can interfere with quality of life and affect sexual intercourse. The majority of surgical conditions of the penis relate to problems with the foreskin and glans. Carcinoma of the penis and Peyronie's disease are rare.

Figure 48 Carcinoma of the penis, revealed with the foreskin retracted.

CAUSES

FORESKIN AND GLANS

- Penile lumps (pearly penile papules, molluscum contagiosam, fordyce spots)
- Phimosis
- Paraphimosis ⚠
- Balanoposthitis
- Balanitis xerotica obliterans
- Herpes genitalis
- Condylomata (warts)
- Trauma (bite)
- Carcinoma (Fig. 48) ⚠
- Erythroplasia of Queyrat (carcinoma in situ)
- Chancre (syphilis)
- Behcet's disease
- Bowen's disease

SHAFT OF THE PENIS
- Peyronie's disease
- Priapism

URETHRA
- Epispadias
- Hypospadias

HISTORY

Foreskin and glans

Penile lumps

Pearly penile papules are small lumps often found in a row which are seperate from warts. Molluscum are pearly spots with a central umbilicated area common in children. Fordyce spots are simply visible sebaceous glands that occur during adolescence.

Phimosis

In most cases, phimosis is congenital. The foreskin has been tight since birth and the patient complains that it will not retract over the glans. In children, this may cause pain with ballooning of the foreskin during micturition, with resulting balanoposthitis. In adults, the complaint is that it interferes with sexual intercourse.

Paraphimosis

The foreskin is pulled back over the glans while washing and then is not returned. It may also occur during sexual intercourse. In hospital practice, it may occur while the patient is being catheterised and the foreskin is not returned to its correct place following this procedure. The foreskin forms a tight constriction around the glans, interfering with venous return and causing swelling of the glans and foreskin. The patient presents with considerable pain and a swollen glans penis.

Balanoposthitis

This is inflammation of the glans and foreskin. The patient complains of an attack of inflammation of the foreskin and glans. It may be associated with poor hygiene, but in children it is often associated with phimosis and collection of urine under the foreskin. In diabetics, it is often due to *candida*.

Balanitis xerotica obliterans

Also known as lichen sclerosus et atrophicus. The patient will complain of thickening and tightening of the foreskin, and the inability to retract it. This is often seen in uncircumsised men.

Herpes genitalis

The patient will complain of painful vesicles on the foreskin or glans penis. Primary infection is often severe with accompanying fever. There will usually be a history of sexual contact.

Condylomata (warts)

The patient may present with warts on the glans and contiguous surface of the prepuce. They are usually of venereal origin.

Trauma

There may be a history of trauma. Love bites may be responsible.

Carcinoma

This usually presents in old age. It is virtually unknown in those who are circumcised. Most patients present with a lump or an ulcer which may be painful. In uncircumcised patients who cannot retract the foreskin, there may be a bloodstained purulent discharge from under the foreskin.

Erythroplasia of Queyrat

The patient will present having noticed a dark, velvety, red, flat patch on the skin of the glans. This can be associated with HPV.

Syphilitic chancre

A chancre presents as a painless hard ulcer on the penis.

Behcet's disease

This a multi-system disease associated with oral and genital ulcers as well as anterior uveitis.

Bowen's disease

This can present as a form of squamous cell carcinoma via a red scaly patch in the penile shaft.

Shaft

Peyronie's disease

The patient may have noticed a subcutaneous lump along the penis. He may complain that when he has an erection, the penis appears bent.

Priapism

The patient will present with a persistent painful erection. This is unassociated with sexual desire. There may be a history of leukaemia, sickle cell disease, disseminated pelvic malignancy, or the patient may be on haemodialysis. Priapism may also result from alprostadil overdose for erectile dysfunction. Recreational drugs including cocaine, cannabis and ecstasy may also cause this.

Urethra

Epispadias

This is rare. The patient, a baby or child, usually presents with the urethra opening on the dorsal surface of the glans penis.

Hypospadias

This is more common than epispadias, the patient presenting with the urethral opening on the ventral or undersurface of the penis. In both epispadias and hypospadias, the patient will complain of a problem with micturition.

EXAMINATION

Foreskin and glans

Penile lumps

Pearly penile papules are often small symmetrical lumps. Molluscum are pearl white spots seen in clusters with a central depression. Fordyce spots appear on the shaft of the penis and are prominent when the skin is stretched.

Phimosis

The foreskin is tight and has a pinhole orifice. It will be impossible to retract it over the glans penis. There may be associated balanoposthitis.

Paraphimosis

The diagnosis is usually obvious. The glans penis is painful, swollen and oedematous and there is a deep groove just proximal to the corona glandis, where there is a tight constricting ring of skin.

Balanoposthitis

There is inflammation of the glans (balanitis) and often associated inflammation of the foreskin (posthitis). There may be a discharge from under the foreskin. In the case of candidiasis, there are itchy red patches on the glans. There may be evidence of poor personal hygiene.

Balanitis xerotica obliterans

The foreskin is thickened, with loss of elasticity and fibrosis. It is usually not possible to retract it over the glans.

Herpes genitalis

Initially, there will be itchy vesicles, but these develop into shallow, painful erosions. There may be associated painful inguinal lymphadenopathy.

Condylomata (warts)

There will be a bunch of warts, usually around the junction between the foreskin and the glans and extending onto the glans.

Trauma

Appearance will depend upon the type of trauma. Teeth marks may be apparent.

Carcinoma

The lesion is usually at the junction of the foreskin and glans. There will be a lump or ulcer. If there is an ulcer, it will have raised everted edges and a necrotic base. It feels hard. The inguinal lymph nodes may be affected, either by metastases or by secondary infection. In patients in whom the foreskin cannot be retracted, it may be necessary to carry out circumcision to make the diagnosis.

Erythroplasia of Queyrat

There is a dark-red, flat, velvety, indurated patch on the glans penis. It is a premalignant condition and represents carcinoma in situ.

Syphilitic chancre

There will be a painless, hard ulcer with a sloping edge. The inguinal nodes will be enlarged, rubbery, discrete and non-tender.

Behcet's disease

Look for ulcers in the mouth or penis. Also consider the systemic nature of this disease and examine joints and gastrointestinal and neurological systems.

Bowen's disease

An ulcer may appear as velvety maculopapular lesion.

Shaft

Peyronie's disease

There are plaques of fibrosis in the corpora cavernosa. These may be felt as hard lumps along the corpora cavernosa. The patient will volunteer the information that the penis becomes bent on erection.

Priapism

The diagnosis will be obvious, there being a painful erection.

Urethra

The diagnosis of epispadias and hypospadias will be obvious. In hypospadias, the opening of the urethra may be anywhere along the line of the urethra, from a few millimetres from the tip of the penis to the perineum. In epispadias, which is rare, the urethral opening is on the dorsal surface of the glans penis.

GENERAL INVESTIGATIONS

- **FBC, ESR**
  WCC ↑ infection, leukaemia (associated with priapism).
  ESR ↑ malignancy.
- **Swab**
  C&S. Microscopy. Balanitis – bacterial or fungal.
- **Blood glucose**
  Diabetes – *candida* balanitis.

SPECIFIC INVESTIGATIONS

- **Sickle cell test**
  Sickle cell disease with priapism.
- **Syphilis serology (e.g. VDRL)**
  Syphilitic chancre.

- **Electron microscopy**
  Identification of herpes virus in vesicular fluid.

- **PCR**
  For rapid diagnosis of herpes.

- **Biopsy**
  Erythroplasia of Queyrat. Carcinoma. Condylomata.

- **Circumcision**
  Diagnostic and management if tight phimosis prevents retraction of foreskin.

- Always take a full sexual history. Enquire about foreign travel and sexual encounters. If STD is suspected, refer to a GUM clinic.

- A persistent solitary mass or ulcer needs thorough investigation as malignancy is likely, especially in the absence of an STD.

- Recurrent candidal balanitis may reflect underlying diabetes. Check the blood sugar.

POLYURIA

The volume of urine produced per day varies in each individual and is affected by the amount of fluid intake, physiological requirements and insensible losses. Polyuria is arbitrarily defined as urine output of more than three litres in 24 hours.

CAUSES

DIURETICS

THERAPEUTIC
- Loop – e.g. furosemide, bumetanide
- Thiazide – e.g. bendroflumethiazide, metolazone, indapamide
- Amiloride

OSMOTIC
- Hyperglycaemia
- Hypercalcaemia
- Mannitol
- Urea

DIABETES INSIPIDUS

CRANIAL
- Head injuries
- Neurosurgery
- Brain tumours (especially of pituitary)
- Idiopathic deficiency of ADH production
- Inherited (dominant or recessive)
- Pituitary granulomas, e.g. sarcoidosis, TB ● *(more common where TB is endemic)*
- Opiates

NEPHROGENIC
- Drugs
  - Lithium
  - Demeclocycline
- Hypokalaemia
- Chronic tubulointerstitial nephritis
- Recovering acute tubular necrosis
- Recovering obstructive uropathy
- Chronic hypercalcaemia
- Inherited (X-linked)

EXCESSIVE FLUID INTAKE

- Drug-induced thirst – anticholinergics
- Psychogenic polydipsia
- Hypothalamic disease

HISTORY

General

Polyuria is often accompanied by polydipsia, and, as with all water-losing states, severe thirst is often a side effect. Frequency of micturition (frequent passing of small amounts of urine) should be differentiated from polyuria (frequent passing of large amounts of urine). Diabetes insipidus may be hereditary and other family members may be affected.

Drug history

A detailed drug history is invaluable, as a significant number of drugs precipitate polyuria by various mechanisms. Therapeutic diuretics are used in a range of disorders, such as hypertension and cardiac failure. Opiates inhibit ADH secretion and may produce cranial diabetes insipidus, whereas drugs such as lithium and demeclocycline may produce nephrogenic diabetes insipidus. A side effect of anticholinergics is dryness of the mouth; patients may therefore ingest excessive quantities of water, causing polyuria. Nephrotoxic drugs, such as aminoglycosides, ciclosporin, NSAIDs and ACE inhibitors, may precipitate acute tubular necrosis, which can result in severe polyuria in the recovery phase.

Past medical history

Hyperglycaemia causes an osmotic diuresis; therefore polyuria and polydipsia are common presenting features of diabetes mellitus. Malignancy and hyperparathyroidism are common causes of chronic hypercalcaemia, which can cause polyuria by an intrinsic osmotic effect or by precipitation of nephrogenic diabetes insipidus. Cranial diabetes insipidus can result from severe, blunt head injuries, craniopharyngiomas, pineal gland tumours or as a transient postoperative complication following neurosurgery. Renal ischaemia from conditions such as sepsis and haemorrhage predisposes to acute tubular necrosis. Chronic tubulointerstitial nephritis can result from reflux nephropathy, polycystic kidney disease, gout and multiple myeloma.

GENERAL INVESTIGATIONS

- Urine dipstick
  +++ glucose with diabetes mellitus.
- 24-hour urine collection
  >3 litres confirms polyuria and helps differentiate from urinary frequency.

- **U&Es**
  Plasma urea and creatinine levels ↑ renal failure. Sodium ↑ with uncompensated polyuria (inadequate water intake). Sodium ↓ with urea/creatinine ↓ indicates polydipsia as the primary cause. Potassium ↓ may cause nephrogenic diabetes insipidus.
- **Urine and plasma osmolality**
  Urine osmolality low and plasma osmolality normal in pituitary and nephrogenic diabetes insipidus. Urine osmolality low and plasma osmolality normal to low in compulsive water drinking.
- **Serum calcium**
  ↑ calcium causes osmotic diuresis and chronic tubulointerstitial nephritis.
- **Serum glucose**
  ↑ diabetes.

SPECIFIC INVESTIGATIONS

- **CT/MRI head**
  Tumours, hypothalamic disease.
- **Renal biopsy**
  Acute tubular necrosis, chronic tubulointerstitial nephritis.

- **Polyuria accompanied by polydipsia is often the first presentation of both type 1 and type 2 diabetes mellitus. Urgent investigation is required.**
- **Diabetes mellitus is not the only cause of polyuria accompanied by thirst. If urinalysis is negative for sugar, diabetes insipidus or hypercalcaemia is a possible diagnosis.**

POPLITEAL SWELLINGS

Popliteal swellings are common. The majority are easily diagnosed on clinical examination alone.

Figure 49 Femoral angiogram of a patient who presented with a pulsatile, expansile swelling in the right popliteal fossa. There is a popliteal aneurysm (arrow).

CAUSES

SUPERFICIAL

- Sebaceous cyst
- Lipoma
- Varix of the short saphenous vein

DEEP

- Lymphadenopathy
- Semi-membranosus bursa
- Baker's cyst
- Popliteal artery aneurysm (Fig. 49) ⚠

BONY

- Exostoses
- Osteogenic sarcoma ⚠

HISTORY

Superficial

Sebaceous cyst

A sebaceous cyst will present as a firm swelling in the skin, often with a distinct punctum (opening). It may be tender if it becomes inflamed and there may be a discharge from it.

Lipoma

This presents as a soft, fluctuant and often lobulated swelling in the subcutaneous tissue.

Varix of the short saphenous vein

This presents as a soft swelling behind the knee, usually associated with varicose veins of the short saphenous system.

Deep

Lymphadenopathy

There may be several palpable lumps within the popliteal fossa. The patient will usually draw attention to a lesion distally, either on the leg or on the foot, usually on the lateral margin of the foot or the back of the leg. Other groups of nodes may be enlarged.

Semi-membranosus bursa

The patient complains of a swelling behind the knee that interferes with knee movement, particularly flexion.

Baker's cyst

A Baker's cyst is a pulsion diverticulum of the knee joint caused by chronic disease within the joint. The patient will usually give a history of a painful knee joint and may have osteoarthritis or rheumatoid arthritis. Occasionally the cyst ruptures and the patient complains of severe pain in the calf, which has to be carefully distinguished from venous thrombosis.

Popliteal artery aneurysm

These often get quite large before they are noticed. The patient may be aware of a pulsatile swelling behind the knee but often notices it when crossing the legs, the upper of the crossed limbs moving with each pulse.

Bony

Exostoses

Exostoses may grow in the region of the epiphyseal cartilage of the femur. There is a well-defined bony swelling in the popliteal fossa.

Osteogenic sarcoma

This may affect either the lower end of the femur or the upper end of the tibia. There is a diffuse swelling around the knee joint. Pain may be a presenting symptom. There may also be general malaise and weight loss. Occasionally, pulmonary metastases have occurred at presentation, and there may be cough and haemoptysis.

EXAMINATION

Superficial

Sebaceous cyst

There will be a small, well-defined swelling in the skin with a punctum. If it is infected, the surrounding skin will be red and there may be discharge.

Lipoma

There will be a soft, lobulated swelling in the popliteal fossa.

Varix of the short saphenous vein

This is common. There will be a soft, compressible dilatation at the termination of the short saphenous vein. There may be an expansile cough impulse. A fluid thrill will be palpable when the short saphenous vein lower down the leg is tapped.

Deep

Lymphadenopathy

There may be a number of discrete glands palpable or they may be firm and matted together. Check for a lesion distally on the leg or foot, e.g. malignant melanoma. Check for lymphadenopathy elsewhere.

Semi-membranosus bursa

The swelling lies above the level of the knee joint line, slightly to the medial side of the popliteal fossa. It tends to be firm in consistency and transilluminates.

Baker's cyst

Baker's cysts occur more often in elderly patients with longstanding arthritis or in younger patients with rheumatoid arthritis. The lump is below the level of the knee joint and deep to gastrocnemius. It may transilluminate. Pressure over the lump may reduce it into the knee joint. Examination of the knee joint reveals changes consistent with arthritis, i.e. limited movements, crepitus and occasionally an effusion.

Popliteal artery aneurysm

An expansile, pulsatile mass will be palpable in the popliteal fossa. They are often bilateral. Check the distal circulation. Popliteal aneurysms may thrombose with distal ischaemia, or may throw off small emboli causing ischaemic toes or ischaemic ulcers on the tips of the toes. Palpate the abdomen: there is an association between popliteal aneurysms and abdominal aortic aneurysms.

Bony

Exostoses

A bony mass may be felt in the popliteal fossa.

Osteogenic sarcoma

The overlying skin may be reddened, with dilated subcutaneous veins. There may be tenderness. The swelling is usually smooth until it spreads into the surrounding tissues, when it becomes irregular. The swelling feels firm but is not usually bony hard.

GENERAL INVESTIGATIONS

■ FBC, ESR
Hb ↓ lymphadenopathy, e.g. part of generalised lymphadenopathy associated with reticulosis. WCC ↑ reticulosis. ESR ↑ reticulosis, osteogenic sarcoma with secondaries.

■ US
Lipoma. Semi-membranosus bursa. Baker's cyst. Popliteal artery aneurysm.

■ Knee X-ray
Exostoses. Osteoarthritis (Baker's cyst). Rheumatoid arthritis (Baker's cyst). Osteogenic sarcoma – bone destruction, grows out of cortex, elevating periosteum with reposition of subperiosteal bone (Codman's triangle), radiating spicules of bone ('sunray' spicules).

SPECIFIC INVESTIGATIONS

■ Duplex Doppler
Varix of short saphenous vein. Popliteal artery aneurysm.

■ CT
Shows invasion of osteogenic sarcoma. Lung secondaries.

■ MRI
Baker's cyst. Bone tumour.

■ Arteriography (i.e. MR angiography)
Popliteal aneurysm. Distal circulation.

- There is an association between popliteal artery aneurysms and abdominal aortic aneurysms. Always examine the abdomen.

- If the lump is thought to be a gland, always examine the sole of the foot, between the toes and under the toenails to exclude a primary lesion, e.g. melanoma.

- Vague generalised swelling around the knee in a young patient may suggest an osteogenic sarcoma.

SECTION A

PRURITUS

Pruritus is itching of the skin. There are a vast number of dermatological causes of pruritus, which are usually visible on inspection. However, the following are causes of generalised pruritus in the absence of skin disease.

CAUSES

- Obstructive jaundice
- Chronic renal failure
- Liver disease
- Stroke

HAEMATOLOGICAL DISEASE

- Iron deficiency
- Polycythaemia ruba vera

INTERNAL MALIGNANCY

- Bronchial carcinoma ⚠
- Hodgkin's lymphoma ⚠

ENDOCRINE DISEASE

- Hyperthyroidism
- Hypothyroidism
- Diabetes mellitus

INFECTION

- HIV
- Hepatitis C

DRUGS

- Oral contraceptive pill (cholestasis)
- Opiates (histamine release)
- Alcohol and drug withdrawal

HISTORY

When approaching a patient with generalised pruritus, enquiries are made regarding the site and duration of symptoms. Occasionally, the onset of pruritus will correlate with the initiation of drug treatment, allowing you to exclude the offending medication. It may also occur as a side effect of alcohol or drug withdrawal. Conversely, a history of alcohol excess may be seen in liver disease. Pruritus after a hot bath classically occurs with polycythaemia. Iron deficiency, even in the absence of anaemia, can cause pruritus; therefore symptoms of blood loss in each system should be carefully elicited.

Haemoptysis, chronic cough and weight loss in smokers may be due to underlying bronchial carcinoma, which is an important subgroup of internal malignancies that present with pruritus. The presence of localised lymphadenopathy, fever, night sweats and weight loss should lead to the consideration of Hodgkin's lymphoma. Patients with obstructive jaundice (p. 236) may present with pruritus (due to the accumulation of bile salts), even while the jaundice is not clinically apparent. With complete obstruction, patients may notice pale stools and dark urine (features of pancreatic cancer).

Lethargy, anorexia, nocturia, oliguria, polyuria, haematuria, frothy urine from proteinuria, skin fragility, oedema and bone pains are some of the multisystemic features suggestive of chronic renal disease. Interestingly, pruritus seldom occurs with acute renal failure.

As pruritus may be due to thyroid disease, clinical assessment of the thyroid status is an important aspect of the history. Features of hyperthyroidism are tremor, heat intolerance, palpitations, increased appetite with weight loss, anxiety and diarrhoea. Features of hypothyroidism are cold intolerance, mental slowing, weight gain, constipation and menorrhagia. In patients with suspected HIV pruritus along with rashes, lymphadenopathy, recurent infections, malaise and myalgia may be present, whilst in hepatitis C pruritus may accompany fever and arthralgia.

EXAMINATION

Inspection

Wide, staring eyes with lid lag and tremor may be present with thyrotoxicosis (hyperthyroidism). Pallor of the conjunctivae may be evident in severe anaemia, whereas, with polycythaemia, conjunctival insufflation and facial plethora occur. The sclera should also be examined for the presence of jaundice. Sallow skin with easy bruising and uraemic frost may be seen with chronic renal failure. Spoon-shaped nails of iron deficiency may be accompanied by angular cheilitis. Clubbing may be due to bronchial carcinoma. Signs of liver disease include spider naevi, bruising and palmar erythema.

GENERAL EXAMINATION

Asymmetrical, non-tender, localised lymphadenopathy in the absence of infection is suggestive of Hodgkin's lymphoma. The thyroid gland is palpated for abnormalities, such as enlargement, nodularity and asymmetry. A respiratory examination is performed; features of bronchial carcinoma include monophonic inspiratory wheeze (partial endoluminal bronchial obstruction), lobar collapse of the lung, pleural effusion and Horner's syndrome for apical lung tumours. Chest wall tenderness may also occur as a result of tumour infiltration. Splenomegaly and hepatomegaly may occur with Hodgkin's lymphoma and polycythaemia rubra vera.

GENERAL INVESTIGATIONS

- **Urine dipstick**
  Protein and blood with chronic renal disease.

- **FBC and blood film**
  Microcytic hypochromic anaemia with iron deficiency, normochromic normocytic anaemia with Hodgkin's, ↑ Hb with polycythaemia.

- **U&Es (including calcium/phosphorous)**
  Urea and creatinine ↑ renal failure.

- **Glucose**
  ↑ with diabetes mellitus.

- **LFTs**
  Bilirubin ↑, alkaline phosphatase ↑ with obstructive jaundice.

- **TFTs**
  TSH ↓ and T_4 ↑ thyrotoxicosis; TSH ↑ and T_4 ↓ hypothyroidism.

- **CXR**
  Bronchial carcinoma, hilar lymphadenopathy with Hodgkin's disease.

SPECIFIC INVESTIGATIONS

- **Excisional biopsy of lymph node**
  Hodgkin's disease: Reed–Sternberg cells.

- **US abdomen**
  Dilated bile ducts with obstructive jaundice, the site and cause of obstruction may be visualised. The size of the kidneys may be decreased with chronic renal disease, and multiple cysts visible with polycystic kidney disease.

- **Iron studies (serum iron, serum ferritin, protoporphyrin)**
  Serum iron ↓, serum ferritin ↓, free erythrocyte protoporphyrin ↑ iron deficiency.

- **CT chest and abdomen**
  Hilar lymphadenopathy in lymphoma. Chest lesion in bronchial carcinoma.

- **Persistent pruritus may be the presenting symptom of lymphoma or other malignancy. Always examine the abdomen and lymph nodes.**

- **HIV/hepatitis C could present with generalised pruritus along with other systemic symptoms. A careful sexual history should be considered.**

PRURITUS ANI

Pruritus ani is itching around the anal canal. It is a common symptom and in approximately half of the cases, no cause can be found.

Figure 50 Anal warts (condylomata acuminata).

CAUSES

ANAL DISCHARGE

- Haemorrhoids
- Fistula-in-ano
- Skin tags
- Warts (Fig. 50)
- Carcinoma ⚠
- Polyps
- Gonococcal proctitis

FAECAL SOILING

- Incontinence
- Poor hygiene
- Diarrhoea

SKIN DISEASE

- Candidiasis
- Tinea cruris
- Lichen sclerosus
- Contact dermatitis
- Scabies
- Psoriasis
- Eczema

PARASITES

- Threadworms

PSYCHOGENIC

- Anxiety

HISTORY

Anal discharge

Any cause within the anus or lower rectum that produces moisture and sogginess of the anal skin may cause pruritus ani. Patients may volunteer the information that they have haemorrhoids or perianal warts. They may have noticed an anal discharge, which soils the underwear. Check for a history of anal sexual exposure.

Faecal soiling

The patient may complain of incontinence. This may be associated with poor hygiene. Chronic diarrhoea may be responsible. There may be an underlying cause for the chronic diarrhoea, e.g. colitis or Crohn's disease. Excessive sweating in hot weather may be associated with pruritus ani.

Skin diseases

If the patient is diabetic or immunosuppressed, candidiasis may be responsible. Recent oral antibiotic therapy may result in candidiasis. Check whether the patient has an itchy rash anywhere else. This may be particularly so with scabies or eczema. Contact dermatitis may result from the use of deodorants or a change in washing powder for the underwear. Psoriasis is not usually itchy but sometimes considerable itching occurs, especially if the area becomes infected. Lichen sclerosus is uncommon, occurring chiefly in women, when it may involve both the vulva and the perineum. In men, this may be associated with balanitis xerotica obliterans; so enquire if there is any abnormality of the foreskin.

Parasites

Threadworms usually occur in children. The parents may have noticed them.

Psychogenic

Idiopathic pruritus may occur in people with anxiety states. An itch–scratch cycle may occur, which is difficult to break.

EXAMINATION

Anal discharge

Inspection of the anus may show skin tags, the external opening of a fistula-in-ano, perianal warts or haemorrhoids. Digital rectal examination may reveal a carcinoma of the anal canal or fibrous anal polyps. Proctoscopy and sigmoidoscopy will confirm any associated anal or rectal lesion. Take a swab if purulent discharge.

Faecal soiling

Soiling of the underwear may be apparent. General poor hygiene may also be apparent in the patient. Carry out a digital rectal examination to check for sphincteric tone.

Skin diseases

Candidiasis may occur in those on long-term antibiotics, diabetics and the immunosuppressed. Tinea cruris is more common in men. The infection often involves the groin and perineum in addition to the perianal areas. The patient may also have co-existing tinea pedis. With lichen sclerosus, there are well-defined plaques of superficial atrophy of the epidermis with a whitish colour. In the male, check the penis for balanitis xerotica obliterans. With contact dermatitis, there may be changes in the skin in other areas apart from the perianal area. With scabies, there are usually lesions on other parts of the body. Burrows 5–10 mm deep appear as long ridges, which may be 'S'-shaped. Isolation of the organism with a pin and examination under the microscope will confirm the diagnosis. With psoriasis, there will usually be lesions on other areas of the body, and this will also be so with eczema.

Parasites

Threadworms may be visible around the anus.

Psychogenic

There may be an obvious history of psychiatric illness or the patient may appear anxious or depressed.

GENERAL INVESTIGATIONS

- **FBC, ESR**
  These are usually normal.
- **Urinalysis**
  Positive for sugar – diabetic.

- ■ Blood glucose
  Diabetic.

SPECIFIC INVESTIGATIONS

- ■ Stool culture
  Ova, parasites and cysts, cause of diarrhoea.
- ■ Anal swab
  Gram stain – Gram-negative intracellular diplococci in gonorrhoea.
- ■ Skin scrapings
  For mycotic infection, microscopy and culture.
- ■ Nocturnal 'Sellotape swab'
  Threadworms.
- ■ Biopsy
  Anal carcinoma. Lichen sclerosus.

- • Always perform a digital rectal examination.
- • Perianal candidiasis suggests diabetes. Check the blood sugar.
- • Perianal warts imply an STD. Refer to a GUM clinic.
- • Suspicious anal lesions should be biopsied to exclude anal cancer.

PYREXIA OF UNKNOWN ORIGIN

Most pyrexias result from a clearly defined illness, e.g. acute pyelonephritis or acute appendicitis, or from self-limiting viral infections, e.g. common cold. Pyrexia of unknown origin is defined as a temperature >38.3°C on several occasions, accompanied by more than three weeks of illness and failure to reach a diagnosis after one week of inpatient investigation. Most cases of pyrexia of unknown origin are unusual presentations of common diseases, e.g. tuberculosis, endocarditis, rather than rare or exotic illnesses.

CAUSES

BACTERIAL

- Abscess, e.g. subphrenic, pelvic
- Subacute bacterial endocarditis
- TB
- Brucellosis
- Typhoid
- Leptospirosis
- Q fever
- Cat scratch disease

VIRAL

- Influenza
- Infectious mononucleosis syndromes
- HIV

FUNGAL

- Candidiasis
- Aspergillosis
- *Pneumocystis jirovecii* (formerly *carinii*)

PROTOZOAL

- Malaria ● *(common in Africa)*
- Amoebiasis
- Toxoplasmosis

NEOPLASIA

- Hypernephroma
- Lymphoma
- Hepatoma
- Acute leukaemia

CONNECTIVE TISSUE DISEASE

- Rheumatoid arthritis
- SLE
- Polyarteritis nodosa and other vasculitis
- Temporal arteritis

GRANULOMATOUS DISEASE

- Crohn's disease
- Sarcoidosis

OTHERS

- Post-immunisation
- Drug induced
- Familial Mediterranean fever
- Munchausen's disease (factitious)

HISTORY

A full and extensive history should be taken, noting especially travel abroad, contact with infection, contact with animals, bites, abrasions, rashes, diarrhoea. Check the drug history, including non-prescription drugs and drug abuse. Check for any recent history of surgery, particularly abdominal surgery. Is there any history of recent immunisations? Has the patient experienced night sweats, weight loss and general malaise?

EXAMINATION

A full physical examination should be carried out. This should be directed at every system of the body, checking particularly for lymphadenopathy and hepatosplenomegaly. Rectal and vaginal examination should be carried out.

INVESTIGATIONS

It may be necessary to carry out numerous and repeated investigations. It may also be necessary to withhold any drugs one at a time, to see if the temperature settles.

GENERAL INVESTIGATIONS

- FBC, CRP/ESR
  Hb ↓ malignancy, anaemia of chronic disease, e.g. rheumatoid arthritis. WCC ↑ infection, leukaemia. Lymphocytes ↑ viral infection. Platelets ↓ leukaemia. CRP/ESR ↑ malignancy, connective tissue disease, TB.

- U&Es
  Connective tissue disease affecting the kidneys.

- LFTs
  Biliary tract or liver disease, e.g. cholangitis, hepatitis.

- Blood glucose
  Diabetes – infections are more common in diabetics.

- Blood culture
  Repeat cultures separated by time and location should be taken.
  Streptococcus viridans is classical for infective endocarditis. Isolation
  of coliforms suggests the possibility of intra-abdominal sepsis.

- Viral antibodies
  Hepatitis B, hepatitis C, EBV (~90% of infectious mononucleosis),
  CMV (~7% of infectious mononucleosis), HIV.

- Sputum culture
  Microscopy for mycobacteria and C&S.

- Urine microscopy and culture
  Microscopic haematuria in endocarditis. Haematuria in
  hypernephroma and blood dyscrasias. White cells – infection.
  Granular or red cell casts – renal inflammation, e.g. connective
  tissue disease. Proteinuria suggests renal disease.

- Stool culture and microscopy
  C&S. Ova, parasites and cysts on microscopy.

- CXR
  TB. Atypical pneumonia. Pneumonitis associated with HIV and
  Pneumocystis jiroveci. Secondary deposits. Hilar glands associated
  with sarcoidosis, TB and lymphoma.

- ECG
  Cardiac disease.

SPECIFIC INVESTIGATIONS

- Rheumatoid factor
  Rheumatoid arthritis.

- Serological tests
  Q fever, brucellosis, leptospirosis.

- Autoantibodies
  Connective tissue disease.

- Mantoux test
  TB.

- Antistreptolysin O titre
  Rheumatic fever.

- Bone marrow aspirate
  Leukaemia. Myeloma.

- Lumbar puncture
  White cells and organisms – meningitis. Blood – subarachnoid
  haemorrhage. Protein – Guillain–Barré syndrome.

- US abdomen
  Intraperitoneal abscesses.

- **Echocardiogram**
  Infective endocarditis.
- **Labelled white cell scan**
  Localised infection/abscess.
- **Liver biopsy**
  Hepatitis.
- **Renal biopsy**
  Glomerular disease. Malignancy.
- **Muscle biopsy**
  Myositis.
- **CT**
  Infection. Malignancy.
- **Diagnostic laparoscopy**
  This may be necessary to exclude intra-abdominal sepsis.

- **Pyrexia of unknown origin presents a diagnostic challenge. Clinical signs are often non-specific and may fluctuate in severity and alter with chronicity.**
- **Empirical treatment is not advocated in cases of pyrexia of unknown origin with the following exceptions: cases meeting the criteria for culture-negative endocarditis; those suggestive of cryptic disseminated TB and in which temporal arteritis is suspected.**

RECTAL BLEEDING

Rectal bleeding is a common symptom. The majority of patients with rectal bleeding have a simple condition such as haemorrhoids, but the symptoms should always be taken seriously and investigated. Rectal bleeding with a change in bowel habit or weight loss should be regarded as due to colorectal cancer until proved otherwise.

Figure 51 Carcinoma of the rectum. An ulcerated carcinoma arising from the lower rectum close to and invading the anal canal. Note the raised everted edges.

CAUSES

ANUS

- Haemorrhoids
- Fissure-in-ano
- Carcinoma ⚠
- Trauma ⚠

COLON AND RECTUM

- Carcinoma (Fig. 51) ⚠
- Polyps
- Diverticular disease
- Inflammatory bowel disease
  - Ulcerative colitis
  - Crohn's disease
- Ischaemic colitis ⚠
- Rectal prolapse
- Angiodysplasia
- Irradiation colitis or proctitis
- Solitary rectal ulcer

SMALL BOWEL

- Meckel's diverticulum
- Intussusception ⚠
- Mesenteric infarction ⚠
- Aortoenteric fistula ⚠

UPPER GASTROINTESTINAL TRACT

- Massive haemorrhage, e.g. duodenal ulcer ⚠

OTHERS

- Anticoagulants
- Bleeding diatheses

HISTORY

Anus

Haemorrhoids

Piles occur at any age. Bleeding from piles is noted either on the toilet paper or as splashes in the toilet after defecation. Uncomplicated piles are not painful.

Fissure-in-ano

Fissure-in-ano is most common under the age of 40 years. It is quite common in children. The patient experiences pain on defecation, which may persist for minutes or hours afterwards. Constipation is usually a precipitating cause, the constipation being made worse by the fissure as the patient avoids defecation because of pain. Blood is noticed on the toilet paper or streaked on the stool.

Carcinoma of the anal canal

Carcinoma of the anal canal usually occurs in the elderly. It presents with pain on defecation and streaking of blood on the stools and blood on the toilet paper. Initially, in the early stages, it may be mistaken for a fissure-in-ano.

Trauma

There may be a history of a penetrating injury to the anal canal. Sexual abuse or homosexual practices may be relevant.

Colorectal

Carcinoma

With colonic carcinoma, the blood may be mixed with the stool. There is usually a history of accompanying change in bowel habit and colicky abdominal pain. With rectal cancer, the blood is usually streaked on the stool and there may be a history of tenesmus, i.e. a sense of incomplete evacuation of the rectum.

Polyps

The history may be similar to that of carcinoma.

Diverticular disease

Bleeding associated with diverticular disease is typically acute, massive and fresh. There may be a past history of diverticular disease.

Inflammatory bowel disease

With ulcerative colitis and Crohn's disease, there is often sudden onset of diarrhoea with watery, brown motions containing mucus and fresh blood. There is usually colicky abdominal pain. With ulcerative proctitis, the patient may complain of tenesmus.

Ischaemic colitis

This usually occurs in the elderly. There is colicky abdominal pain associated with the passage of dark-red venous blood PR.

Angiodysplasia

The patient is usually elderly. There is bleeding PR, which may be torrential but is more often repeated small bleeds.

Irradiation proctitis or colitis

There will be a history of irradiation, often for carcinoma of the cervix. The patient passes blood and mucus PR and complains of tenesmus.

Rectal prolapse

The patient will be aware of something hanging out of the back passage that comes down on defecation. Bleeding is due to trauma.

Solitary rectal ulcer

Bleeding occurs after defecation, usually in small volumes. This may be associated with mucus discharge and a feeling of a lump in the anus.

Small bowel

Meckel's diverticulum

This usually results in painless bleeding in young adults. The blood tends to be dark red and may on occasions have the characteristics of melaena.

Intussusception

This usually occurs in infants, but may rarely occur at any age. The child has colicky abdominal pain and draws the legs up, screams and passes a stool consisting of mixed blood and mucus ('redcurrant jelly' stool).

Mesenteric infarction

The patient is usually elderly, or a younger patient who has a history of heart disease (embolism). The patient develops severe central abdominal, colicky pain associated with diffuse tenderness and later collapse and shock.

Aortoenteric fistula

This usually occurs following repair of an infrarenal aortic aneurysm with a Dacron graft. The Dacron graft becomes infected; the fistula forms between the aorta and duodenum. Depending on the speed of the bleed, there may be either melaena or profuse red rectal haemorrhage with shock.

Upper gastrointestinal tract

Massive haemorrhage from the upper gastrointestinal tract, e.g. bleeding oesophageal varices, duodenal ulcer, may present with bright-red bleeding PR. This is due to extremely fast intestinal transit and the patient will always be shocked.

Others

Check for a history of anticoagulants. The patient may have a bleeding disorder. Check for bleeding from other sites or spontaneous bruising.

EXAMINATION

Anus

Haemorrhoids

There may be obvious prolapsed haemorrhoids; however, sigmoidoscopy and proctoscopy are usually required to make the diagnosis.

Fissure-in-ano

Separate the buttocks. A chronic fissure-in-ano with a sentinel pile may be seen in the midline posteriorly, or more rarely, in the midline anteriorly. Digital rectal examination, if attempted, will be extremely painful.

Carcinoma

This may show a hard ulcer in the anal canal with everted edges; however, in the early stages, carcinoma of the anal canal may be difficult to distinguish from a chronic fissure-in-ano. Biopsy should be undertaken.

Trauma

Bruising may be apparent around the anal canal. There may be a split in the skin or mucosa. Digital rectal examination will be painful.

Colon and rectum

Carcinoma

An abdominal mass may be palpable. There may be signs of intestinal obstruction. Digital rectal examination may reveal a hard, irregular, ulcerating mass.

Polyps

A polyp may be palpable in the rectum. There may be no findings on physical examination.

Diverticular disease

The patient may be tender in the left iliac fossa. Often, there are no abdominal findings.

Inflammatory bowel disease

There may be a palpable abdominal mass with Crohn's disease. There may be localised abdominal tenderness. If toxic dilatation has occurred, the abdomen will be distended and tender, and there may be signs of peritonitis if perforation has occurred.

Ischaemic colitis

Physical examination may show left-sided abdominal tenderness and the patient may be shocked.

Angiodysplasia

There may be little to find other than rectal bleeding. There are usually no abdominal signs.

Irradiation colitis or proctitis

There may be some abdominal tenderness. Digital rectal examination will reveal a granular mucosa and blood on the glove.

Rectal prolapse

There will be obvious prolapse of the rectum with ulcerated, bleeding rectal mucosa.

Solitary rectal ulcer

There are no abdominal findings. Digital rectal examination may give the impression of a polypoid swelling just inside the rectum, which may be mistaken for carcinoma. Proctoscopy will reveal redness and oedema of the mucosa and, in about 50% of patients, frank ulceration will be noted.

Small bowel

Meckel's diverticulum

There will usually be nothing to find on abdominal examination.

Intussusception

A mass may be palpable in the right iliac fossa. Eventually, as the intussusception proceeds, the right iliac fossa becomes 'empty'.

Mesenteric infarction

The patient may be in atrial fibrillation and this suggests embolism. There will be diffuse abdominal tenderness, later accompanied by collapse and shock.

Aortoenteric fistula

There will usually be the long midline scar of a recent aortic aneurysm repair. Otherwise, there will be little to find on abdominal examination.

Upper gastrointestinal tract

Massive haemorrhage

There may be signs of liver failure associated with a massive bleed from varices. There may be epigastric tenderness associated with duodenal ulceration.

Others

With anticoagulants, there may be bleeding from other orifices, as may also occur with bleeding diatheses. Look for signs of bruising. Rectal bleeding from collagen diseases is rare. Polyarteritis nodosa is probably the most common. Bleeding is due to necrotising vasculitis and there may be signs of vasculitis elsewhere, e.g. skin.

GENERAL INVESTIGATIONS

- **FBC, ESR**
  Hb ↓ may occur in almost any type of rectal bleeding. WCC ↑ inflammatory bowel disease, ischaemic colitis, aortoenteric fistula. ESR ↑ carcinoma, collagen disease.

- **U&Es**
  Urea and creatinine raised with uraemic bleeding. The urea may be raised due to absorption of blood from the bowel. Usually in this case, the creatinine is normal.

- **LFTs, coagulation screem**
  Liver failure associated with oesophageal varices. In addition, a coagulation should be considered if on anticoagulants.

- **Venous lactate**
  Raised lactate with ischaemic colitis.

- **Sigmoidoscopy/proctoscopy**
  Anorectal tumours. Haemorrhoids. Distal colitis. Solitary rectal ulcer. Biopsy.

SPECIFIC INVESTIGATIONS

- **Colonoscopy (inc virtual colonscopy)**
  Diverticular disease. Colonic tumours. Angiodysplasia. Colitis.

- **CT Angiography (in the bleeding phase)**
  Angiodysplasia. Bleeding Meckel's diverticulum.

- **Upper GI endoscopy**
  If a major upper GI bleed is suspected.

- **Examination under anaesthesia (EUA)**
  Haemorrhoids. Fissure-in-ano. Prolapse.

- **Labelled red cell scan**
  Angiodysplasia. Meckel's diverticulum.

- **Technetium scan**
  Meckel's diverticulum.

- Always do a digital rectal examination and sigmoidoscopy.
- Change of bowel habit and weight loss in association with rectal bleeding require urgent investigation.
- In a child presenting with rectal bleeding with no obvious cause, always consider non-accidental injury.

SCALP LESIONS

Lesions on the scalp are common; the most common are sebaceous cysts, which are often multiple.

Figure 52 A large epidermal cyst (sebaceous cyst) of the scalp.

CAUSES

TRAUMATIC

- Haematoma
- Cephalhaematoma

CYSTIC

- Sebaceous cysts (epidermal cysts) (Fig. 52)

NEOPLASTIC

BENIGN

- Ivory osteoma

MALIGNANT

Primary

- Basal cell carcinoma ⚠
- Squamous cell carcinoma ⚠
- Malignant melanoma ⚠
- Leukaemia
- Myeloma

Secondary

- Breast
- Bronchus
- Thyroid
- Prostate
- Kidney

INFECTIVE

- Scalp abscess
- Tinea capitis
- Cock's peculiar tumour

OTHER

- Psoriasis
- Seborrhoeic dermatitis

HISTORY

Traumatic

Check for a history of trauma. A boggy haematoma may overlie a skull fracture. A cephalhaematoma is seen in a newborn baby. It follows a traumatic delivery. The haematoma is below the periosteum of the skull.

Sebaceous cyst

These may be multiple. The patient usually notices them when combing the hair. These may get infected resulting in an abscess.

Neoplastic

With an ivory osteoma, the patient may notice a rock-hard swelling on the scalp. The patient is usually a young adult and is asymptomatic. Malignant ulcers may occur on the scalp. The patient will notice a lesion when combing the hair and bleeding may occur. These lesions present earlier in bald patients. Bony tenderness and swelling may be a presenting symptom of secondary deposits. There may be a history of a primary, or a careful history must be taken to establish the site of a primary.

Infective

With Cock's peculiar tumour, the patient may notice a sore, bleeding lesion on the scalp. Cock's peculiar tumour is due to a sebaceous cyst suppurating and granulation tissue appearing on its surface. It may be mistaken for a squamous cell carcinoma. Tinea capitis usually occurs in childhood. There is an itchy, red, scaly patch on the scalp and the hairs break easily, leaving patches of stubble.

Other

Psoriasis may affect the scalp. There is usually a history of lesions elsewhere on the body. Seborrhoeic dermatitis presents with a fine, scaly rash on the scalp. Hair growth is usually normal with both these lesions.

EXAMINATION

Traumatic

A knock on the head may cause a boggy haematoma. CT of the head may be required to exclude an underlying fracture. Cephalhaematoma occurs in the newborn; the haematoma spreads beneath the periosteum of the skull and is therefore limited by the skull suture lines.

Sebaceous cyst

Sebaceous cysts are spherical, tender, firm swellings in the scalp. They may be multiple. A punctum may be visible with sebaceous cysts on the scalp.

Neoplastic

An ivory osteoma is a bony, hard, smooth swelling, arising from the outer table of the skull. The skin is freely mobile over it. A squamous cell carcinoma presents as an ulcer with a hard, everted edge. A malignant melanoma is usually pigmented, ulcerated and bleeds. In both these conditions, cervical lymphadenopathy may be present. A basal cell carcinoma is a raised ulcer with a rolled edge with a pearly appearance, often with superficial telangiectasia. Lesions in the skull may be secondaries from lung, breast, thyroid, prostate and kidney. Each of these areas should be examined for a possible primary. Myeloma may present with painful lesions in the skull. There may be areas of localised tenderness.

Infective

Cock's peculiar tumour presents as an open, granulating sebaceous cyst. It appears angry and swollen and may be mistaken for a squamous cell carcinoma. In tinea capitis, there are red, scaly patches on the scalp, with broken hairs giving a stubbled appearance.

Other

With psoriasis, there are well-demarcated areas of scales heaped up over red plaque. The hair grows normally through the plaques. Check for psoriatic lesions elsewhere. Seborrhoeic dermatitis shows fine scales but the hairs remain intact.

GENERAL INVESTIGATIONS

The diagnosis of most of these lesions is made on clinical examination alone.

- ■ FBC, ESR, CRP
  WCC & CRP ↑ in infected cyst. Hb ↓ malignancy. WCC ↑ leukaemia.
  ESR ↑ myeloma and other malignancies.

- ■ Scalp scrapings
  Fungal infection, e.g. tinea capitis.

- ■ Biopsy
  Malignant lesions. Cock's peculiar tumour.

SPECIFIC INVESTIGATIONS

- ■ CXR
  Primary tumour. Secondary malignancy, e.g. secondaries from malignant melanoma.

- ■ Skull X-ray
  Fracture. Ivory osteoma. Pepper-pot skull – myeloma. Secondary deposits – osteolytic from lung, breast and thyroid. Osteosclerotic from prostate and occasionally kidney.

- ■ Serum protein electrophoresis
  Monoclonal gammopathy with myeloma.

- ■ Bone scan
  Bony secondaries.

- • The scalp is a common site of tumour, especially in elderly, bald men and those with outside occupations. Biopsy is essential to confirm the diagnosis.

SCROTAL PAIN

This may be due to lesions on the scrotal skin, within the scrotum, or may, rarely, be due to referred pain. It is important to make rapid diagnosis of emergencies, such as torsion and gangrene, and swiftly referred for surgery.

Figure 53 Fournier's scrotal gangrene. This 64-year-old diabetic presented with scrotal pain and high pyrexia. Within a few hours of admission, black necrotic areas appeared on the scrotum.

CAUSES

SKIN

- Infected sebaceous cyst
- Irritation (urine/faeces in the incontinent)
- Dermatitis
- Herpes simplex
- Behçet's disease
- Fournier's gangrene (Fig. 53) ⚠

INTERNAL SCROTAL SWELLINGS

- Strangulated hernia ⚠
- Testicular torsion ⚠
- Epididymo-orchitis
- Torsion of testicular appendage ⚠
- Haematocele
- Varicocele

REFERRED

- Groin strain
- Ilioinguinal nerve entrapment after hernia repair
- Idiopathic cord neuralgia
- Spinal nerve irritation

HISTORY

Skin

Irritation

The patient may have noticed a skin lesion, which is itchy, sore or painful. In the elderly, confused and incontinent, pain and soreness may be due to the irritant effect of faeces and urine with superadded infection.

Sebaceous cyst

Previous history of a superficial swelling may suggest an infected sebaceous cyst. There may be a history to suggest contact dermatitis. Painful vesicular lesions may suggest herpes. Behçet's syndrome may cause painful ulcerative lesions of the scrotum and the patient may also have similar lesions on the penis. Fournier's gangrene usually has acute onset in a young, healthy male with rapid progression to gangrene of the skin. There is often absence of a discernible cause.

Internal scrotal swellings

Indirect inguinal hernia

There may be a previous history of an inguinal hernia descending into the scrotum. Sudden onset of colicky abdominal pain and irreducibility may suggest the development of a strangulated inguinal hernia.

Testicular torsion

Sudden onset of pain, redness and swelling in the scrotum or groin of a teenager or young male suggests a diagnosis of testicular torsion. It is rare over 25 years of age. This may come on during vigorous exercise, straining, lifting or even masturbation. The pain may also radiate to the lower abdomen. This may be accompanied by nausea and vomiting. Always ascertain the exact time of onset of symptoms. To ensure testicular salvage, surgery should be performed within 6–8 hours of onset of symptoms. This is a surgical emergency and needs urgent surgery.

Epididymo orchitis

Gradual onset of unilateral pain, redness, swelling and tenderness will suggest epididymo-orchitis. Check for symptoms of urinary tract infection, e.g. dysuria or frequency, which may accompany epididymo-orchitis. Orchitis may be associated with mumps and this may be apparent, the patient complaining of bilateral painful parotid and submandibular glands, together with painful cervical lymphadenopathy and constitutional illness.

Haematocele

This is a collection of blood between the layers of the tunica vaginalis. A history of trauma will suggest haematocele.

Varicocele

A dull ache, often poorly localised, to the scrotum or groin. The patient (or partner) may notice varicose veins in the scrotum. Subfertility may be a presentation and is associated with bilateral varicoceles. A varicocele is more common on the left.

Referred pain

Rarely, the patient may complain of pain in the scrotum, with no visible or palpable abnormality. Check for a history of previous inguinal hernia repair, which may have resulted in ilioinguinal nerve entrapment. Idiopathic cord neuralgia may occur but is rare. Occasionally 'groin strain' may cause scrotal pain. Referred pain from spinal lesions may rarely cause scrotal pain.

EXAMINATION

Skin

A red, scaly lesion will suggest dermatitis. There may be superadded infection. In the elderly and incontinent, the diagnosis of irritation from urine or faeces will usually be apparent. An infected sebaceous cyst will present as a localised, tender, red swelling on the scrotum. There may be purulent discharge. Herpes simplex will present with vesicular lesions. They may be present elsewhere, e.g. on the penis. Behçet's disease will present with painful ulcerative lesions on the scrotum as well as on the penis. There may be other signs of Behçet's disease, e.g. arthritis, keratitis, iritis, mouth ulcers. With Fournier's gangrene, there is usually a tense, glossy oedema developing over the scrotum. Crepitations develop later before subcutaneous gangrene occurs. The gangrene may spread over the inguinal area and the lower abdominal wall. In the advanced case, the skin will have completely disappeared, leaving the testes hanging naked in the scrotum.

Internal scrotal swellings

Inguinal hernia

There may be a tense, tender scrotal mass, which is impossible to 'get above'. This would suggest a strangulated hernia.

Testicular torsion

The presence of an enlarged tender testicle drawn up towards the groin suggests testicular torsion. The scrotal skin is usually hot, red and oedematous.

Epididymo-orchitis

An enlarged tender testis with scrotal redness and oedema suggests epididymo-orchitis. The erythema may be initially confined to the epididymis; however it may spread to involve the entire testis. The parotid and submandibular glands should be checked to exclude mumps. Occasionally, torsion of a testicular appendage may occur and cause pain and scrotal swelling out of all proportion to the size of the lesion, which may be less than a few millimetres in diameter.

Haematocele

A tender swelling with scrotal bruising and oedema following trauma will suggest a haematocele.

Varicocele

A varicocele may not be obvious until the patient has been standing up for 10–15 seconds. Classically, it feels like a 'bag of worms' with the warm blood filling dilated veins, which are palpable through the scrotal skin. It is more common on the left-hand side. Rapid onset of a left-sided varicocele may be associated with carcinoma of the left kidney, the tumour growing down the left renal vein and obstructing the left testicular vein. Examine the abdomen for a left renal mass.

Haematocele

There is a tense, tender, fluctuant swelling. There may be obvious scrotal bruising. The testis cannot be felt separately as the blood surrounds it within the layers of the tunica vaginalis.

Referred pain

Check for the scar of an inguinal hernia repair. In ilioinguinal nerve entrapment, there will be anaesthesia/paraesthesia below the scar and on the anterior aspect of the scrotal skin. In the rare case where scrotal pain may be referred from a spinal lesion, a full neurological examination should be carried out. Examine the lumbosacral spine for localised tenderness.

GENERAL INVESTIGATIONS

- **FBC, ESR, CRP**
  WCC & CRP ↑ infection. ESR ↑ infection, tumour.
- **MSU**
  Urinary tract infection associated with epididymo-orchitis.
- **Swab**
  Ulcer, C&S.
- **US testes**
  Testicular lesion. Haematocele.

SPECIFIC INVESTIGATIONS

- **Laser Doppler***
  Check for testicular blood flow. Absent in testicular torsion.

- **Exploratory surgery**
  Diagnostic between torsion and infection. There is rarely the time or equipment to carry out laser Doppler or a technetium scan. If a testicular torsion is not dealt with within six hours of onset, there is likely to be permanent damage to the testis. If there is any doubt in the diagnosis, assume that it is torsion and explore the scrotum surgically.

- **Technetium scan**
  Testicular torsion (no outline of testis) versus epididymo-orchitis (good testicular blood flow).

- **US abdomen**
  Left renal carcinoma (varicocele).

- **Lumbosacral spine X-ray**
  Referred pain due to degenerative disease or metastases.

- **MRI**
  Spinal lesion.

*There is rarely time or equipment to carry out these investigations. If there is any doubt about the diagnosis, assume that it is torsion and explore the scrotum surgically.

- **It is difficult, if not impossible, to distinguish between torsion and epididymo-orchitis. Urgent referral and surgical exploration are required.**

SCROTAL SWELLINGS

Scrotal swellings are a common presenting complaint in the outpatient clinic. It is also important to distinguish between those swellings that have underlying serious pathology (testicular tumour) and those that are simple and benign (epididymal cysts).

Figure 54 Epididymal cyst. The swelling is being transilluminated. *A 3 cm soft rounded swelling of the upper pole of epididymis can be seen. The fact that it transilluminates confirms the presence of an epididymal cyst containing clear fluid. A spermatocele, because of its opaque contents, does not transilluminate.*

CAUSES

- Sebaceous cyst
- Indirect inguinal hernia
- Hydrocele
- Epididymal cyst (spermatocele) (Fig. 54)
- Epididymo-orchitis
- Testicular torsion ⚠

- Testicular tumour ⚠
- Varicocele
- Haematocele
- Sperm granuloma
- TB ● *(common where TB is endemic)*
- Gumma

HISTORY

Please also refer to the chapter on scrotal pain.

Sebaceous cyst

The patient may complain of several painful lumps on the scrotal skin. There may be a history of one or more of them becoming red, inflamed and tender with discharge.

Indirect inguinal hernia

The patient will be often aware of a lump in their groin. They may be able to reduce it. The hernia may present with a painful, irreducible swelling and signs of intestinal obstruction.

Hydrocele

An idiopathic hydrocele usually presents as a painless scrotal swelling, which may become quite large. They usually occur over the age of 50 years. Occasionally, there may be pain and discomfort if there is underlying testicular disease. A younger patient presenting with a hydrocele should raise the suspicion of an underlying malignancy.

Epididymal cyst

This presents as a painless scrotal swelling. Epididymal cysts may slowly enlarge over many years. They may be bilateral.

Testicular tumour

Teratomas occur between 18 and 30 years, seminomas between 30 and 45 years. The common presentation is a feeling of heaviness in the scrotum accompanied by a painless swelling. Occasionally, symptoms are due to secondary deposits, e.g. abdominal pain from enlarged retroperitoneal lymph nodes. Occasionally, distant lymphadenopathy, e.g. cervical, may be a presenting symptom.

Sperm granuloma

This may develop 2–4 months after vasectomy. The patient will complain of a small tender nodule at the site of vasectomy.

TB

This is now rare in the UK. A scrotal lump with associated dull, aching pain is the usual presentation. There may be a history of pulmonary or renal TB. There may be malaise, weight loss, haemoptysis or haematuria.

Gumma

This is extremely rare. There is a painless swelling of the testis. It needs to be distinguished from a testicular tumour. Other signs of syphilis may be present.

EXAMINATION

Sebaceous cyst

A small swelling or multiple small swellings occur in the scrotal skin. They are tense and spherical. Because of the thinness of the scrotal skin stretched over the swelling, the cheesy yellow material contained within them can be seen. There may be a small punctum surmounting the cyst.

Indirect inguinal hernia

Hernias that descend in the scrotum are invariably indirect. They may be reducible. It is impossible to get above the swelling. There is an expansile cough impulse, and bowel sounds may be heard over the hernia.

Hydrocele

A hydrocele is usually unilateral. It may become very large. A hydrocele is fluctuant, transilluminates and is dull to percussion. If large enough, there may be a fluid thrill. The testis cannot be palpated separately from the hydrocele. It is possible to get above the swelling except with infantile hydroceles, when the fluid extends up to the deep inguinal ring.

Epididymal cyst

An epididymal cyst usually occurs above and behind the testis. The testis can be palpated separately from it. An epididymal cyst frequently feels lobulated because often the fluid is in locules. They are fluctuant. Those containing clear fluid transilluminate. Those containing a milky opalescent fluid are called spermatoceles and do not transilluminate.

Testicular tumour

There is a firm, irregular swelling in the scrotum. Often the patient notices the lump when it is very small, but in other cases it may become very large before the patient presents. Rarely the tumour has been allowed to advance so far that it is attached to the scrotal skin. Check for palpable para-aortic nodes. Examine the cervical nodes, especially in the left supraclavicular fossa. Testicular tumours metastasise to the para-aortic nodes, to the mediastinal nodes, and occasionally into the cervical nodes. Inguinal nodes are not involved unless the tumour has invaded the scrotal skin, which is rare.

Sperm granuloma

There is a small, tender, painful nodule at the site of previous vasectomy.

Tuberculosis

The swelling is usually confined to the epididymis, where there is a hard lump. The spermatic cord and vas are thickened. Occasionally, a sinus may have formed. Check the chest for signs of pulmonary TB. Check the neck for scars (lymph node drainage for cold abscess) or lymphadenopathy.

Gumma

A gumma is a painless swelling of the whole testis. Other signs of syphilis may be present.

GENERAL INVESTIGATIONS

■ **FBC, ESR, CRP**
Hb ↓ chronic disease, e.g. TB. WCC & CRP ↑ inflammation, e.g. epididymo-orchitis, torsion. ESR ↑ TB, syphilis, tumour.

■ **Tumour markers**
AFP, βhCG, LDH.

■ **MSU**
UTI associated with epididymo-orchitis.

■ **US**
Solid versus cystic. Hydrocele versus epididymal cyst. Always arrange an ultrasound of the underlying testis in the young patient with a lax hydrocele as there may be an underlying tumour.

SPECIFIC INVESTIGATIONS

■ **CXR**
TB. Secondary deposits from testicular tumour.

■ **US abdomen**
Carcinoma of left kidney invading the left renal vein, associated with left varicocele.

■ **EMSU**
TB.

■ **VDRL**
Gumma.

■ **MRI**
Abdominal and chest MRI scan may confirm lymphadenopathy associated with secondary deposits from testicular tumours.

- A hydrocele in a fit young male should raise the suspicion of an underlying malignancy. Arrange a US scan.
- A feeling of heaviness, discomfort or a dragging sensation in the scrotum may be presenting symptoms of testicular cancer. Examine the testes carefully. If any doubt, arrange a US scan.

SHOCK

Shock is an abnormality of the circulation that results in inadequate organ perfusion and tissue oxygenation.

CAUSES ⚠ (ALL CAUSES OF SHOCK REQUIRE EMERGENCY ASSESSMENT)

HYPOVOLAEMIC

- Haemorrhage
- Burns
- Gastrointestinal losses

CARDIOGENIC

- Myocardial infarction
- Acute valvular damage
- Arrhythmia

DISTRIBUTIVE

- Sepsis
- Anaphylaxis
- Neurogenic shock (spinal injury)

OBSTRUCTIVE

- Massive pulmonary embolism
- Tension pneumothorax
- Cardiac tamponade

HISTORY

Trauma

Trauma is a pertinent feature in the history, as haemorrhage invariably accompanies penetrating trauma. The site and approximate amount of blood loss should be assessed. Blunt trauma to the chest is associated with tension pneumothorax, myocardial contusion and cardiac tamponade. Trauma to the pelvis and long bones can result in closed fractures, causing significant haemorrhage that may not always be apparent to the observer. Thermal injury can occur with patients involved in fires, water-heater explosions and gas explosions. Acute onset of paralysis following trauma may be due to spinal or peripheral nerve injury. Disruption to the descending sympathetic pathways with spinal injuries results in loss of vasomotor tone and consequently hypotension.

Dyspnoea

Although tachypnoea is a physiological accompaniment to blood loss, when dyspnoea is the predominant symptom you should consider pulmonary oedema from the causes of cardiogenic shock. In addition, dyspnoea is also a prominent feature of all the causes of obstructive shock.

Chest pain

The consequences of blunt trauma to the chest have been described above. In the absence of trauma, the presence of chest pain should lead you to consider myocardial infarction (central crushing) and pulmonary embolism (pleuritic).

Precipitating factors

Occasionally, patients may be aware of allergens that provoke anaphylaxis. In the community, food products (shellfish, eggs, peanuts) and insect venom (bees, wasps) are common causes. In hospital, penicillin, anaesthetic agents and intravenous contrast media are the major provoking factors. Detailed systemic enquiry for presence of infection may elucidate the offending focus for patients in septic shock. A history of profuse vomiting, diarrhoea or intestinal obstruction (vomiting, constipation, colicky abdominal pain and distension) would indicate gastrointestinal losses as the cause for hypovolaemia.

EXAMINATION

Inspection

A thorough systematic inspection should be undertaken; burns and sites of bleeding from penetrating trauma may be obvious. Cyanosis is a feature of large pulmonary emboli and tension pneumothoraces. Patients with anaphylaxis often exhibit angio-oedema and urticaria.

Temperature

Patients in shock are generally cold and clammy. With septic shock, however, the skin is warm to the touch and the patient is usually pyrexial.

Pulse

A tachycardia is the earliest measurable indicator of shock; however, it may not be elevated in cases of neurogenic shock. The character of the pulse is usually weak. The rhythm may suggest an arrhythmia as the precipitating factor in cardiogenic shock. Pulsus paradoxus (decrease in amplitude of the pulse on inspiration) is consistent with cardiac tamponade.

JVP

A low JVP is a useful discriminator for hypovolaemic shock, as it will usually be elevated with all causes of cardiogenic and obstructive shock.

Auscultation

Bronchospasm, and consequently wheezing, may be prominent in anaphylactic shock. Unilateral absent breath sounds indicate a pneumothorax, while muffled heart sounds are features of cardiac tamponade. The presence of a new murmur can be due to acute valvular insufficiency as a cause for cardiogenic shock.

GENERAL INVESTIGATIONS

- **Pulse oximetry**
  Although low saturation per se is not very discriminatory, severe impairment of oxygen saturation is associated with pulmonary embolus and pneumothorax. This may be confirmed with ABGs.

- **FBC**
  With blood loss, a low Hb may be noted, although this will not be evident immediately. A raised WCC occurs with infection. Unfortunately, it will also be raised in most causes of acute physiological stress.

- **U&Es**
  With significant gastrointestinal losses, low serum sodium and potassium accompanied by raised urea and creatinine are the usual abnormalities.

- **ECG**
  The ECG may reveal myocardial infarction or the presence of an arrhythmia as the precipitating aetiology. Electrical alternans (alternating large and small QRS complexes) is a specific indicator of pericardial tamponade. Widespread low-amplitude complexes are common in significant pericardial effusion.

- **CXR**
  May reveal a pneumothorax with deviation of the trachea (although the diagnosis of a tension pneumothorax should be clinical and relieved before a chest X-ray is performed). The cardiac silhouette may be globular in the presence of a pericardial effusion; however, tamponade is still possible with a normal-appearing chest film.

SPECIFIC INVESTIGATIONS

- **Blood cultures**
  Blood and site-specific cultures are essential in suspected septic shock. The underlying organism may be isolated.

- **Echocardiography**
  An echocardiogram will be able to demonstrate valvular dysfunction, the presence of tamponade and massive pulmonary embolism (when right heart failure is present).

- **CT pulmonary angiography**
  For the diagnosis of pulmonary embolism in the presence of shock. Emergency therapeutic measures (such as thrombolysis) may require a formal contrast pulmonary angiogram.

■ CT/MRI spine
May be required to assess the extent and confirm the level of injury.

- When assessing patients in shock, it is important to appreciate that low blood pressure is a relatively late feature.

- In patients with massive haemorrhage, low blood count is also a late feature and cannot be relied upon to assess the initial degree of blood loss.

SPLENOMEGALY

The spleen must be enlarged to about three times its normal size before it becomes clinically palpable. The lower margin may feel notched on palpation. The spleen may become so massive in size that it is palpable in the right iliac fossa. Massive splenomegaly in the UK is likely to be due to chronic myeloid leukaemia, myelofibrosis or lymphoma. Splenomegaly may lead to hypersplenism, i.e. pancytopenia as cells become trapped and destroyed in an overactive spleen.

Figure 55 MRI (sagittal section) of a patient with gross splenomegaly due to chronic myeloid leukaemia. The spleen (arrow) fills virtually the whole of the abdominal cavity. Because of the size of the spleen, the patient could not sit upright.

CAUSES

INFECTIVE

BACTERIAL
- Typhoid
- Tuberculosis
- Leptospirosis

Septicaemia

Abscess

VIRAL

Infectious mononucleosis syndromes (EBV/CMV)

PROTOZOAL

Malaria ● *(common in Africa)*

PARASITIC

Hydatid cyst

INFLAMMATORY

Rheumatoid arthritis (Felty's syndrome)

Sarcoidosis

Lupus

Amyloid

NEOPLASTIC

Metastases

Primary tumours

Leukaemia (Fig. 55)

Lymphoma

Polycythaemia vera

Myelofibrosis

HAEMOLYTIC DISEASE

Hereditary spherocytosis

Acquired haemolytic anaemia

Thrombocytopenic purpura

STORAGE DISEASES

Gaucher's disease

DEFICIENCY DISEASES

Severe iron-deficiency anaemia

Pernicious anaemia

SPLENIC VEIN HYPERTENSION

Cirrhosis

Splenic vein thrombosis

Portal vein thrombosis

NON-PARASITIC CYSTS

HISTORY

Infective

Most infective causes present with fever, malaise and anorexia. With typhus, there will be a history of foreign travel. With typhoid, there will be a history of malaise, headache, fever, cough and diarrhoea. Epistaxis and abdominal pain may occur. TB usually presents with weight loss, night sweats and a cough. If septicaemia is responsible, there will usually be an obvious cause, and the patient may already be hospitalised. With splenic abscess, there may be a history of endocarditis, lung abscess, drug abuse or it may occur if immunocompromised. With malaria, there is usually a history of travel to an area where it is endemic. The patient usually presents within two months of travel abroad with malaise, myalgia, sweating, coldness, followed by rigors, high fever and drenching sweats. Hydatid disease occurs most frequently in rural sheep-farming regions, e.g. Wales. The commonest presentation is with a cyst in the lung causing dyspnoea, haemoptysis or anaphylaxis.

Inflammatory

Rheumatoid arthritis may be apparent. Sarcoidosis may present with lymphadenopathy, fever and malaise, as well as hepatosplenomegaly. Lupus may present with protean manifestations with cutaneous, musculoskeletal, renal, pulmonary and haematological problems. Amyloid may be primary or secondary. There may be cutaneous, cerebral, cardiac or endocrine manifestations. With secondary amyloidosis, there may be a history of chronic infection, e.g. TB or inflammatory disease, e.g. rheumatoid arthritis. There may also be a history of neoplasis. Secondary amyloidosis usually affects the kidney and liver as well as the spleen.

Neoplastic

There will often be generalised signs of malignancy. Often, there will be general malaise with weight loss, and with lymphoma, there will be a history of night sweats. There may also be a tendency to spontaneous bruising. Primary tumours of the spleen and splenic metastases are rare.

Haemolytic disease

Haemolytic disease usually presents with the symptoms of anaemia, namely tiredness and malaise. Jaundice may be present, although is often not very deep, merely giving a lemonish tinge to the skin. With excessive breakdown of red blood cells, pigment stones may form in the gall bladder and the disease may present with acute cholecystitis.

Storage diseases

Apart from variable hepatosplenomegaly, these may present with neurological problems, skeletal deformities or mental deterioration.

Deficiency diseases

There may be a history of pernicious anaemia. Splenomegaly is usually mild. With iron-deficiency anaemia, there may be dietary deficiency, malabsorption or blood loss. Check for a history of blood loss.

Splenic vein hypertension

There may be an obvious history, with cirrhosis and signs of liver failure. Isolated splenic vein thrombosis is rare.

Non-parasitic cysts

These are rare but may arise from organised haematomas, infarcts or inflammation. They are usually isolated findings when the patient is being investigated for other conditions.

EXAMINATION

General

The spleen appears from below the tip of the left tenth rib and enlarges towards the umbilicus. It is firm and smooth and usually has a notch on its upper edge. It moves with respiration, is dull to percussion and it is impossible to get above it.

Infective

With typhoid, there is moderate splenomegaly, the patient being pyrexial with a tender abdomen and with rose spots on the trunk. Again with TB, the splenomegaly is only moderate. There may be chest signs. With septicaemia, there is usually an obvious cause and again there is only moderate splenomegaly. With splenic abscess, again there is only moderate splenomegaly and the spleen may be tender and feel irregular. With glandular fever, the patient will be pyrexial with lymphadenopathy. Splenomegaly is moderate. With leptospirosis ictohaemorrhagica, the patient is usually ill with pyrexia, jaundice and purpuric rash. There may be signs of meningitis. There also may be tender muscles (myositis). There may be signs of acute renal failure. With malaria, there is often anaemia, jaundice and hepatosplenomegaly. With hydatid disease, the liver is usually more affected than the spleen. There may be hepatomegaly in addition to splenomegaly.

Inflammatory

With inflammatory disease, the spleen is rarely grossly enlarged. Changes of rheumatoid arthritis may be apparent elsewhere in the body. With sarcoidosis, there may be lymphadenopathy as well as hepatosplenomegaly. With lupus, there may be cutaneous manifestations as well as musculoskeletal, renal and pulmonary manifestations.

Neoplastic

There may be massive splenomegaly associated with chronic myeloid leukaemia, myelofibrosis and lymphoma. Other signs such as lymphadenopathy and spontaneous bruising may be present.

Haemolytic disease

The patient may have a mild jaundice together with moderate splenomegaly. A purpuric rash may be apparent with thrombocytopenic purpura.

Storage diseases

These are rare. There may be signs of cardiac failure, skeletal deformity or neurological deficits.

Splenic vein hypertension

Signs of liver failure, e.g. spider naevi, liver palms, caput medusae and jaundice, may be present.

Non-parasitic cysts

The only finding may be splenomegaly.

GENERAL INVESTIGATIONS

- FBC, ESR, blood film
  Hb ↓ anaemias. Hb ↑ polycythaemia. WCC ↑ infection, leukaemia, abscess. ESR ↑ infection, malignancy. WCC ↓, platelets ↓ hypersplenism. PCV ↑ polycythaemia. MCV ↑ pernicious anaemia. Blood film – spherocytosis, malaria.

- U&Es
  Urea ↑, creatinine ↑ renal failure, e.g. with leptospirosis, amyloid, septicaemia.

- LFTs
  Cirrhosis

SPECIFIC INVESTIGATIONS

- Rheumatoid factor
  Rheumatoid arthritis.

- Serum iron and serum ferritin
  ↓ iron-deficiency anaemia.

- Parietal cell antibodies
  Pernicious anaemia.

- Serum vitamin B_{12}
  Pernicious anaemia.

- Blood culture
  Septicaemia. Leptospirosis. Typhoid.

- Stool culture
  Typhoid.

- Urine culture
  Typhoid. Leptospirosis.

- CSF culture
  Leptospirosis.

- ■ **Bone marrow aspirate**
  Myelofibrosis. Polycythaemia. Leukaemia. Gaucher's disease.
- ■ **Ultrasound**
  Cause of splenomegaly, e.g. cyst, tumour, diffuse enlargement. Cirrhosis of the liver.
- ■ **CT**
  Causes of splenomegaly, e.g. cyst, tumour, diffuse enlargement, cirrhosis.

> • **The spleen may enlarge massively. Palpation for suspected splenomegaly should begin in the right lower quadrant.**

STEATORRHOEA

Steatorrhoea refers to the passing of excessive amounts of fat in the faeces.

CAUSES

LIPASE DEFICIENCY

- Impaired secretion – chronic pancreatitis
- Inactivation – excess gastric acid

BILE DEFICIENCY

- Underproduction – liver disease
- Obstruction – obstructive jaundice ⚠

MUCOSAL DISEASE

- Coeliac disease
- Ileal resection
- Crohn's disease

IMPAIRED FAT TRANSPORT

- Abetalipoproteinaemia

LYMPHATIC DEFICIENCY

- Lymphoma ⚠
- Whipple's disease

DRUGS

- Orlistat

HISTORY

Patients with steatorrhoea often pass bulky, sticky and greasy stool that floats and is often difficult to flush away. Diarrhoea is the usual accompanying symptom (p. 90) for most of the causes. Jaundice with pale stools and dark urine implies obstruction to the flow of bile, which is essential for the absorption of fat and fat-soluble vitamins. The causes and diagnostic approach to jaundice are found on p. 236.

Abdominal pain

Vague epigastric abdominal pain experienced by patients with chronic pancreatitis may radiate to the back and is usually worse with food. Epigastric pain exacerbated by food may be a symptom of Zollinger–Ellison syndrome, which results in excessive gastric acid production (lowering the pH of gastric chyme), inactivating lipase. It usually presents with symptoms of peptic ulceration refractory to medical treatment. Abdominal pains associated with Crohn's disease are often felt in the right iliac fossa due to regional ileitis.

Associated symptoms

Patients with coeliac disease may also suffer with growth retardation and nutritional deficiencies, causing anaemia and muscle wasting. Other symptoms may include bone fracture due to demineralisation, cerebellar ataxia and peripheral neuropathy. Joint pains, pyrexia, skin pigmentation and peripheral lymphadenopathy are among the varied symptoms of Whipple's disease, resulting from infection with the bacterium *Tropheryma whipplei*. Steatorrhoea is the primary manifestation of intestinal lymphoma. It may be accompanied by abdominal pains and pyrexia and occasionally present with intestinal obstruction. Mouth ulcers, perianal abscesses, right iliac fossa pains and blood PR are some of the symptoms experienced by patients with Crohn's disease. Ataxia and night blindness from retinitis pigmentosa may result from abetalipoproteinaemia, which is caused by the absence of apolipoprotein B and therefore results in defective chylomicron formation.

Past medical history

Previous surgical resection involving the terminal ileum will predispose an individual to malabsorption of fat due to decreased enterohepatic circulation of bile salts. Moreover, with decreased length of absorptive intestine, intestinal transit time decreases and there is a decrease in concomitant fat absorption. Conditions associated with intestinal stasis, hypomotility and decreased gastric acid secretion predispose to intestinal bacterial overgrowth and increased degradation of bile salts.

Drug history

Ask about Orlistat medication used in the treatment of obesity (prevents absorption of fats from the diet).

EXAMINATION

Steatorrhoea is often associated with malabsorption and therefore patients may appear emaciated. Mouth ulcers may be due to Crohn's or coeliac disease. Clubbing is associated with Crohn's, liver cirrhosis, coeliac disease and cystic fibrosis, which is associated with pancreatic exocrine insufficiency. Jaundice may be present with bile duct obstruction and liver disease. Bruising may result from impaired clotting due to vitamin K deficiency. The classical rash of dermatitis herpetiformis may be seen with coeliac disease. Erythema nodosum is a feature of Crohn's disease and may be accompanied by right iliac fossa tenderness, perianal abscesses and fistulae. Hepatomegaly may be found in liver disease, and splenomegaly with intestinal lymphoma.

GENERAL INVESTIGATIONS

- **Faecal fat estimation**
  Stool collections over a period of three days are performed with a diet consisting of $\geq$50 g fat per day. The normal value of faecal fat is <7 g per day.

- **FBC and blood film**
  WCC $\uparrow$ with active inflammation. Acanthocytes are present on the blood film with abetalipoproteinaemia.

- **ESR & CRP**
  $\uparrow$ with acute Crohn's disease.

- **LFTs**
  Bilirubin and alkaline phosphatase $\uparrow$ obstructive jaundice. Transaminases $\uparrow$ liver parenchymal disease. Albumin $\downarrow$ malabsorption syndromes.

- **Blood glucose**
  $\uparrow$ with diabetes, a complication of chronic pancreatitis.

- **Serum amylase**
  Usually normal with chronic pancreatitis, but may be elevated if associated with recurrent acute attacks of pancreatitis.

- **AXR**
  Calcification with chronic pancreatitis.

SPECIFIC INVESTIGATIONS

- **Antigliadin, antiendomysial and antireticulin antibodies**
  To detect coeliac disease.

- **Jejunal biopsy**
  Subtotal villous atrophy and crypt hyperplasia with coeliac disease, which are reversible on a gluten-free diet. Dilated lymphatics and periodic acid-Schiff-positive macrophages in Whipple's disease. Absent villi with lymphocytic infiltration of the lamina propria and histological evidence of malignancy with intestinal lymphoma.

- **Tropheryma whipplei serology**
  Positive in Whipple's disease

- **^{14}C-labelled bile acid breath tests**
  Screening test for bacterial overgrowth.

- **Serum gastrin assay**
  Zollinger–Ellison syndrome.

- **Small bowel enema**
  Strictures, skip lesions, fissures and fistulae with Crohn's disease.

- **Colonoscopy**
  Mucosal hyperaemia, friability, ulceration and contact bleeding with Crohn's disease.

- **CT abdomen**
  Abdominal lymphadenopathy with lymphoma.

- Always take a careful history as the patient may actually complain of diarrhoea. In steatorrhoea, the stool is classically described as pale, fatty and offensive and difficult to flush away. Clear distinction between diarrhoea and steatorrhoea is important.

STRIDOR

Stridor is a high-pitched inspiratory sound produced by upper airway obstruction.

CAUSES

CONGENITAL

- Laryngomalacia (congenital flaccid larynx)

ACQUIRED

- Foreign body ⚠
- Infection ⚠
  - Epiglottitis (green in countries without universal Hib vaccination)
  - Retropharyngeal abscess
- Iatrogenic
  - Post-tracheostomy stenosis
  - Post-intubation stenosis
  - Post-radiotherapy stenosis
  - Post-thyroid surgery
- Goitre
- Laryngeal oedema ⚠
  - Anaphylaxis
  - Inhalational injury
- Cricoarytenoid rheumatoid arthritis
- Relapsing polychondritis
- Fractured larynx ⚠

MALIGNANCY

- Intraluminal obstruction
  - Larynx
  - Trachea
  - Bronchus
- External compression
  - Malignant nodes

BILATERAL VOCAL CORD PALSY

- Brainstem stroke
- Thyroid carcinoma
- Oesophageal carcinoma

HISTORY

Onset

Instantaneous onset of stridor usually implies an inhaled foreign body. This is accompanied by violent bouts of coughing, and a clear history may be obtained from a witness. Stridor indicates partial obstruction, as complete occlusion of the upper airway is silent. Stridor that develops over a period of a few seconds to minutes may be due to laryngeal oedema from an anaphylactic reaction. This may be accompanied by urticaria and facial oedema. Enquiries should immediately determine known allergens and treatment can be initiated without delay. The most common cause of infantile stridor is laryngomalacia. During inspiration, there is extreme infolding of the epiglottis and aryepiglottic folds due to inadequate cartilaginous support. Head flexion aggravates the stridor, whereas patency of the airway is improved by the prone position and head extension. The stridor gradually resolves in most infants within 2–3 months.

Precipitating factors

Iatrogenic causes of stridor may have clear precipitating factors. Tracheal stenosis may complicate a long period of intubation or tracheostomy. Upper airway obstruction occurring immediately after thyroid surgery may be due to laryngeal oedema, haematoma and bilateral recurrent nerve injury. Patients who have been rescued from fires may suffer inhalation injuries due to the high temperature of inhaled gases.

Associated symptoms

Respiratory obstruction may occur with massive enlargement of the tonsils, e.g. in glandular fever, or when complicated by a retropharyngeal abscess. Patients may notice swelling of the neck in the presence of a goitre and may be euthyroid or complain of symptoms of abnormal thyroid function (p. 169). Symptoms of joint pains, stiffness and deformities occur with rheumatoid arthritis. Associated stridor can result from cricoarytenoid involvement. Weight loss can be an accompanying feature of malignancy. Hoarseness of the voice is an early symptom of laryngeal carcinoma; stridor occurs as a late feature. Chronic cough with haemoptysis in a chronic smoker usually heralds the onset of bronchial carcinoma. The location of the carcinoma may alter the quality of the wheeze. Partial intraluminal upper airway obstruction from bronchial carcinoma produces stridor, whereas partial lower airways obstruction produces the inspiratory monophonic wheeze. Rapid progressive painless dysphagia occurs with oesophageal carcinoma.

EXAMINATION

Inspection

With acute partial upper airway obstruction, patients will often appear very distressed. Immediate assessment for generalised urticaria, facial oedema, hypotension and widespread wheezing will allow the diagnosis of anaphylaxis to be made and appropriate treatment initiated. Soot on the face and singed nasal hair from thermal exposure may be present with inhalational injuries. A large goitre will be visible on inspection. Bilateral symmetrical deforming arthropathy involving the small joints of the hands (MCP, PIP) is suggestive of rheumatoid disease. Clubbing may be present in the fingers with bronchial carcinoma.

The cause of stridor may be visible on inspection of the throat. Further information is obtained on inspection using indirect laryngoscopy. With bilateral vocal cord palsy, the cords lie in a cadaveric position. A small glottic aperture is seen and does not widen on attempted inspiration. Supraglottic and glottic carcinomas may be readily visible.

Palpation and auscultation

The presence of cervical lymphadenopathy may be due to infection or carcinoma of the larynx, pharynx, bronchus or oesophagus. A goitre may also be palpable in the neck, skewing the trachea to one side due to compression effects. The chest is examined for monophonic wheezing, collapse of a segment, pleural effusion and rib tenderness, which are the thoracic manifestations of bronchial carcinoma.

GENERAL INVESTIGATIONS

General investigations should be tailored to the clinical findings.

- **FBC**
  WCC ↑ infection.
- **CRP/ESR**
  ↑ with infection and malignancy.
- **TFTs**
  ↑, ↓ or normal with goitres.
- **Lateral soft-tissue neck X-ray**
  Radio-opaque foreign bodies.
- **CXR**
  Both frontal and lateral views are required to identify radio-opaque foreign bodies. Bronchial carcinoma may present as a central mass, peripheral mass, collapse of a segment, consolidation of a lobe or as a pleural effusion. Hilar lymphadenopathy may be apparent, causing external compression of trachea or bronchus.

SPECIFIC INVESTIGATIONS

- **Fibreoptic laryngoscopy**
  Visualisation of the vocal cords, tumour masses, tracheal stenosis and allows biopsies to be taken.
- **Bronchoscopy**
  To screen for lesions in the distal trachea and proximal airways.

- ■ **Upper GI endoscopy**
  To determine the presence of carcinoma that may be infiltrating both recurrent laryngeal nerves when associated symptoms of dysphagia are present.

- ■ **FNAC of a goitre**
  To determine the underlying aetiology of a goitre.

- ■ **CT neck and thorax**
  Define the extent and assist in staging of laryngeal carcinoma, thyroid carcinoma, oesophageal carcinoma and bronchial carcinoma.

- Stridor can be a symptom of impending airways obstruction and asphyxia. Urgent cricothyroidotomy may be required.

- The toxic child with stridor, severe sore throat, respiratory distress and difficulty in swallowing has acute epiglottitis until proved otherwise. Urgent admission and treatment are required.

- If the onset of stridor is very sudden, consider an inhaled foreign body.

SWEATING ABNORMALITIES

Excessive sweating is often brought to the attention of the physician when it becomes socially unacceptable. The underlying cause ranging from trivial to serious.

CAUSES

EXCESSIVE SWEATING

- Primary hyperhidrosis
- Hypoglycaemia

INFECTIONS
- Any systemic infection

MALIGNANCY
- Brain tumours ⚠
- Hodgkin's lymphoma

ENDOCRINE
- Diabetic autonomic neuropathy
- Menopause
- Thyrotoxicosis
- Carcinoid syndrome ⚠
- Phaeochromocytoma ⚠

PSYCHIATRIC
- Substance dependency/withdrawal
- Anxiety states

DEFICIENT SWEATING

- Heat stroke
- Miliaria
- Hypohidrotic ectodermal dysplasia
- Sympathetic tract lesions

HISTORY

Apart from heat stroke, the causes of deficient sweating are rare and usually arise from congenital disorders of the sweat glands, such as hypohidrotic ectodermal dysplasia, a condition associated with poor hair and teeth formation. Absent sweating can also be caused by miliaria, which is caused by plugging or rupture of the sweat ducts.

Excessive sweating is commonly encountered as it is a physiological accompaniment to pain, nausea, vomiting (p. 464) and shock (p. 389). The causes in the absence of these symptoms have been listed above. Excessive sweating may be episodic or constant. Episodic bouts of

SECTION A

sweating may be due to hypogylcaemia, phaeochromocytoma, carcinoid syndrome or menopause. Patients with hypogylcaemia often complain of associated tremor, dizziness, anxiety and hunger. Paroxysmal release of catecholamines by phaeochromocytomas may produce attacks of sweating, hypertension, palpitations, headaches and anxiety. It usually comes to medical attention presenting as a result of hypertension. Carcinoid syndrome is produced by a variety of hormones secreted by enterochromaffin tumours, originating from the small bowel in the presence of hepatic metastases. Episodic sweating is associated with brick-red flushing, diarrhoea, wheezing and occasionally right-sided heart lesions.

Hot flushes and sweating may also be prominent symptoms experienced by women reaching the menopause; the aetiology has often been attributed to alterations in the concentrations of female reproductive hormones.

Patients with night sweats may complain of waking up with their clothes and bed sheets drenched in perspiration. Classically, these features are reported with TB and Hodgkin's disease. The accompanying symptoms of pulmonary TB include weight loss, cough and haemoptysis. With Hodgkin's disease, patients may complain of localised lymphadenopathy, weight loss, pruritus, fever and malaise.

Constant sweating and heat intolerance are features of thyrotoxicosis. This may result from increased metabolic rate and may be accompanied by symptoms of increased appetite with weight loss, emotional lability, diarrhoea and palpitations. Rarely, excessive sweating may result from tumours encroaching on the hypothalamus.

Enquiries should be undertaken regarding substance dependency, as withdrawal states can produce severe sweating and hallucinations.

EXAMINATION

A psychological examination is required if an anxiety disorder is suspected. The following are specific features in the examination that may suggest an underlying cause.

Temperature

The presence of pyrexia (p. 365) would suggest infection as the underlying cause for sweating. However, it can also occur with Hodgkin's disease.

Inspection

Wide, staring eyes with lid lag may result from thyrotoxicosis, causing sweating; in addition, the presence of exophthalmos or ophthalmoplegia specifically indicates Graves' disease as the underlying cause. Episodic brick-red flushing of the face may be experienced with carcinoid syndrome.

Palpation and auscultation

The thyroid is palpated to exclude enlargement of the gland. Regional lymph nodes are examined for enlargement, which may be due to infection or malignancy. A tachycardia is present with thyrotoxicosis and systemic infection. A rapid pulse may also be palpated during paroxysmal attacks with phaeochromocytoma, and the blood pressure will be markedly elevated. With primary pulmonary TB, pleural effusion or segmental collapse may be the only features found on examination. Detection of a new or changing heart murmur may imply endocarditis. However, either stenosis or regurgitation of the tricuspid or pulmonary valve has been reported with carcinoid syndrome. The presence of splenomegaly on abdominal examination may be due to Hodgkin's disease.

GENERAL INVESTIGATIONS

- FBC and blood film
  WCC ↑ infection.
- ESR and CRP
  ↑ with infection, malignancy and lymphoma.
- TSH and free T$_4$
  TSH ↓ and T$_4$ ↑ with thyrotoxicosis.
- BM stix
  Identify hypoglycaemia and initiate immediate treatment.
  Glucose may be ↑ with phaeochromocytoma.

SPECIFIC INVESTIGATIONS

- CXR
  TB, bronchial carcinoid, chest infection.
- Mantoux test/ELISpot assay
  Diluted Mantoux test if no previous BCG immunisation has been performed to screen for TB. Serological testing is now available for TB.
- Urinary 5HIAA
  ↑ with carcinoid tumours.
- Urinary catecholamines and metanephrines
  ↑ with phaeochromocytoma.
- Lymph node USS, FNA and excision biopsy
  Assess lymph node and facilitate assessment. Reed–Sternberg cells with Hodgkin's disease.
- MRI head
  Hypothalamic tumours.

- Drenching night sweats are serious as the underlying diagnosis may be lymphoma or chronic infection such as TB. Urgent investigation is required.

SYNCOPE

Syncope is the transient loss of consciousness due to impaired cerebral blood flow.

CAUSES

CARDIOVASCULAR

- Myocardial infarction (when complicated by arrhythmia or cardiogenic shock) ⚠
- Pulmonary embolism ⚠
- Aortic stenosis
- Carotid sinus hypersensitivity
- Hypertrophic obstructive cardiomyopathy

VASOVAGAL SYNCOPE
- Situational syncope
- Micturition syncope
- Cough syncope

ORTHOSTATIC HYPOTENSION
- Prolonged bedrest
- Drug-induced
- Hypovolaemic
- Autonomic failure

ARRHYTHMIA
- Supraventricular tachycardia
- Ventricular tachycardia ⚠
- Sick sinus syndrome
- AV nodal block (Mobitz type 2 or 3rd degree block) ⚠

NEUROLOGICAL

- Seizure
- Functional syncope

METABOLIC ⚠

- Hypoxia
- Hypoglycaemia

HISTORY

Vasovagal syncope (the common faint) is the most common cause of syncope. It is associated with peripheral vasodilatation and a vagally mediated slowing of the heart rate. It may be precipitated by situations such as fear, emotion, prolonged standing or pain. The patient may complain of nausea, weakness and blurred vision, and appear pale with bradycardia on examination. Palpitations (p. 342) preceding collapse may suggest a tachyarrhythmia, whereas sudden brief syncope without prodrome followed by rapid return to full consciousness is suggestive of a bradyarrhythmia. Situational syncope are faints classified according to the precipitating factors and are often due to an excessive vagal response to the offending stimuli.

Orthostatic hypotension is a drop in blood pressure on standing. This causes a transient decrease in cerebral perfusion and therefore loss of consciousness. Prolonged bedrest can result in the deconditioning of the baroreceptors in the body, resulting in a postural drop of blood pressure. A drug history may exclude offending medication such as antihypertensives and opiates. Hypovolaemia is also a cause of postural hypotension (see Shock, p. 389); it is associated with pallor, tachycardia and a low urine output. Disease states such as diabetes mellitus, Parkinson's plus syndromes and Guillain–Barré syndrome can result in autonomic failure and inability of the body to maintain an appropriate blood pressure.

Cardiac outflow obstruction, which occurs with aortic stenosis and hypertrophic obstructive cardiomyopathy, will result in syncope on effort as the cardiac output cannot be increased on demand.

In carotid sinus syndrome, the receptors of the carotid sinus are more sensitive than normal, thus minor stimulation, such as turning the head or pressure from a tight collar, may elicit the carotid sinus reflex and precipitate syncope.

Seizures are paroxysmal discharges in the cortex, which are sufficient to produce clinically detectable events, e.g. convulsions, loss of consciousness or behavioural symptoms. Although it is not strictly syncope, atonic seizures may present in a similar fashion, with a sudden loss of muscle tone and collapse. Patients may be incontinent during a seizure and drowsy or confused during the post-ictal phase.

Functional syncope tends to be very dramatic with normal examination findings during the attack.

Hypoglycaemia causes faintness and even results in loss of consciousness. It tends to be more common with insulin-treated diabetics but may also occur in normal individuals after an alcohol binge. Symptoms usually occur when the glucose is below 2.5 mmol/L.

EXAMINATION

Appearance

Vasovagal syncope often results in pallor of the complexion and clamminess. Convulsions may occur.

Blood pressure

Should be taken supine and standing, only then will a postural drop be noted.

Pulse

During the attack of syncope, taking the pulse is a good way to detect an arrhythmia. Bradycardia is the usual finding in vasovagal syncope. AV nodal block may be associated with significant bradycardia, transient asystole or ventricular standstill. The sick sinus syndrome is associated with alternating episodes of bradycardia and tachycardia. Shock, supraventricular and ventricular tachycardias may result in very rapid heart rates.

Pressure on the carotid sinus, located at the bifurcation of the carotid arteries, will cause syncope in patients with carotid sinus syndrome.

Auscultation

A soft second heart sound and an ejection systolic murmur radiating to the carotids characterises aortic valvular stenosis. An ejection systolic murmur can also be auscultated in hypertrophic obstructive cardiomyopathy, where the outflow of blood from the left ventricle is obstructed owing to hypertrophy of the cardiac muscle.

GENERAL INVESTIGATIONS

- **Finger prick blood glucose test**
  Testing the blood for glucose is a simple and very rapid way of obtaining a blood glucose level. More accurate readings can be confirmed with a serum sample.

- **FBC**
  Will indicate anaemia when haemorrhage is the underlying cause of hypovolaemia. Septic shock with peripheral vasodilatation may be associated with an elevated white cell count.

- **U&Es**
  Electrolyte abnormalities will predispose to seizures.

- **Serum lactate**
  Usually raised following a true epileptic seizure.

- **Blood glucose**
  Hypoglycaemia.

- **ECG**
  When obtained during an attack, an ECG may reveal an arrhythmia. Pulseless ventricular tachycardia should be treated as ventricular fibrillation and cardiac resuscitation should commence. Q waves and ST elevations may be seen with myocardial infarction.

SPECIFIC INVESTIGATIONS

- **EEG**
  Although epilepsy is essentially a clinical diagnosis, seizures associated with specific electrical changes in the cortex can be used to confirm the diagnosis. A negative EEG does not, however, exclude epilepsy.

- **24-Hour ECG**
  May be able to document arrhythmias associated with episodes of syncope.

- **Echocardiography**
  Allows assessment of the aortic valve and diagnosis of hypertrophic obstructive cardiomyopathy.

- **CT pulmonary angiography**
  Allows diagnosis of the majority of acute pulmonary emboli.

- **Tilt table testing**
  This is usually reserved for patients with recurrent syncope of indeterminate cause. In patients with vasovagal syncope, a 60° tilt will produce hypotension, bradycardia and syncope within 30 minutes.

- Syncope should never be ignored due to the potential serious consequences of this symptom. Any suggestion of a cardiac cause requires urgent investigation and treatment.

- When assessing a patient with syncope always remember to check blood glucose.

THIRST

Thirst as a symptom, is usually associated with two other symptoms, i.e. drinking excessive amounts of water (polydipsia) and excessive urination (polyuria).

CAUSES

INADEQUATE FLUID INTAKE

- General debility/frailty
- Neurological disease
- Anorexia

EXCESSIVE FLUID LOSS

- Vomiting
- Fever
- Diarrhoea
- Bleeding (i.e. loss of blood volume)
- Excessive sweating
- Burns

ENDOCRINE AND METABOLIC

- Diabetes mellitus
- Chronic renal failure
- Liver failure
- Diabetes insipidus (cranial and nephrogenic)

DRUGS

- Diuretics (especially overdose)
- Ecstasy

CAUSES OF DRY MOUTH

- Sjögren's syndrome
- Drugs, e.g. anticholinergics, monoamine oxidase inhibitors
- Post head and neck radiotherapy

PSYCHIATRIC

- Psychogenic polydipsia

DIET

- Salty foods
- Spicy foods

HISTORY

It is important to distinguish between thirst and a dry mouth. Enquire about the onset of thirst, whether it is acute or chronic. Key features of a dry mouth may include change in taste, soreness and difficulty swallowing. Take a full dietary history, including salt intake and ingestion of spicy foods. The patient may be palliative and entering the terminal phase with reduced oral intake. A history of tiredness, lethargy with weight loss will suggest diabetes mellitus. Check for signs of infection. Check for a history of vomiting or diarrhoea as well as muscle cramps and weakness. A full drug history should be taken, as some drugs, e.g. anticholinergics, can result in dryness of the mouth and therefore patients may ingest excessive quantities of water, giving rise to polyuria. A history of any salivary gland swelling in association with dry eyes, dry mouth and arthritis should be sought, which would suggest Sjögren's syndrome. A history of any blood loss should be sought.

Malignancy and primary hyperparathyroidism are common causes of chronic hypercalcaemia, which can lead to polyuria by an intrinsic osmotic effect or by precipitation of nephrogenic diabetes insipidus. Cranial diabetes insipidus can result from severe, blunt head injuries, craniopharyngioma, pineal gland tumours or as a transient postoperative complication following neurosurgery. Full psychological assessment may be required if psychogenic polydipsia is suspected.

EXAMINATION

Check the temperature. Look for signs of dehydration, e.g. dry coated tongue, loss of skin turgor. Look for evidence of recent weight loss. Look for signs of Sjögren's syndrome, i.e. symmetrical enlargement of the salivary glands both parotid and submandibular. Check for systemic signs including dry eyes and arthritis or signs of drug toxicity.

GENERAL INVESTIGATIONS

- **Urinalysis**
  Diabetes. Glucose and ketones in the urine.
- **FBC**
  PCV ↑ dehydration. Hb ↓ anaemia (blood loss). WCC ↑ infection.
- **U&Es and LFTs**
  Renal failure. Renal failure.
- **Serum calcium**
  ↑ Ca – causes osmotic diuresis.
- **Blood sugar**
  ↑ diabetes mellitus.

SPECIFIC INVESTIGATIONS

- **PTH**
  ↑ hyperparathyroidism.

- **Drug screen**
  Lithium level.

- **Water deprivation tests (see Polyuria on p. 351)**
  Differentiate between diabetes insipidus and primary polydipsia.

- **Desmopressin stimulation test**
  Urine osmolality ↑ cranial diabetes insipidus. No urine osmolality
  rise in nephrogenic diabetes insipidus.

- **CT/MRI**
  Cranial diabetes insipidus, e.g. tumour/CVA.

- **US**
  Renal failure.

- **Renal biopsy**
  Renal failure.

- It is important to distinguish between true thirst and a
  dry mouth.
- Thirst in an acute illness may be due to dehydration. However,
  it may also herald acute onset of diabetes. Always carry out
  an appropriate history and a urinalysis to exclude diabetes
  mellitus.

THROAT DISORDERS

A sore throat is an extremely common symptom, especially in children and young adults. Persistent sore throat in an elderly patient is a cause for concern, as it may indicate the presence of neoplasia.

Figure 56 Tonsillitis. Bacterial tonsillitis with exudative pus coating inflamed tonsils.

CAUSES

INFECTIVE

- Tonsillitis (Fig. 56)
  - Bacterial, e.g. *streptococcus*, gonococcus
  - Viral, e.g. glandular fever (infectious mononucleosis)
- Pharyngitis/laryngitis
  - Viral
  - Fungal
- Quinsy (peritonsillar abscess) ⚠
- Measles (on the increase)

INFLAMMATORY

- Thyroiditis

NEOPLASTIC

- Carcinoma ⚠
  - Tonsil
  - Posterior third of the tongue
  - Larynx ● *(common in Far East including Hong Kong, Singapore)*
- Haematological disorders (e.g. lymphoma)

NEUROLOGICAL

- Glossopharyngeal neuralgia

REFERRED PAIN
●   Angina
●   Oesophageal spasm

OTHER
●   Muscle strain
●   Tobacco
●   Allergy
●   Reflux oesophagitis
●   AIDS

HISTORY

Infective

Symptoms include sore throat dysphagia, referred pain to ear, headache and malaise. A history of oral sex may suggest oropharyngeal gonorrhoea. Quinsy is a peritonsillar abscess. Initially, there is usually a history of acute tonsillitis but the patient becomes more ill with a high temperature, dysphagia and referred pain to the ear. In glandular fever, the patient can present with a severe membranous tonsillitis but usually has more systemic symptoms including malaise and lymphadenopathy elsewhere. Measles can present as a sore throat as well as Koplik spots, fever and conjunctivitis.

Inflammatory

Subacute thyroiditis presents with a swelling of the thyroid, with neck pain, fever, weakness and malaise, although this is a rare condition.

Neoplastic

Carcinoma of a tonsil presents with painful ulceration and induration. There is often referred pain to the ear and the patient may spit blood. Occasionally, the presenting symptom is a lump in the neck representing metastatic cervical lymphadenopathy. Carcinoma of the posterior third of the tongue may present with a feeling of soreness in the throat with difficulty in swallowing. Supraglottic carcinoma presents with a feeling of a lump in the throat but there is usually a change in voice and early cervical lymphadenopathy. Lymphoma of the tonsil rarely causes pain but may present with enlargement of one tonsil. Patients with other haematological disorders may present with a sore throat resulting from infection as a consequence of neutropenia. Also, ask about relevant drugs the patient may be taking including DMARDs and carbimazole.

Neurological

Glossopharyngeal neuralgia has a sharp stabbing pain at the root of the tongue, radiating into the throat and ear, triggered by swallowing or touching the pharynx.

Referred pain

Angina may cause pain in the throat, although it is usually associated with exercise. There may also be pain in the chest, radiating into the jaw and down the left arm. Occasionally, diffuse oesophageal spasm gives rise to chest pain radiating into the throat and jaw.

Other

Sore throat may occur with AIDS. It may be due to a variety of infective organisms, e.g. viral or fungal. Reflux oesophagitis may cause a burning pain in the throat or a sensation of a lump in the throat. Muscle strain can occur from prolonged talking without rest. Tobacco use in heavy smokers may develop chronic pharyngitis with pain. Allergies to dust or pollen may present with post-nasal drip, runny eyes and general irritability.

EXAMINATION

Infective

With tonsillitis, there is usually pyrexia, foetor and pus exuding from the tonsillar crypts. The pharyngeal mucosa is often inflamed with cervical lymphadenopathy. However check for lymphadenopathy elsewhere, and splenomegaly, which may be associated with glandular fever. Scoring systems may be used to assess for likelihood of streptococcal infection (e.g. FEVERPain or Centor criteria). Quinsy is associated with trismus and the tonsil is pushed downwards and medially by the quinsy. The uvula is usually oedematous.

Inflammatory

Thyroiditis presents with a tender, diffuse swelling in the thyroid gland, which moves on swallowing. It is rare.

Neoplastic

Carcinoma of the tonsil presents as a hard, ulcerated swelling on the tonsil. Cervical lymphadenopathy may be present. In carcinoma of the posterior third of the tongue and supraglottic larynx, there is usually an indurated ulcer. Laryngoscopy is required as part of the examination. Check for cervical nodes and other sites for metastases, e.g. lung, liver. Lymphoma usually presents as a painless enlargement of the tonsil. Haematological disorders may present with lymphadenopathy and hepatosplenomegaly. Agranulocytosis results in ulceration and membrane formation on the tonsils and oral mucosa.

Neurological

The diagnosis of glossopharyngeal neuralgia is usually made from the history. Touching the palate may trigger the symptoms.

Referred pain

Angina and oesophageal spasms are usually diagnosed from the history.

Others

Pharyngitis and tonsillitis may occur as part of AIDS, due to either viral or fungal infections. Other signs of AIDS include malaise, fever, weight loss, chest infections, Kaposi's sarcoma. Diagnosis of reflux oesophagitis is usually made on a history. In tobacco, there may be evidence of staining on the hands and fingernails whilst in allergies the patient may be sneezing, have runny eyes and post-nasal drip.

GENERAL INVESTIGATIONS

- FBC, ESR
  Hb ↓ malignancy. WCC ↑ infection. Blood disorder. Lymphocytosis in glandular fever. ESR ↑ malignancy. Infection. Thyroiditis.

- Throat swab
  Culture and sensitivity – *streptococcus* and gonococcus.

- Viral antibodies
  Glandular fever (i.e. monospot test).

- ECG
  Cardiac ischaemia.

- CXR
  Metastases.

SPECIFIC INVESTIGATIONS

- Laryngoscopy
  Infection. Malignancy.

- OGD
  Oesophagitis. Hiatus hernia.

- HIV testing
  HIV

- Biopsy
  Benign versus malignant.

- CT Neck
  Tumour. Spread of tumour.

- Viral culture
  Measles

- Throat swabs are useful particularly in the management of recurrent or persistent cases.
- Occasionally, a sore throat may be the first symptom of a more serious disorder, e.g. diabetes, agranulocytosis or malignancy.
- Prolonged and persistent sore throat in an elderly patient is a cause for concern as it may be an indication of malignancy.

TIREDNESS

Tiredness or physical fatigue with no obvious cause is a very common complaint. It is normal to feel tired at times, e.g. after working long hours, unaccustomed exertion or sleepless nights. However, it is important to differentiate between tiredness due to excessive normal activities and tiredness due to disease.

CAUSES

POST-VIRAL FATIGUE SYNDROMES

ACUTE
- Infectious mononucleosis
- Viral hepatitis

CHRONIC
- Chronic post-viral fatigue syndrome (CFS)

ENDOCRINE
- Hypothyroidism
- Diabetes mellitus
- Hyperthyroidism
- Addison's disease

MAJOR ORGAN FAILURE
- Cardiac failure
- Renal failure
- Liver failure

NEOPLASTIC
- Malignancy ⚠

CHRONIC INFECTION
- TB
- HIV
- Brucellosis

CHRONIC INFLAMMATORY DISEASE
- Rheumatoid arthritis
- Polymyalgia rheumatica
- Crohn's disease
- SLE

CHRONIC NEUROLOGICAL DISORDERS

- Multiple sclerosis
- Myasthenia gravis
- Restless legs

DRUGS

- Beta blockers
- Diuretics

DRUG ABUSE

- Alcohol
- Benzodiazepines

OTHERS

- Stress, e.g. overwork, family commitments
- Depressive illness
- Anaemia
- Coeliac disease
- Pregnancy
- The over-training syndrome
- Carbon monoxide poisoning

HISTORY

The history is most important in the diagnosis. It is necessary to define exactly what is meant by tiredness or fatigue. Fatigue is sometimes known as 'tired all the time syndrome'. Take a full history to decide whether tiredness is of a physical, psychological or social nature. Note the duration of the problem. Is it getting worse? Was there any precipitating factor? Ask about previous levels of energy and how this compares with the present. Consider asking about symptoms relating to other systems including gastro-intestinal, urinary and obstetric. Has the patient noticed any other changes, e.g. in appetite, increased urine output or thirst or sleep disturbances? Has there been any recent change in medication, e.g. beta blockers causing lethargy? Chronic fatigue syndrome is more common in teenagers and young adults, especially students with a history over several months. It is uncommon after early middle age. Depression is more common in women aged 30 and over, whilst in the middle-aged and elderly the symptoms are more likely to represent underlying organic disease.

A history of previous illnesses such as infectious mononucleosis or influenza should be sought. Weight loss may suggest malignancy or depression with episodes of fever, suggesting chronic infection, e.g. TB. Cold intolerance suggests myxoedema a feature of thyroid disease. Heat intolerance suggests thyrotoxicosis. In chronic fatigue syndrome, the illness may fluctuate from week to week and may occasionally be relieved by rest. In malignancy, the symptoms are progressive and deterioration occurs. The same is true for endocrine disorders. Tiredness associated with depression may fluctuate considerably with changing circumstances.

Ask about the patient's lifestyle. Is there an excessive consumption of alcohol? Alcohol itself may cause tiredness, but if alcohol is being used as a coping mechanism for stress-related illness, it is likely to aggravate rather than alleviate the problem. Ask about recreational drugs. Ask about work. Have the patient's work circumstances changed and are they working very long hours together with home commitments? Take a full neurological history to exclude conditions such as multiple sclerosis and myasthenia gravis. Restless legs often involves involuntary leg movement mainly at night with an aching sensation. The patient often has poor sleep as a result. Also, ask about joint pain and swelling in the history of inflammatory disease. Ask about excessively hard training in runners, weight trainers and athletes. The over-training syndrome may lead to persistent fatigue. Carbon monoxide poisoning is rare but does occur occasionally and it is appropriate to take a history about any change of health of other members of the household as carbon monoxide poisoning would be likely to affect them also. In coeliac disease, this may present as tiredness, bowel changes, anaemia and weight loss.

EXAMINATION

Meticulous examination is essential. Look at the patient. Is the patient someone who looks systemically unwell or has lost weight? Is there any evidence of anxiety, tiredness or sleep deprivation? Pyrexia may indicate the presence of systemic illness, e.g. TB, HIV. In chronic fatigue syndrome and in depression, there will be no abnormal physical signs. A slight tachycardia may occur with anxiety and stress. Check for clinical signs of anaemia. Check for signs of hyperthyroidism or hypothyroidism. Anaemia and thyrotoxicosis will produce a bounding, hyperdynamic pulse. In malignancy, there may be enlarged lymph nodes or the liver may be palpable. A detailed neurological examination may also be required to exclude neurological disease as a cause of symptoms. Postural hypotension may occur in Addison's disease. Restless legs may be visible during examination with involuntary movement.

GENERAL INVESTIGATIONS

- Urinalysis
  Diabetes. Renal disease.
- FBC
  Hb ↓ anaemia. WCC ↑ infection.
- ESR
  ↑ infection, inflammatory disease, malignancy.

- U&Es
  Chronic renal failure. Addison's disease.
- LFTs
  Alcohol abuse, hepatitis, malignancy.
- CXR
  TB. Malignancy. Cardiac failure.

SPECIFIC INVESTIGATIONS

- TFTs
  Hypothyroidism. Hyperthyroidism.
- Monospot test
  Infectious mononucleosis.
- Autoantibody and complement screen
  Connective tissue disease. SLE.
- Coeliac screen (ttg-IgA)
  Coeliac disease.

- Only 20–30% of cases will have an identifiable physical cause whilst up to 50% of cases have a psychological cause, with tiredness often presenting as a sign of depression.
- Tiredness as a single presenting symptom in the absence of other symptoms is unlikely to have a physical cause.
- Patients presenting with tiredness and other symptoms including weight loss, lymphadenopathy and focal neurological signs need to be investigated thoroughly.

TOE LESIONS

Lesions of the toes are extremely common. They are caused by a variety of conditions ranging from simple ingrowing toenails to severe pain and ulceration caused by ischaemia. Deformities of the toes are also exceptionally common, particularly in the elderly.

Figure 57 Ingrowing toenails of both great toes. The patient had suffered repeated infections. There is overgrowth of granulation tissue and a purulent discharge. Bilateral avulsion of the toenail and ablation of the germinal matrix cured the condition.

CAUSES

TOENAILS

- Ingrowing toenail (Fig. 57)
- Subungual haematoma
- Warts/verrucas
- Subungual melanoma ⚠
- Subungual exostosis
- Onychogryphosis
- Onychomycosis

DEFORMITIES

- Hallux valgus
- Hallux rigidus
- Hammer, claw or mallet toe

ULCERS

ISCHAEMIC

Large vessel disease
- Atherosclerosis
- Embolism

Small vessel disease
- Diabetes
- Raynaud's
- Buerger's
- Vasculitis (e.g. scleroderma, SLE, rheumatoid)

NEUROPATHIC

Peripheral nerve lesions
- Diabetes
- Nerve injuries
- Leprosy ● *(common where leprosy is endemic)*

Spinal cord lesions
- Spina bifida
- Spinal injuries
- Syringomyelia

NEOPLASTIC
- Skin tumours (perineural invasion)

DISCOLORATION
- Chilblains
- Ischaemia

HISTORY

Nails

Ingrowing toenail usually presents with pain at the sides of the nail and often with infection and local inflammation. With infection, the toe is painful and throbs, especially in bed at night. With subungual haematoma, there is a history of injury to the nail. Bleeding occurs beneath the nail, which is extremely painful, and occasionally the patient may faint with the pain. Subungual melanoma can be easily missed and presents with pigmentation under the nail. With subungual exostosis, there is lifting of the nail with deformity. Onychogryphosis is a 'ram's horn' deformity of the nail. The nail thickens and curves over the end with one end growing faster than the other. It is common in the elderly but may occur in young people after injury to the nailbed.

Deformities

A patient with hallux valgus normally presents with a 'bunion'. The first metatarsal deviates medially. It is more common in females.

The patient may complain that the great toe overrides the second toe. Unsuitable, tight footwear may be a precipitating cause. Hallux rigidus is osteoarthritis of the first MTP joint. It occurs in young adults. The patient complains of pain on walking, especially when 'pushing off', and stiffness in the joint. Hammer toe usually affects the second toe. The patient complains of a deformed toe and may also complain of painful callosities that have developed where the deformed toe presses against the footwear. With clawed toes. The tips of the toes may develop painful callosities.

Ulcers

Ulcers are usually ischaemic (painful) or neuropathic (painless). Check for a history of intermittent claudication, smoking, Raynaud's disease, cardiac disease and diabetes. With neuropathic ulcers, there may be a history of diabetes, nerve injuries and spinal cord lesions. Ulcers usually occur on the pressure points over the tips of the toes. Neoplastic ulcers on the toes are extremely rare.

Discoloration

Painful discoloration, either red or shiny, white, blue or black (gangrene), suggests ischaemia. Conversely, chilblains occurs in childhood and early adult life, usually in females. They are more likely in those with outdoor occupations precipitated by the cold. Painful swelling occurs on the toes, which may become itchy and erythematous. They are often multiple and may develop into shallow ulcers.

EXAMINATION

Nails

With ingrowing toenails, there is often a serous discharge or purulent discharge from the nailfold. The toe becomes red and swollen. Granulation tissue may be apparent at the nailfold. Subungual haematoma is usually obvious. Occasionally, however, the patient forgets the injury and presents with a brownish discoloration under the nail and this has to be distinguished from a melanoma. Haematoma is usually reddish-brown colour with sharp edges, the melanoma being brownish-grey with an indistinct edge. A haematoma grows out with the nail whilst a melanoma does not. With suspected melanoma, examine the regional lymph nodes and liver for secondaries. Subungual exostosis results in deformity of the nail, which is pushed up and deformed. The swelling between the toe and the end of the nail eventually becomes obvious. Onychogryphosis is obvious with a very thick discoloured nail, which curves and claws over at the end (ram's horn deformity).

Deformities

With hallux valgus, the first metatarsal bone deviates medially, the great toe laterally. There may be a thickened bursa over the medial aspect of the joint. The great toe may override the second toe. In hallux rigidus, there is a stiff, painful, enlarged, first MTP joint. With hammer toe, the second toe is usually affected. There is a fixed flexed deformity of the PIP joint and compensatory hyperextension of the adjacent joint. Check for the presence of corns and callosities. In claw toes, both IP joints are flexed and in mallet toes only the DIP is flexed (see Foot deformities, p. 153).

Ulcers

Punched out, painful ulcers over pressure points suggest ischaemic ulcers. Check for discoloration of the toe, capillary return and absence of foot pulses. Neuropathic ulcers are painless; the circulation is usually good but sensation is absent or blunted locally. Carry out a full neurological examination in this instance.

Discoloration

With ischaemic toe, it may be shiny red, blue, white or black with gangrene. Examine the pulses. Chilblains are usually reddish-blue, with oedema and blistering occuring which bursts, leaving superficial ulcers.

GENERAL INVESTIGATIONS

- ■ FBC, ESR
  Hb ↓ anaemia of chronic disease, e.g. rheumatoid arthritis, SLE.
  WCC ↑ infection, CRP/ESR ↑ vasculitis, e.g. rheumatoid arthritis, SLE.

- ■ U&Es
  Chronic renal failure with connective tissues diseases.

- ■ Blood glucose
  Ischaemia due to small vessel disease in diabetes.

- ■ X-rays
  Subungual exostosis. Hallux rigidus.

SPECIFIC INVESTIGATIONS

- ■ Antibody screen
  Connective tissue disease.

- ■ Doppler studies
  Ischaemia.

- ■ Arteriography
  Arterial disease.

- ■ MRI spine (or MRI foot)
  Spinal cord lesions with neuropathy.

- ■ Nerve conduction studies
  Peripheral neuropathy.

- ■ Excision biopsy
  Malignant lesions, e.g. subungual melanoma.

- A pigmented lesion below the nail (subungual) may be a haematoma or melanoma. Check carefully for a history of trauma. A haematoma grows out with the nail; a melanoma does not.

- Arteriopaths who develop painful toes need urgent investigation. It may be due to the development of critical limb or digit ischaemia or may be embolic (remember the 6Ps of critical limb ischaemia).

TONGUE DISORDERS

Tongue disorders are extremely common, ranging from minor furring of the tongue to extensive inflammation and even malignancy. Tongue disorders can also be a manifestation of systemic disease.

Figure 58 Ulcerating squamous cell carcinoma on the lateral margin of the tongue.

CAUSES

FURRING

- Gastrointestinal disease
- Dehydration
- Smokers
- Antibiotics

COLOUR CHANGE

- White patches, e.g. leucoplakia, thrush
- Pallor (anaemia)
- Blue (central cyanosis)
- Red (pernicious anaemia, vitamin deficiency)
- Black (black hairy tongue)
- Pigmented (Addison's disease)

SWELLING (MACROGLOSSIA)

- Down's syndrome
- Trauma, e.g. hot liquids, corrosive substances
- Myxoedema
- Allergy
- Infiltration, e.g. amyloid, lymphoma
- Congenital hypothyroidism
- Acromegaly

GLOSSITIS

- Smoking
- Spices
- Spirits
- Sepsis
- Sharp teeth
- Geographic tongue
- Syphilis (tertiary syphilis)
- Scarlet fever

ULCERATION

- Aphthous ulcer
- Dental trauma
- Carcinoma (Fig. 58)
- Chancre
- Gumma

WASTING

- Bulbar palsy
- Hypoglossal nerve palsy
- Motor neuron disease

OTHER

- Burning mouth syndrome
- Oral Lichen planus
- Sjogren's syndrome

HISTORY

Furring

A history of gastrointestinal disease, dehydration, smoking or antibiotics.

Colour change

White patches on the tongue are suggestive of leucoplakia or candidiasis, the last being associated with antibiotic therapy, chemotherapy or immunosuppression. Hairy leucoplakia is associated with EBV and is found almost exclusively in patients with HIV. A pale tongue may indicate anaemia, a blue tongue central cyanosis. The patient may present with a red, painful tongue, which may occur in pernicious anaemia or other forms of vitamin B deficiency. A black hairy tongue may be the result of environmental factors including smoking, mouth hygeine and diet. Pigmentation may be a sign of Addison's disease.

Swelling

The patient may present with a swollen tongue, which may or may not be painful. Difficulty in articulation or swallowing may be apparent. Congenital hypothyroidism will be obvious (extremely rare nowadays), as will Down's syndrome. A swollen tongue may be a presentation of myxoedema in thyroid disease. Other symptoms of myxoedema may be present, e.g. slowness, weight gain, dry skin, hoarse voice, constipation, lethargy, dislike of cold weather. Acromegaly may be obvious, the patient having noticed an increase in shoe size, change in voice and jaw changes. Infection (see below) may present with swelling, as may allergies or trauma, especially burns with hot fluids or caustic substances. Infection will result in a painful tongue.

Glossitis

There is a sequence of chronic inflammatory, degenerative and hypertrophic changes in the tongue, which terminate in the development of a carcinoma. There may be a history of the six Ss: syphilis, smoking, sharp tooth, spirits, spices and sepsis. The patient is usually over the age of 50 and presents with a tongue that has become shiny or white, or has developed a lump on the tongue. There is usually no pain and no interference with eating. A geographic tongue is often named so due to its map like appearance with patients reporting red and white patches as well as a burning sensation after food. In scarlett fever, there is usually a history of fever, sore throat, rash and a strawberry tongue.

Ulceration

Ulceration is common. Aphthous ulcers are painful and are often associated with chronic disease. Dental trauma from a sharp tooth or ill-fitting dentures may cause ulcers. Chancre and gumma associated with syphilis are rare. Carcinoma has a peak incidence at 60–70 years and presents with a painless persistent ulcer on the tongue, often at the margins on the dorsal surface. Carcinoma of the posterior third of the tongue may present with referred pain to the ear, the pain being referred from the lingual branch of the trigeminal nerve, which supplies the tongue, to the ear, via the auriculotemporal nerve.

Wasting

Wasting of the tongue is caused by paralysis of the hypoglossal nerve. Check for a history of recent trauma or surgery to the neck, which may have damaged the hypoglossal nerve. Atrophy of the tongue occurs on the same side as the lesion. In motor neuron disease, there is usually a history of progressive decline with muscle wasting, fasciculations and weakness.

Other

In burning mouth syndrome, this is a burning sensation in the absence of any obvious cause. Lichen planus is a chronic inflammatory disorder that can affect the mouth with pain and burning. In Sjogren's the patient may complain of dry mouth, eyes as well as tongue.

EXAMINATION

Furring

Examination will reveal uniformed furring of the tongue. Note its colour. Look for signs of gastrointestinal disease including the hands, eyes and abdomen.

Colour change

This will usually be obvious. White patches on the tongue may be due to leucoplakia. The white plaques may fissure with time. This can be a pre-malignant condition. Other white patches may be due to candidal infection (thrush). Unlike leucoplakia, these white plaques may be rubbed off, revealing ulcerated buccal mucosa underneath. Colour changes may be uniform (pallor and cyanosis) or patchy (the pigmentation of Addison's disease). In pernicious anaemia, the tongue is red, bald and painful. A black hairy tongue is often a spot diagnosis.

Swelling

The tongue is large and tends to protrude in Down's syndrome. Other signs of Down's syndrome will be apparent, e.g. epicanthic folds, single palmar crease. Look for signs of congenital hypothyroidism, e.g. stunted growth, relatively large head, thick eyelids, thick broad nose, thick lips, widely spaced eyes. With myxoedema, there will be dry skin, dry hair, goitre, slow relaxing reflexes, congestive cardiac failure and non-pitting oedema. With acromegaly, there will be large feet, prognathism, thick spade-like hands, deep voice and possible cardiac failure. In generalised infections, the tongue will be red and swollen. Allergies may present with a swollen tongue, lips, larynx, bronchospasm and rash. There will usually be a history of exposure to an allergen. The ingestion of corrosive or hot fluids will result in inflammation not only to the tongue but also to the rest of the mouth and the pharynx.

Glossitis

Examination reveals a thin, grey transparent film on the tongue in the early stages. Leucoplakia occurs next and eventually overt carcinoma develops. A classic strawberry tongue can be a sign of scarlet fever, especially in the presence of a rash. In a geographic tongue, this is erythematous with white-grey borders.

Ulceration

Aphthous ulcers start as tender vesicular lesions with a hyperaemic base, which ulcerate leaving a small, white, circular, deep, painful ulcer. Dental trauma will usually result in ulcers at the lateral margins of the tongue adjacent to a sharp tooth. Chancres and gummas are rare, as is tuberculous ulcer of the tongue. A carcinomatous ulcer usually occurs on the upper surface of the tongue, most often at the lateral margins. It feels hard, has an everted edge, is friable and bleeds. Local lymph nodes may be palpable, due to either secondary infection or metastases.

Wasting

Ask the patient to protrude the tongue. Wasting will be noted on the affected side and the tongue deviates to the side of the lesion. Check for scars on the neck to suggest hypoglossal nerve damage. In motor neuron disease, consider a full neurological examination to examine for weakness, muscle wasting and fasciculations.

Other

In burning mouth syndrome, there may an erythematous patch or no signs at all. In oral lichen planus look for an itchy rash as well as nail changes (e.g. nail plate thinning).

GENERAL INVESTIGATIONS

- **FBC, ESR, CRP**
  Hb ↓ anaemia (microcytic, macrocytic). WCC ↑ infection. ESR and CRP ↑ infection, malignancy.
- **Serum vitamin B$_{12}$**
  Reduced in pernicious anaemia.
- **TFTs**
  T$_4$ ↓, TSH ↑ in myxoedema.
- **Swab**
  Culture and sensitivity. Infection. Syphilis. Bacterial, viral and fungal infections.

SPECIFIC INVESTIGATIONS

- **VDRL**
  Syphilis.
- **Serology**
  Parietal cell antibodies in pernicious anaemia.
- **HIV test**
  Hairy leucoplakia.
- **CT/MRI**
  Pituitary tumour in acromegaly.

- Oral glucose tolerance test with growth hormone and IGF-1 measurement
  Acromegaly.
- ACTH stimulation tests
  Addison's disease.
- Tongue biopsy
  Carcinoma.

- A persistent mouth ulcer, mass or unexplained red/white patches requires further investigation for malignancy, especially in smokers.
- Candidal infection may have an underlying cause including diabetes or an immunosupressive disease (e.g. HIV).

TREMOR

A tremor is an involuntary rhythmic oscillation of a body part and usually refers to the movements around the small joints of the hands.

CAUSES

RESTING TREMOR

- Parkinsonian tremor

ACTION TREMOR

- Idiopathic
- Benign essential tremor
- Physiological
- Anxiety
- Exercise
- Chronic respiratory disease
- Thyrotoxicosis

INTENTION TREMOR

- Cerebellar disease

DRUGS

- Caffeine
- Alcohol (including alcohol withdrawal)
- Drug withdrawal (benzodiazepines, opiates)
- Beta agonists
- Lithium
- Phenytoin
- Ciclosporin
- Anti-psychotic medications

HISTORY

Tremor is divided into three groups: (1) resting tremor; (2) an action tremor, which is evident when the hand is held in a sustained position or against gravity; and (3) an intention tremor, which is present during movement. Physiological causes of tremor usually have clear precipitating factors, such as anger and exercise.

An action tremor that resolves when the limb is fully supported against gravity is characteristic of benign essential tremor; in addition, it may also be relieved by alcohol and is attenuated during movement. Up to one-third of patients with benign essential tremor have a family history of it. In addition to tremor, patients with thyrotoxicosis may also complain of heat intolerance, palpitations, increased appetite with weight loss, anxiety and diarrhoea.

A detailed drug history will easily allow you to identify any drug that may potentially cause tremor. Enquiries should also include the amount of coffee and alcohol intake.

Associated symptoms of slowness, difficulty initiating and stopping walking, muscle rigidity and muscle fatigue (especially with writing) may be present with Parkinson's disease, the most common cause of a parkinsonian tremor. A history of cognitive impairment, hallucinations and autonomic dysfunction should be sought to assess for Parkinson's plus syndromes. With cerebellar disease, difficulties may be experienced with balance and coordination.

EXAMINATION

Tremor

Observe the patient at rest: the presence of a pill-rolling tremor is suggestive of a parkinsonian tremor. Thyrotoxic patients will be thin, with wide, staring eyes, lid lag, a goitre and exophthalmos with Graves' disease.

The arms are then held outstretched; all other causes of tremor will now be visible. Fine tremors can be accentuated by placing a piece of paper on the outstretched hands. The arm should be fully supported and this will cause resolution of benign essential tremor. An intention tremor is demonstrated by the finger–nose test; a tremor is markedly increased when the finger approaches the target. In addition, there may also be past-pointing, where the finger overshoots the target.

General

Following this evaluation, further examination may be required to determine the underlying cause. The gait is assessed (p. 165) and differences between the parkinsonian and ataxic gait of cerebellar disease will be obvious (the Parkinson's plus syndrome multiple system atrophy may have features of both). Eye movements should be assessed looking for gaze palsies (progressive supranuclear palsy) and nystagmus (cerebellar dysfunction). Further features of cerebellar dysfunction are scanning speech, dysdiadochokinesia and pendular reflexes. When thyrotoxicosis is suspected, the thyroid gland is palpated, eye movements assessed and the thyroid gland auscultated for a bruit associated with Graves' disease. Features of prolonged alcohol excess may be present (signs of chronic liver disease) and alcohol may lead to cerebellar degeneration.

GENERAL INVESTIGATIONS

- TSH and free T_4
  ↓ TSH and ↑ T_4 with thyrotoxicosis.

- **LFTs**
  Abnormalities of synthetic liver function may be present in chronic alcohol excess.

- **ABGs**
  Hypoxia and CO_2 retention in respiratory disease.

SPECIFIC INVESTIGATIONS

- **CT/MRI head**
  For the evaluation of patients with impaired coordination suggestive of cerebellar disease.

- **DaTscan**
  Dopamine uptake scan used to distinguish Parkinson's disease from vascular or drug-induced parkinsonism, or essential tremor, when the diagnosis is unclear.

- The tremor of Parkinson's disease is often subtle and therefore other features of this condition should be sought.

- Always consider alcohol excess as a possible cause of tremor.

URETHRAL DISCHARGE

Any inflammatory condition within the urethra may cause a discharge. It is important to diagnose sexually transmitted diseases so that appropriate treatment is given, not only to the patient but also to sexual contacts via contract tracing.

CAUSES

- Prostatitis
- Non-gonococcal urethritis
  - Chlamydia trachmatis
  - UTI
  - HSV
  - Adenovirus
  - Trichomonas vaginalis
  - Mycoplasma genitalium
- Gonococcal urethritis
- Rare causes
  - Coliforms
  - *Haemophilus ducreyi* (chancroid)
  - TB
  - Syphilis (chancre)
- Reiter's disease
- Traumatic
  - Instrumental
  - Accidental
  - Foreign body
- Chemical (e.g. soaps)
- Neoplastic

HISTORY

General

For any sexually transmitted disease, check for a history of sexual contact, time of last sexual intercourse, contraceptive methods, number and duration of relationships, sexual practices and unusual sexual practices.

Prostatitis

Urethral discharge is rare with acute prostatitis, but with chronic prostatitis, there may be a clear white urethral discharge. The patient may also complain of suprapubic pain, low back pain, perineal discomfort and pain referred to the testicles.

Non-gonococcal urethritis

The patient complains of urethral discharge, which may be thinner than with gonorrhoea. The presentation may be less acute than with gonorrhoea. Chlamydia is one of the most common causes and often asymptomatic in a large proportion of patients. If symptoms are present, they include a clear discharge, pain or burning sensation during micturition. Similar symptoms are found in mycoplasma but patients often report more symptoms. In UTI, there will also be a history of increased frequency with lower abdominal pain. A history of cold sores may be apparent as well as a tingling, burning or pain when passing urine in HSV. Adenovirus usually has a history of a flu-like symptoms, whilst in trichomonas vaginalis there is a yellow/green frothy discharge.

Gonococcal urethritis

The patient will complain of a thickish, purulent urethral discharge and dysuria. Prostatitis and epididymitis may occur, the patient complaining of deep perineal pain or scrotal swelling.

Rare causes

Infection with *Haemophilus ducreyi* causes chancroid or soft sore. It is a tropical infection causing painful genital ulcers and swelling of the inguinal glands. The soft sores may affect the terminal urethra, resulting in dysuria and a profuse, thin, watery discharge. TB of the urethra is very rare. It is usually secondary to TB elsewhere in the genitourinary tract. A syphilitic chancre is now rare but presents as a painful swelling involving the terminal urethra.

Reiter's disease

The patient is usually a young male with recent non-specific urethritis, or it may follow a recent infection. Apart from a urethral discharge, there may be a history of conjunctivitis and joint pains.

Trauma

Urethral instrumentation or prolonged catheterisation may cause urethritis. There will be a clear history of this. Foreign bodies may be introduced by the patient. The variety of these defies description! Other foreign bodies include stones passing from the bladder or fragments of urethral catheters. The patient may be too embarrassed to confess that s/he has introduced a foreign body into the urethra.

Chemical

Chemical urethritis is more common in females. There may be a history of change of soap or bath oils.

Neoplastic

Urethral carcinoma is rare. The patient will complain of dysuria and bloodstained urethral discharge.

EXAMINATION

Prostatitis

There may be a tender, occasionally boggy prostate on digital rectal examination.

Non-gonococcal urethritis

Pus may again be seen at the external urethral meatus. Check for prostatitis and epididymitis. It is important to remember in chlamydia there may be very few signs as many patients are asymptomatic. In HSV, look for cold sores, painful genital ulcers and even gingivostomatitis. In trichomonas vaginalis, there will be evidence of vulvovaginitis and a strawberry cervix in women. Ask about pain and swelling of the joints as well in mycoplasma.

Gonococcal urethritis

Often a bead of pus may be seen at the external urethral meatus. It is appropriate to check for evidence of proctitis or anal discharge (homosexuals). There may be evidence of prostatitis, there being a tender, boggy prostate on digital rectal examination. Palpation of the scrotum may reveal epididymitis.

Rare causes

Other forms of urethritis may show a discharge at the external urethral meatus. With chancroid, there may be sores on the genitals with sores around the meatus. Check for inguinal lymphadenopathy. Urethral TB is very rare. Check for evidence of TB elsewhere, e.g. lungs, kidneys, epididymis. With a syphilitic chancre, the meatus is oedematous and swollen. There may also be inguinal lymphadenopathy.

Reiter's disease

Examine for conjunctivitis and arthritis. There may be co-existent plantar fasciitis and Achilles tendonitis. Examine for abscesses on the soles of the feet and palms of the hands (keratoderma blenorrhagica).

Traumatic

Feel along the course of the urethra for tenderness or palpable stone or foreign body.

Neoplastic

A hard lump may be felt along the course of the urethra. Pressure on it may cause a bloodstained urethral discharge.

GENERAL INVESTIGATIONS

- FBC, ESR
  WCC ↑ in infection, e.g. gonorrhoea. ESR ↑ inflammation, e.g. syphilis.

- ■ Urethral swab
  Microscopy and culture and sensitivity of urethral discharge. This may grow gonococcus, *Chlamydia trachomatis, Trichomonas* spp., *Ureaplasma urealyticum*. Secondary infection, e.g. with *candida* or coliforms, may occur. *Haemophilus ducreyi* may be grown in chancroid. Dark-ground microscopy may reveal treponemes in syphilis.

- ■ Urinalysis and culture
  Bacterial infections causing UTI.

- ■ NAAT
  Neisseria gonorrhoeae, chlamydia trachomatis.

SPECIFIC INVESTIGATIONS

- ■ Mantoux test
  TB.

- ■ Prostatic examination
  C&S of discharge in chronic prostatitis. Symptoms elicited on examination.

- ■ VDRL
  Syphilitic chancre.

- ■ Cystourethroscopy
  Foreign body. Urethral carcinoma.

- • Always take a full sexual history, if STD is suspected, and refer to a GUM clinic for full assessment and contact tracing.

- • Consider full STD screen in suspected and confirmed STD cases including HIV and syphilis.

URINARY INCONTINENCE

Urinary incontinence is the involuntary loss of urine from the bladder. This has profound implications for patients quality of life including at times and places which are inconvenient, inappropriate and socially embarrassing. Stress incontinence is loss of urine during coughing or straining. Urge incontinence is the inability to maintain urinary continence in the presence of frequent and persistent urges to void. Overflow incontinence occurs when the detrusor muscle becomes flaccid and often insensitive to stretch as the bladder distends. Weakness of the sphincter mechanism eventually leads to overflow, with urine leaking out through the urethra.

CAUSES

STRESS INCONTINENCE

PELVIC FLOOR INJURY
- Childbirth
- Obesity
- Prostatectomy
- Hysterectomy

URGE INCONTINENCE

DETRUSOR INSTABILITY
- Constipation
- Excess alcohol/caffeine
- Cystitis
- Stones
- Prostatectomy
- Post-radiotherapy
- Tuberculous-cystitis
- Interstitial nephritis
- Tumour

OVERFLOW INCONTINENCE

LOWER MOTOR NEURONE LESIONS
- Diabetes
- Sacral nerve injury (e.g. pelvic surgery)
- Cauda equina injury ⚠

CHRONIC OUTFLOW OBSTRUCTION
- Prostatic enlargement

NEUROLOGICAL

UPPER MOTOR NEURONE LESION

- Disc lesions
- Stroke
- Head injury
- Spinal cord injury above sacral centre
- Spinal tumours
- Parkinson's disease
- Multiple sclerosis
- Syringomyelia

ANATOMICAL

- Ectopia vesicae
- Ectopic ureter
- Vesicovaginal fistula

OTHER

- Nocturnal enuresis
- Medications (ACE-I, HRT, diuretics)

HISTORY

Stress incontinence

History of multiple childbirth and current pregnancy. Difficult delivery. Recent prostatectomy or hysterectomy due to bladder damage. History of loss of urine during coughing and straining. Increased abdominal pressure as a result of obesity may also cause this.

Urge incontinence

The patient is unable to maintain urinary continence in the presence of frequent and persistent urges to void. Clarify how much alcohol or caffeine the patient drinks as this may be a cause. Recurrent attacks of cystitis with dysuria and frequency. Past history of pelvic radiotherapy. History of TB. History of ureteric colic. Persistent suprapubic discomfort and haematuria is often associated with a stone. Persistent haematuria can also be associated with a tumour. Ask about bowel habit in cases of suspected constipation.

Overflow incontinence

The patient may still be able to void reasonably normally but feels the bladder is not emptying and leakage continues. Check for a history of spinal injury involving lumbar vertebra (sacral centre, cauda equina). History of pelvic surgery, e.g. abdominoperineal resection of rectum with damage to pelvic nerves. History of diabetes. History of prostatism with chronic retention with overflow.

Neurological

With upper motor neurone lesions, there may be a history of spinal trauma affecting the cord above the sacral centre. Also ask about a history of head injury, stroke, multiple sclerosis, Parkinson's disease and syringomyelia.

Anatomical

Ectopia vesicae will be obvious at birth with an abdominal wall defect and abnormal ureter opening into an exposed bladder mucosa on the lower abdominal wall. Duplex ureter may be associated with an ectopic opening of the ureter into the vagina recurrent UTI and incontinence. Vesicovaginal fistula may follow pelvic surgery or pelvic radiotherapy. Rarely, ureterovaginal fistula may occur from an erosion of a ureteric calculus into a vaginal fornix. With duplex ureter, vesicovaginal fistula or ureterovaginal fistula, urine dribbles from the vagina continuously.

Other

Nocturnal enuresis occurs in up to 5% of 10-year-old children. Bed-wetting after puberty usually indicates the presence of an unstable bladder or other pathology. Do not forget to ask about medications the patient may be on, including ACE-I, HRT or diuretics.

EXAMINATION

Stress incontinence

Observe leakage when patient coughs. A cystocele or complete prolapse may be seen. Assess BMI.

Urge incontinence

There may be little to find on examination.

Overflow incontinence

There may be a palpable bladder. Carry out a full neurological examination. Digital rectal examination may reveal prostatic hypertrophy.

Neurological

Reflex emptying of the bladder occurs. Carry out a full neurological examination.

Anatomical

Ectopia vesicae – ureters opening into bladder mucosa on the abdominal wall. With vesicovaginal fistula, examination with a vaginal speculum may indicate the site of the fistula.

GENERAL INVESTIGATIONS

- FBC
  WCC ↑ in infection.

- Urinalysis and MSU
  C&S for infection.

- Intravenous urogram
  Assess upper tracts, obstruction, bladder lesions, fistula.

SPECIFIC INVESTIGATIONS

- Cystoscopy
  Bladder stone. Neoplasia.

- Cystography
  Vesicovaginal fistula.

- Urodynamics
  Uroflowmetry – measures flow rate. Cystometry – detrusor contractions. Videocystometry – leakage of urine on straining in stress incontinence – urethral pressure profiles – sphincter function and outlet obstruction.

- CT spine
  Cord lesion. Spinal tumour.

- MRI spine
  Cord lesion. Disc lesion. Spinal tumour. Syringomyelia.

- Recurrent incontinence suggests a fistula, chronic outflow problems or a neurological cause.

- Incontinence with leg weakness or saddle anaesthesia suggests spinal cord compression. Urgent neurosurgical referral is required.

- In patients with incontinence and persistent haematuria consider malignancy in the absence of UTI.

URINARY RETENTION

Retention of urine may be acute, chronic or acute-on-chronic. Patients with acute retention present as surgical emergencies. Acute retention is the sudden inability to pass urine, with the presence of painful bladder. Chronic retention is the presence of an enlarged, painless bladder with or without difficulty in micturition, which may be accompanied by overflow.

Figure 59 MRI (sagittal section) of a patient who presented with acute urinary retention. The bladder (short arrow) is distended and there is an enlarged benign prostate (longer arrow).

CAUSES

LOCAL

URETHRAL LUMEN OR BLADDER NECK
- Stones
- Blood clot

- Tumours
- Urethral valves

URETHRAL OR BLADDER WALL
- Urethral trauma ⚠
- Urethral stricture
- Urethral tumour

OUTSIDE THE WALL
- Prostatic enlargement (Fig. 59)
- Faecal impaction
- Pregnant uterus
- Pelvic tumour

GENERAL

POSTOPERATIVE

Neurogenic
- Spinal cord injuries ⚠
- Diabetic autonomic neuropathy
- Spinal cord disease
  - Multiple sclerosis
  - Spinal tumour
  - Tabes dorsalis

Drugs
- Anticholinergic drugs
- Antidepressants
- Alcohol

HISTORY

Local

Check for a history of problems with micturition, e.g. difficulty in starting, poor stream, nocturia, frequency, dysuria. Is there any history of urinary tract infection, urethritis, ureteric colic (to suggest a stone which may have passed into the bladder and then impacted into the bladder neck or urethra) or haematuria? Is there a past history of prolonged catheterisation to suggest a urethral stricture? A history of trauma will be apparent. Has the patient fallen astride an object? Has trauma caused a pelvic fracture? Is the patient constipated, to suggest faecal impaction? A pregnant uterus will be obvious.

General

Postoperative acute retention is common, especially in elderly men. This may be due to anxiety, embarrassment, supine posture, pain, drugs, fluid overload or previous unrecognised prostatism, with minimal symptoms. After urological procedures, it may be due to blood clot in the bladder. Check for a history of neurological disease. Has the patient suffered spinal cord injury? Check the drug history.

EXAMINATION

Local

The patient may have a tender, palpable, painful bladder with sudden onset of retention. In acute retention, the bladder rarely extends far above the pubic symphysis. In chronic retention, the distended bladder is often painless and more markedly distended than in acute retention, often reaching to the umbilicus. With chronic retention, there may be overflow incontinence. Feel along the course of the urethra for a stone or stricture. Perform a digital rectal examination to check for prostatic hypertrophy or pelvic tumour. Following pelvic trauma with urethral injury, there will be a high 'floating' prostate on rectal examination. Check the urethral meatus for ulcer or stone. Examine the patient for signs of uraemia, which may be present with chronic retention.

General

Postoperative retention will be obvious. Occasionally, it is difficult to palpate the bladder because of pain and guarding related to a surgical incision. Neurological causes of acute retention or those related to spinal trauma are often obvious. Carry out a full neurological examination.

GENERAL INVESTIGATIONS

- **FBC, ESR**
  Hb ↓ in chronic renal failure, tumours, haematuria. WCC ↑ infection. ESR ↑ malignancy and infection.

- **U&Es**
  Renal failure. Obstructive uropathy.

- **Mid-stream urine (MSU)**
  Urine dip. Microscopy. Culture and sensitivity for UTI. Cytology to confirm malignancy.

- **Bladder scan**
  Quantify amount of urine in bladder on presentation. Post-micturation scan may help identify chronic retention.

- **CXR**
  Pulmonary oedema (chronic renal failure). Possible tumour metastases.

- **US renal tract**
  Bladder size confirms diagnosis. Dilated upper urinary tract due to back pressure. Pregnant uterus.

SPECIFIC INVESTIGATIONS

- PSA
  Carcinoma of the prostate.
- Urethrography
  Urethral valves. Stricture. Urethral trauma.
- Cystoscopy
  Stone, tumour, stricture.
- Urodynamics
  Identification and assessment of neurological or bladder neck problems.

- Digital rectal examination is mandatory in the patient with retention.
- Faecal impaction in the elderly may be a cause of urinary retention.
- A history suggestive of disc prolapse with urinary retention suggests cord compression. An urgent neurosurgical opinion is required.
- Following catheterisation for chronic retention, do not empty the bladder rapidly. This may result in brisk haematuria from the sudden decompression. Controlled drainage is required.

VAGINAL DISCHARGE

Vaginal discharge can occur at any age but is usually a symptom of reproductive years.

Figure 60 Trichomoniasis. Typical vulvovaginitis, with perfuse foul-smelling purulent frothy discharge.

CAUSES

- Candidiasis
- Bacterial vaginosis
- *Trichomonas* vaginosis (Fig. 60)
- Cervicitis, e.g. gonorrhoea, *Chlamydia*, herpes
- Excessive normal secretions
- Retained foreign body, e.g. tampon, pessary ⚠
- Intrauterine contraceptive device
- Salpingitis
- Infection of Bartholin's glands ⚠
- Neoplasm, e.g. vagina, vulva ⚠
- Pyometra ⚠
- Colovaginal fistula

HISTORY

Obtain a full history of the discharge, including timing, colour, consistency, smell and the presence or absence of itch. Intensive itch suggests thrush. An offensive smell occurs with trichomonal and bacterial vaginosis. Ask whether the patient experiences pain on intercourse. Pelvic pain, tenderness and fever suggest pelvic inflammatory disease. Take a full sexual history (young women, change of partner, multiple partners). Excessive normal secretions just feel wet. There is no discomfort.

EXAMINATION

A red, swollen, sore and itchy vulva suggests candidiasis. The character of the discharge is important. A thick yellow-brown discharge from the cervix occurs with gonorrhoea; a thinner yellow-brown cervical discharge occurs with *Chlamydia*; a thin greeny-yellow and often frothy discharge with an unpleasant fishy smell occurs with trichomoniasis; a thin grey-white fishy smelling discharge suggests bacterial vaginosis; a thick white odourless discharge occurs with candidiasis. Carry out a PV and speculum examination. This will show an inflamed cervix with trichomonal vaginosis and also with cervicitis due to gonococcus, *Chlamydia* and herpes.

GENERAL INVESTIGATIONS

- Triple swabs
  High vaginal swab – bacterial vaginosis, candidiasis, trichomonal vaginalis.
  Endocervical swab – gonorrhoea.
  Endocervical swab – *Chlamydia* DNA amplification for *Chlamydia trachomatis*.
- Vaginal pH testing
  pH > 4.5 in bacterial vaginosis. pH < 4.5 in candidiasis.
- Urine analysis (first catch)
  DNA amplification for *Chlamydia*.
- Gram stain
  Gram stain on cervical or urethral exudate – gram-negative intracellular diplococci in gonorrhoea.

SPECIFIC INVESTIGATIONS

- Hysteroscopy
  Malignancy/menorrhagia.
- Cervical smear test
  Malignancy.
- Barium enema
  Colovaginal fistula.
- MRI
  Colovaginal fistula.

- Malignancy is a likely cause of vaginal discharge in postmenopausal years. Always perform a full pelvic examination.

- Always take a full sexual history and, if sexually transmitted disease is suspected, refer to the GUM clinic for full assessment and contact tracing.

- Vaginal discharge is rare before puberty. Consider foreign body or sexual abuse.

- Recurrent thrush may be a presenting symptom of diabetes mellitus.

VISUAL PROBLEMS

Patients who present with visual disturbance are often very distressed, with their quality of life affected, including their ability to drive. Below is a list of common conditions that may give rise to visual problems, grouped according to symptoms.

Figure 61 Papilloedema. Note the blurring of the optic disc, retinal oedema, flame haemorrhages (small arrow) and exudates (large arrows).

CAUSES

VISUAL DISTURBANCES (FLASHING LIGHTS OR FLOATERS)

- Migraine
- Retinal detachment ⚠
- Vitreous haemorrhage
- Age-related macular degeneration
- Vitreous detachment

BLURRING OF VISION

- Refractive errors (long or short sighted)
- Head injuries

● Acute angle-closure glaucoma ▲

◐ Blunt trauma to the eye

LOSS OF VISION

PARTIAL LOSS

● Homonymous hemianopia – stroke, tumour ▲

● Peripheral field loss – glaucoma, papilloedema

● Central field loss – age-related macular degeneration

◐ Bitemporal hemianopia – pituitary tumour

● Horizontal field loss – retinal vascular occlusion

TOTAL LOSS

Acute

● Amaurosis fugax (thrombosis/embolism) ▲

◐ Papilloedema (Fig. 61)
  - ○ Raised intracranial pressure
  - ● Malignant hypertension

◐ Temporal arteritis ▲

◐ Optic neuritis

◐ Central retinal vein occlusion

◐ Central retinal artery occlusion

◐ Corneal ulcer

◐ Vitreous haemorrhage

◐ Posterior uveitis

◐ Pituitary apoplexy

● Retinal detachment

Gradual

● Cataract

● Glaucoma

● Diabetic retinopathy

● Hypertensive retinopathy

● Age-related macular degeneration

● Retinitis pigmentosa

● Infectious
  - ● Trachoma (*Chlamydia trachomatis*) ● *(common in underdeveloped countries)*
  - ● *Onchocerciasis* (nematode infection) ● *(common in underdeveloped countries)*

● Vitamin A deficiency ● *(common in underdeveloped countries)*

HISTORY

First establish if visual loss is monocular or binocular. Ocular or optic nerve pathology generally causes monocular visual loss, whereas lesions at the optic chiasma or more posteriorly cause binocular loss that will respect the vertical meridian. Loss of central vision may be due to macular or optic nerve pathology. Retinal lesions cause a 'positive' scotoma (the patient is aware that part of the field is obstructed), whereas damage posterior to the retina causes a 'negative' scotoma (the patient does not see that a segment of the visual field is missing). Always ask about pain, as this will help differentiate the cause.

Visual disturbances

Bilateral flashing lights and zigzag lines are often reported by patients suffering with attacks of migraine. This is accompanied by throbbing headache, nausea, vomiting and photophobia. Posterior vitreous detachment, vitreous haemorrhage and retinal detachment are all associated with floaters and flashing lights. Visual acuity and visual fields are normal at first but may be impaired with a large vitreous haemorrhage or advanced retinal detachment, the latter which is a surgical emergency. In age-related macular degeneration, there is a reduction in visual acuity and flashes of light.

Blurring of vision

Errors of refraction (long- or short-sighted) are the most common cause of blurring of vision. This is a common problem and is usually corrected with glasses by optometrists. Head and eye injuries may also give rise to transient blurring of the vision, whilst with acute angle-closure glaucoma, corneal oedema will give rise to the appearances of haloes around lights and is associated with a red and painful eye and difficulty adjusting to night vision.

Loss of vision

Visual loss may be partial or total. The description of the area of partial visual field loss is very informative. Complaints of vertical visual field losses are due to lesions posterior to the optic chiasma and most commonly caused by strokes, although similar effects can be produced by space-occupying lesions such as cerebral tumours. Horizontal visual field losses imply that the cause lies within the retina and is usually due to retinal vascular occlusions. Patients with glaucoma may complain of tunnel vision, and patients with age-related macular degeneration may experience sudden central visual field loss.

Sudden total visual loss is usually due to a vascular aetiology. Amaurosis fugax is sudden transient monocular blindness due to atheroembolism of the ophthalmic artery. Patients classically complain of a 'curtain descending across the field of vision'. With temporal arteritis affecting the ophthalmic artery, sudden onset of blindness can occur in conjunction with the symptoms of temporal headache, jaw claudication and scalp tenderness. It is often associated with polymyalgia rheumatica. Papilloedema may cause transient visual loss, lasting seconds, related to posture.

Monocular blindness due to optic neuritis may occur with multiple sclerosis; it is often associated with retro-orbital pain that worsens with eye movements and starts with a progressive dimming of vision over a few days but can transiently recover. In corneal ulcer, there may be a history of trauma with visual loss and a painful red eye, whilst in pituitary apoplexy, there is acute loss of vision with an underlying headache. In uveitis, this occurs over days with photophobia and a red painful eye.

Diabetic retinopathy is the most common cause of blindness in Western society. In addition, diabetics are also more prone to develop cataracts and glaucoma. In the elderly, gradual onset of visual loss may be due to cataracts, glaucoma or age-related macular degeneration. Owing to the gradual onset of symptoms, these groups of patients may present very late.

EXAMINATION

Visual acuity should be assessed with a Snellen chart. If visualisation of the largest letter is not possible, then assess vision by counting fingers. Further tests to use are those of movement and, finally, the ability to discriminate between light and dark. With refractive errors, vision can be corrected by viewing the Snellen chart through a pinhole. Visual fields are examined by confrontational testing, and the extent of visual field loss can be assessed approximately.

Pupillary response to light (direct and consensual) allows the assessment of the visual pathway. Direct light reflex may be lost in lesions involving the unilateral optic nerve and with central retinal artery occlusion.

Colour vision will be reduced disproportionately compared with visual acuity in optic nerve diseases. This may be assessed with the use of Ishihara colour plates.

Fundoscopy

A wealth of information is obtained on fundoscopy. The red reflex is lost with cataracts. Examination of the retina may reveal background retinopathy with diabetes, consisting of dot and blot haemorrhages with cotton-wool spots. With hypertensive retinopathy, silver wiring, arteriovenous nipping, retinal haemorrhages and eventually papilloedema may be appreciated. Growth of new vessels on the retina indicates proliferative retinopathy. An infarcted retina appears oedematous and pale; the macula appears prominent and red (cherry-red spot). Detached retinal folds may be seen, and clots of blood are visible with vitreous haemorrhage. The margins of the optic disc become blurred with papilloedema and optic neuritis but later may appear pale. A cupped optic disc appearance occurs with chronic glaucoma and optic disc pallor with bayoneting of vessels.

Upon completion of the examination of the eye, a neurological examination should be performed including a cranial nerve examination, followed by a cardiovascular examination to exclude sources of emboli. The rhythm of the pulse is assessed for atrial fibrillation and the heart and carotids are auscultated for murmurs. Blood pressure should be measured to exclude hypertension.

GENERAL INVESTIGATIONS

- ■ **ESR and CRP**
  Temporal arteritis.

- ■ **Blood glucose**
  Glucose ↑ diabetes with vitreous haemorrhage.

- ■ **Intraocular pressure measurements**
  ↑ with glaucoma.

- ■ **Perimetry**
  Formal charting of visual fields. Arcuate scotomas are found
  with glaucoma. Central scotomas may be seen with optic
  neuritis. Bitemporal hemianopias/homonymous hemianopias and
  quadrantanopias in neurological pathology.

- ■ **Fluorescein angiography**
  ARMD, retinal vein/artery occlusion.

SPECIFIC INVESTIGATIONS

- ■ **Gram stain**
  Bacterial infection for corneal ulcer.

- ■ **CT/MRI head**
  Tumours, stroke, multiple sclerosis.

- ■ **Carotid Doppler**
  Atherosclerotic plaque with amaurosis fugax.

- ■ **Temporal artery biopsy**
  Temporal arteritis.

- ■ **US**
  To assess retina if no visualisation of fundus behind cataract or
  vitreous haemorrhage.

- • **Sudden onset of visual disturbance or loss is an opthalmic
  emergency and must be investigated immediately.**

- • **If temporal arteritis is suspected consider treatment
  with corticosteroids.**

VOICE DISORDERS

Voice disorders can be caused by a number of conditions. Change in the quality of the voice ranges from mild hoarseness to aphonia. It is important to exclude laryngeal carcinoma, which is easily treated in the early stages but has a poor prognosis once metastatic spread has occurred.

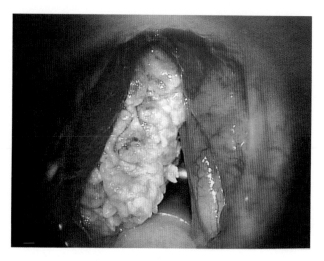

Figure 62 Laryngeal carcinoma. There is a verrucous squamous cell carcinoma of the left vocal fold. The entire length of the vocal fold is involved by this exophytic growth.

CAUSES

INFECTIVE

● Laryngitis

TRAUMATIC

● Blunt trauma

● Excessive vocal use

NEOPLASTIC

● Laryngeal papilloma (due to HPV infection)

● Laryngeal carcinoma (Fig. 62) ⚠

● Leukoplakia

RECURRENT LARYNGEAL NERVE PALSY

- Goitre
- Bronchial carcinoma
- Postoperative – thoracic, parathyroid and thyroid surgery
- Oesophageal carcinoma
- Thoracic aortic aneurysm ⚠

AUTOIMMUNE DISEASE

- Myasthenia gravis
- Parkinson's disease

OTHER

- Psychogenic
- Acid-reflux disease
- Vocal fold nodule
- Vocal fold cyst
- Vocal fold granulomatoma
- Reinke's oedema
- Presbylarynx

HISTORY

Onset

The temporal profile of deterioration in quality of the voice is useful in discriminating between the causes. Infection and excessive vocal use may result in transient deterioration. Progressive deterioration may be due to tumours, recurrent laryngeal nerve palsy. Reinke's oedema is oedema and gelatinous material accumulating along the vocal cord, whilst presbylarynx refers to age-related atrophy of the larynx.

Precipitating factors

Viral infections usually precede and cause acute laryngitis. It is most commonly due to the influenza virus. Smoking and vocal cord trauma from excessive use by singers, or simply excessive shouting, are often enough to precipitate hoarseness. A history of blunt trauma to the larynx may be evident and hoarseness from resulting laryngeal fractures may be the first indication of a precarious airway. A history of GORD due to dietary intake may result in laryngeal irritation. Also ask about alcohol and smoking.

Past medical history

Recurrent laryngeal nerve palsy associated with a goitre is usually due to thyroid malignancy. Tumour infiltration of the recurrent nerve may also result from malignancy occurring in oesophagus and lung. Hoarseness of the voice may be the first complaint of patients with a thoracic aneurysm. Previous thyroid or thoracic surgery may have resulted in vagus or recurrent laryngeal nerve injuries. A history of Parkinson's disease or myasthenia gravis may explain gradual hoarseness and changes in voice quality.

Associated symptoms

Sore throat from pharyngitis may accompany acute laryngitis. Pain referred to the ear or dysphagia can be late presenting features of laryngeal carcinomas. Rapidly progressive dysphagia is also a symptom of oesophageal carcinoma. Nasal voice may be accompanied by ptosis, diplopia and muscle fatigue with myasthenia gravis. Bizarre associated symptoms with impaired voice intensity but normal coughing ability should lead to the consideration of a functional cause; however, this should be a diagnosis of exclusion.

EXAMINATION

Indirect laryngoscopy is performed with a mirror and headlamp. If unsuccessful, the larynx can easily be examined with a flexible fibreoptic laryngoscope under local anaesthetic. A dry erythematous larynx is seen with acute laryngitis. Vocal cord papillomas and supraglottic carcinomas may be readily visible. Recurrent laryngeal nerve injury will result in paralysis of the unilateral vocal cord. Upon observing this, a detailed examination is undertaken to determine the underlying cause. The neck should be examined for the presence of a goitre. Palpable supraclavicular lymphadenopathy may arise from oesophageal carcinoma. The chest is carefully examined for signs of collapse and effusion, which may be secondary to bronchial carcinoma.

GENERAL INVESTIGATIONS

- FBC
  ↑ white count with laryngitis.
- ESR
  ↑ with laryngitis, carcinoma.
- CXR
  Bronchial carcinoma, widened mediastinum with thoracic aneurysm.

SPECIFIC INVESTIGATIONS

- Tensilon test
  Myasthenia gravis.
- Endoscopy
  Oesophageal carcinoma. Cyst. Nodule.
- CT neck
  Diagnosis and staging for laryngeal and thyroid carcinoma.
- CT thorax
  Lung tumours, thoracic aneurysms.

- **Aortography**
  Thoracic aneurysm.
- **FNAC**
  Thyroid carcinoma.

> • Abnormality of the voice in association with dysphagia is of grave concern and urgent assessment for carcinoma is necessary, especially in a smoker.

VOMITING

Vomiting is the forceful ejection of gastric contents through the mouth. It occurs when the vomiting centre in the medulla oblongata is stimulated. This may be due to direct stimulation of the centre (central vomiting) or via afferent fibres (reflex vomiting). Haematemesis (vomiting blood) is dealt with in a separate chapter on p. 185.

Figure 63 Peptic ulcer. There is a benign gastric ulcer on the lesser curvature of the stomach, seen at gastroscopy.

CAUSES

CENTRAL VOMITING

- Drugs, e.g. narcotic analgesics, chemotherapeutic agents
- Acute infections
- Endocrine/metabolic
  - Pregnancy
  - Uraemia

- Diabetic ketoacidosis ⚠
- Hypercalcaemia
- Addison's disease

REFLEX VOMITING

GASTROINTESTINAL DISEASE

Inflammation/irritation
- Appendicitis ⚠
- Cholecystitis
- Pancreatitis ⚠
- Peptic ulceration/acute gastritis (Fig. 63) ⚠
- Peritonitis ⚠
- Biliary colic
- Gastroenteritis
  - Viral
  - Bacteria, e.g. *Campylobacter, Salmonella* spp.
- Drugs, e.g. aspirin, NSAIDs, alcohol, iron, antibiotics
- Emetics, e.g. sodium chloride, ipecacuanha
- Poisons, e.g. arsenic

Obstruction
- Small bowel obstruction ⚠
- Pyloric stenosis
- Large bowel obstruction ⚠

CNS CAUSES
- Raised intracranial pressure ⚠
- Labyrinthine disorders
- Head injury ⚠
- Migraine
- Ménière's disease

PSYCHOGENIC
- Offensive sights and smells
- Psychiatric disorders, e.g. bulimia nervosa, anorexia nervosa

OTHERS
- Myocardial infarction ⚠
- Severe pain, e.g. testicular torsion, fractures ⚠
- Irradiation
- Widespread malignant disease
- Severe coughing, e.g. chronic bronchitis

HISTORY

General

Nature of the vomiting

Bright-red blood, e.g. bleeding peptic ulcer. Altered blood (coffee grounds). Bile (high small bowel obstruction), faeculent (low small or large bowel obstruction). Recently eaten food. Food several days old (pyloric stenosis), projectile vomiting (infantile pyloric stenosis).

Time of vomit

Soon after meal (gastric ulcer, gastric carcinoma). Early morning (pregnancy). Chronic chest infection (after bout of coughing).

Relief of pain by vomiting

Peptic ulcer disease.

Central vomiting

Take a careful drug history. It will be obvious if the patient is having chemotherapy. Check for pregnancy. Endocrine and metabolic disorders will largely be determined by the result of blood tests.

Reflex vomiting

Gastrointestinal

There will usually be a clear history of a gastrointestinal problem, e.g. localised tenderness of peritonitis or colicky abdominal pain associated with obstruction. Take a careful drug history for irritant drugs, e.g. aspirin. Check for abuse of emetics, e.g. bulimia.

CNS

With raised intracranial pressure, there will usually be headache, drowsiness and fits in addition to vomiting. With labyrinthitis, there will be nausea, vomiting, vertigo and often a hearing defect. Ménière's disease presents with vertigo, tinnitus and deafness. The tinnitus is usually constant but more severe before an attack. Tinnitus may precede other symptoms by many months. Attacks of Ménière's disease may last from minutes to hours. Migraine will present with a visual aura with unilateral throbbing headache and sometimes photophobia. With motion sickness, the history is usually obvious.

Psychogenic

Bulimia is eating followed by self-induced vomiting. Vomiting may also occur in anorexia nervosa but failure to eat is usually the prominent feature. Full psychiatric assessment is recommended.

Others

There will usually be severe chest pain in myocardial infarction, and severe pain associated with testicular torsion or trauma. A history of a fracture will be obvious. There may be a history of severe chest infection, e.g. bronchitis or bronchiectasis, associated with coughing bouts followed by vomiting. There may be a recent history of radiotherapy for malignant disease. Widespread malignant disease may cause vomiting.

EXAMINATION

Gastrointestinal

A full gastrointestinal examination should be carried out. Look for signs of localised tenderness or signs of intestinal obstruction.

CNS

With raised intracranial pressure, there will be listlessness, irritability, drowsiness and the pulse rate will be low with a rising blood pressure. Check for papilloedema. Ultimately, coma and irregular breathing will occur. With acute labyrinthitis, there may be nystagmus to the opposite side from the lesion. Sensorineural deafness may occur in purulent labyrinthitis. With Ménière's, there will be rotatory nystagmus and unsteadiness of stance and gait during an attack, together with past-pointing.

Others

With myocardial infarction, there may be signs of acute congestive cardiac failure. With causes of severe pain, attention will normally be drawn to the appropriate area, e.g. scrotum with testicular trauma or torsion. With irradiation, there may be skin signs of recent radiotherapy. With widespread malignant disease, the patient is often cachectic. A site of the primary may be obvious. With severe coughing, chest signs may be obvious.

GENERAL INVESTIGATIONS

- **FBC, ESR/CRP**
  Hb ↓ gastrointestinal disease. Malignancy. Anorexia nervosa.
  WCC ↑ abdominal inflammation. ESR ↑ inflammation. Tumour.

- **U&Es**
  Dehydration. Uraemia. Hyperkalaemia occurs in Addison's disease.

- **LFTs**
  Biliary tract disease.

- **Serum amylase**
  Pancreatitis.

- **Urinalysis**
  Glucose and ketones in diabetes; blood, white cells and protein suggest UTI, blood may indicate kidney stone.

- **CXR**
  Congestive cardiac failure – pulmonary oedema. Malignancy.
  Pneumonia. Bronchiectasis.

- **ECG**
  Myocardial infarction.

- **AXR**
  Obstruction.

SPECIFIC INVESTIGATIONS

- **Blood glucose**
  Raised in diabetes. Low in Addison's disease.

- **Serum calcium**
  Hyperparathyroidism and other causes of hypercalcaemia.

- **ABGs**
  Diabetic ketoacidosis.

- **βHCG**
  Pregnancy.

- **Toxicology screen**
  Drug causes of vomiting.

- **Barium enema**
  Malignancy. Diverticular disease.

- **Small bowel enema**
  Gastrointestinal disease, e.g. Crohn's disease.

- **OGD**
  Peptic ulcer disease. Malignancy.

- **US**
  Gastrointestinal disease, e.g. gallstones.

- **CT**
  Abdominal malignancy. Cerebral haemorrhage.

- **MRI**
  Intracranial lesion associated with raised intracranial pressure.

- **Caloric tests**
  Labyrinthitis, Ménière's disease.

- **Audiometry**
  Ménière's disease, labyrinthitis.

- Although vomiting is a frequent symptom, with most cases being self-limiting, it may be a clue to serious pathology. Further investigation is required urgently if there are any associated systemic signs, e.g. neurological, abdominal.

- Diabetics need careful monitoring, as vomiting may lead to poor sugar control.

WEIGHT GAIN

Weight gain is extremely common and the most frequent cause is simple obesity. Excessive weight gain itself has deleterious effects on general health. With the exception of simple obesity and pregnancy, other conditions only account for <1% of patients presenting with weight gain.

Figure 64 (A,B) Cushing's syndrome. Note central obesity, typical facial features and a 'buffalo hump'.

CAUSES

INCREASED FAT

- Simple obesity
- Hypothyroidism
- Cushing's syndrome (Fig. 64)

- Polycystic ovarian syndrome
- Hypothalamic disease

INCREASED FLUID

- Cardiac failure
- Hepatic failure with ascites
- Renal failure (e.g. nephrotic syndrome)
- Lymphatic obstruction

INCREASED MUSCLE

- Athletes, e.g. weightlifters
- Androgenic steroids
- Growth hormone

OTHER

- Pregnancy
- Depression
- Drugs, e.g. insulin gliclazide and corticosteroids
- Tiredness
- Premenstrual syndrome

HISTORY

General

Enquire about the possibility of pregnancy and any changes in dietary habits that may result in simple weight gain as well as a sedentary lifestyle. Rapid weight gain is often secondary to increased fluid, as opposed to an increase in dry weight. A drug history is taken to exclude the use of anabolic steroids and growth hormone, especially in body builders. Enquire about a family history, diet and amount of activity in relation to simple obesity. With regard to sleep, some evidence is emerging that patients who have reduced sleep are likely to be overweight.

Cushing's syndrome

Patients with Cushing's syndrome present with moon face, 'buffalo hump' (deposits of fat on the back of neck and shoulders), hair growth, acne, abdominal striae, muscle weakness, back pain, amenorrhoea, thin skin, bruising and depression. A drug history should be taken to exclude exogenous corticosteroids as the cause.

Hypothyroidism

With hypothyroidism, patients may complain of lethargy, anorexia, cold intolerance, goitre, dry hair, dry skin, constipation and menorrhagia.

Polycystic ovarian syndrome

Women with this condition present with hirsutism, obesity and menstrual irregularities. It is also associated with insulin resistance.

Hypothalamic disease

Prior history of neurosurgery, craniopharyngioma or other brain tumours may have resulted in damage to the hypothalamus. As it is the regulatory centre for appetite, uncontrolled excessive eating may result.

Cardiac failure

Fluid retention from cardiac failure may be accompanied by symptoms of exertional dyspnoea, orthopnoea, paroxysmal nocturnal dyspnoea. Ascites and peripheral oedema may also result from congestive heart failure (specifically right-sided heart failure).

Renal failure

Patients with renal failure may present with lethargy, fragile pigmented skin, peripheral oedema, periorbital oedema, thirst and polyuria.

EXAMINATION

Inspection

The distribution of body fat should be noted. Patients with Cushing's syndrome have truncal obesity with proximal muscle wasting. Hirsutism is a feature of both polycystic ovarian syndrome and Cushing's syndrome. With hypothyroidism, there may be loss of the outer third of the eyebrows and a 'peaches and cream' complexion.

Inspection of the trunk may reveal thin skin with easy bruising in both Cushing's syndrome and renal failure. In addition, striae and thoracic kyphosis may be present with Cushing's caused by wedge fractures caused by osteoporosis.

Proximal muscle weakness is found in both Cushing's syndrome and hypothyroidism. Check for the physique of a 'body builder'.

Palpation and auscultation

Peripheral oedema may be a feature of fluid overload seen in renal, hepatic and cardiac failure. Non-pitting oedema is characteristically found with hypothyroidism. The JVP should be examined and will be elevated with congestive cardiac failure. The pulse is taken and bradycardia may be noted with hypothyroidism. The blood pressure is measured and hypertension may occur as a complication of Cushing's disease. A third heart sound may be present with cardiac failure, and widespread pulmonary crepitation suggests pulmonary oedema from cardiac failure or from fluid overload in renal or hepatic failure.

Further examination of the abdominal system may reveal the presence of ascites (p. 27), which may result from liver disease, malignancy or cardiac failure. A complete neurological examination may also be performed to screen for neurological deficits, which will warrant diagnostic imaging to look for lesions involving the hypothalamus. If there is any suspicion that a patient is taking body-building drugs, e.g. anabolic steroids, check for testicular atrophy and prostatic hypertrophy.

GENERAL INVESTIGATIONS

- **Urine dipstick**
  +++ glucose – diabetes from Cushing's syndrome or as a complication of obesity. +++ protein is present with nephrotic syndrome. Blood may be present in renal disease.
- **U&Es**
  K^+ ↓ Cushing's. Urea and creatinine ↑ renal failure.
- **LFTs**
  Liver disease.
- **TFTs**
  Hypothyroidism.
- **Random cortisol**
  ↑ evening levels may suggest Cushing's syndrome but is not the gold standard diagnostic test.

SPECIFIC INVESTIGATIONS

- **24-Hour urinary free cortisol**
  ↑ with Cushing's.
- **24-Hour urine collection for protein**
  >3.5 g with nephrotic syndrome.
- **Low-dose dexamethasone test**
  Failure of cortisol suppression with Cushing's.
- **US abdomen and pelvis**
  Renal disease, polycystic ovaries, ascites.
- **Echocardiography**
  Cardiac failure.
- **CT/MRI head**
  Hypothalamic disease.
- **Renal biopsy**
  Aetiology of renal parenchymal disease.

- **Every opportunity should be taken to identify risk factors in order to reduce weight. Advice regarding diet and exercise is a crucial first step.**

WEIGHT LOSS

Unintentional weight loss is often a manifestation of significant underlying disease and should never be ignored.

Figure 65 Obvious signs of weight loss with widespread muscle and soft-tissue wasting in a malnourished patient.

CAUSES

SYSTEMIC DISEASE

- Malignancy
- Cardiac failure
- Chronic respiratory disease
- Renal failure
- Liver failure
- Malabsorption
- Connective tissue disease (e.g. SLE, rheumatoid arthritis)

ENDOCRINE

- Diabetes mellitus
- Hyperthyroidism
- Addison's disease

INFECTIVE	
	TB ● *(very common in the developing world and on the increase in the developed world)*
	HIV ● *(very common in the developing world)*
●	Helminth (worms) infection ● *(very common in endemic areas)*

PSYCHIATRIC	
●	Depression
	Anorexia nervosa

OTHER	
●	Any terminal illness
●	Substance abuse (e.g. laxatives, amphetamines, opiates)
	Drugs, e.g. excessive thyroxine replacement
●	Malnutrition (Fig. 65) ● *(common in developing countries)*

HISTORY

General

The timeframe and amount of weight loss should be noted. A dietary history is required to determine the amount and type of food ingested. Decreased dietary intake may result from loss of appetite or loss of interest in eating due to depression. On the other hand, patients with thyrotoxicosis lose weight, despite a voracious appetite.

Enquiries should be undertaken regarding perception of body image, as patients with anorexia nervosa believe that they are overweight, despite being severely underweight. Risk factors for HIV should be screened for and a sexual history as well as information regarding intravenous drug use should be obtained. Systemic enquiry is required to identify features suggestive of malignancy or organ failure in each system to account for unintentional weight loss. A butterfly rash may be present in cases of SLE.

Cardiorespiratory system

Dyspnoea, orthopnoea, paroxysmal nocturnal dyspnoea and peripheral oedema are symptoms suggestive of congestive cardiac failure. With longstanding cardiac failure, cardiac cachexia results from loss of total body fat and lean body mass. Currently, the most common aetiology is end-stage heart failure. Dyspnoea without accompanying orthopnoea or paroxysmal nocturnal dyspnoea suggests respiratory disease. With any chronic respiratory disorder, basal metabolic rate is increased as a result of the increased work of breathing. The presence of haemoptysis may be due to malignancy or TB. A long smoking history is a strong predisposing factor for the development of bronchial carcinoma and COPD. Night sweats and weight loss may be accompanying features of both TB and Hodgkin's disease.

Gastrointestinal system

Lethargy, diarrhoea, steatorrhoea (p. 399) and abdominal discomfort are various symptoms suggestive of malabsorption. Jaundice, dark urine, pale stools, itching, prolonged bleeding, abdominal swelling from ascites and confusion are symptoms associated with liver disease. Vague abdominal pains, change in bowel habit, tenesmus, blood or mucus mixed with the stools may be due to gastrointestinal malignancy. Patients with helminth infections, such as ascaris, may complain of perianal itching and notice worms in their faeces. Although this is rare in the UK, it may be encountered in patients returning from foreign travel.

Renal system

Lethargy, anorexia, nocturia, oliguria, polyuria, haematuria, frothy urine from proteinuria, skin fragility, pruritus, oedema and bone pains are some of the multisystemic features suggestive of renal disease.

Haematological system

Localised non-tender lymphadenopathy from Hodgkin's disease may be accompanied by pyrexia and pruritus. Persistent generalised lymphadenopathy, however, is a recognised presenting feature of HIV.

Endocrine system

Polydipsia and polyuria with weight loss may be presenting features of diabetics. Patients with thyrotoxicosis may complain of tremor, staring eyes, heat intolerance, palpitations and diarrhoea. With Addison's disease, anorexia, malaise, nausea, vomiting, diarrhoea or syncope from postural hypotension may be experienced.

Connective tissue diseases

Arthritis is a very common presentation of connective tissue disease, including rheumatoid arthritis and SLE. Patients may also complain of early morning joint stiffness, lethargy and poor mobility.

EXAMINATION

The causes of weight loss are varied. The following specific features identified on examination may be useful in determining an underlying cause.

Inspection

Signs suggestive of endocrine disorder may be obvious; a goitre may be visible with thyrotoxicosis, accompanied by exophthalmos and tremor. Pigmentation of the skin creases and buccal mucosa in a cachectic patient with postural hypotension are the usual findings with Addison's disease. Jaundice, caput medusae, spider naevi and gynaecomastia may be seen with liver disease. Tachypnoea and pursed-lip breathing may be evident with COPD. Clubbing may be a feature of bronchial carcinoma, suppurative lung disease, cirrhosis and inflammatory bowel disease.

The JVP is elevated with congestive cardiac failure. Swelling and deformity of the small joints of the hand may be seen with connective tissue disease. In addition, a rash will frequently be present with SLE.

Palpation and auscultation

Peripheral oedema may be present with cardiac failure, malabsorption, renal and liver disease. Auscultation of the chest may reveal widespread crepitations with pulmonary oedema from cardiac failure, or uniformly decreased breath sounds with COPD. Palpation of the abdomen may reveal hepatomegaly and ascites with liver disease; ascites may also occur with cardiac failure and gastrointestinal malignancies. Lying and standing blood pressure should be measured, as a postural drop is present with Addison's disease. Joint tenderness is present with connective tissue disease.

GENERAL INVESTIGATIONS

- **FBC**
  Hb ↓ chronic disease, malabsorption, renal and liver failure and connective tissue disease. WCC ↑ in infective and inflammatory disease.

- **ESR and CRP**
  ↑ with malignancy and connective tissue disease.

- **U&Es**
  Urea and creatinine ↑ renal failure. Na^+ ↓, K^+ ↑ and HCO_3^- ↓ in Addison's disease.

- **Blood glucose**
  More than 11.1 mmol/L on two separate occasions indicates diabetes mellitus.

- **LFTs & clotting screen**
  Bilirubin ↑, transaminases ↑ and albumin ↓ liver failure.
  PT ↑ liver failure.

- **TSH and free T_4**
  TSH ↓ and T_4 ↑ thyrotoxicosis.

- **Urine dipstick**
  Glucose with diabetes. Protein and blood with renal disorders.

- **CXR**
  Malignancy, TB.

SPECIFIC INVESTIGATIONS

- **Faecal occult blood**
  Colorectal carcinoma.

- **Colonoscopy**
  Colorectal carcinoma, inflammatory bowel disease.

- **Gastroscopy**
  Gastric carcinoma.

- **US/CT abdomen**
  Malignancy, small kidneys with renal failure.
- **ECG +/− echocardiography**
  Ventricular impairment with cardiac failure.
- **Stool cultures**
  Microscopy for helminths and their ova. Helminths may occasionally be visible with the naked eye.
- **Faecal fat estimation**
  ↑ with fat malabsorption.
- **ANA, RF**
  ANA raised in SLE and RF increased in rheumatoid arthritis.
- **HIV antibodies**
  For the diagnosis of HIV.

- **Dramatic weight loss over a short period of time raises the possibility of malignancy. Urgent investigation is mandatory.**

SECTION B

BIOCHEMICAL PRESENTATIONS

HYPERGLYCAEMIA

Hyperglycaemia is defined as a plasma glucose >7.0 mmol/L. By far the most common cause is diabetes mellitus.

CAUSES

ENDOCRINE

- Diabetes mellitus (types 1 and 2)

DRUGS

- Corticosteroids
- Beta blockers
- Thiazide diuretics
- Niacin
- Pentamidine
- Protease inhibitors
- L-asparaginase
- Antipsychotic agents

SYSTEMIC DISEASE

- Cushing's syndrome

SEVERE STRESS ⚠

- Stroke
- Myocardial infarction

PHYSIOLOGICAL

- Infection
- Inflammation

OTHER

- Pregnancy

SYMPTOMS AND SIGNS

The most common symptoms include polydipsia, polyuria, polyphagia, fatigue, weight loss and blurred vision. Acute hyperglycaemia may present as hyperventilation, stupor or coma as part of diabetic ketoacidosis. Recurrent infections are common, especially of the skin and urinary tract.

The patient may have a history of diabetes or the symptoms may be the first presentation of the disease. Type 1 diabetes usually occurs in younger age groups, whereas type 2 generally affects older individuals, with obesity being a common accompanying condition.

A thorough drug history is important. Steroids are used for a large number of conditions and therefore the dose and duration of treatment should be evaluated. The patient may complain of features of Cushing's syndrome such as excessive appetite, weight gain and weakness.

Enquire about recent severe illness such as heart attack or stroke. Enquire about current or recent pregnancy.

Examination may reveal complications of diabetes such as peripheral vascular disease, retinopathy, neuropathy and Charcot joints may be present. Skin infection is common in diabetes, especially boils and abscesses. Obesity is frequent in type 2 diabetics. Look for the features of Cushing's syndrome, including central obesity, moon face, hirsutism, cataracts, weakness, striae and hypertension.

GENERAL INVESTIGATIONS

- Blood glucose test strips
  ↑ glucose.
- Plasma glucose – random and fasting
  ↑ glucose.
- Urinalysis
  ↑ glucose and ketones in diabetic ketoacidosis.
- Oral glucose tolerance test
  ↑ glucose in diabetes.
- HbA_{1c}
  ↑ diabetes.
- VBGs
  Diabetic ketoacidosis.
- U&Es
  ↑ urea and creatinine with diabetic nephropathy.
- FBC
  ↑ WCC in infection and inflammation.
- βHCG
  Pregnancy.

- Diabetic ketoacidosis is an emergency which is identified by clinical features and a significantly raised blood sugar level with glucose and ketones in the urine. This may be the first presentation of diabetes or may occur with established diabetes.

- Causes for diabetic ketoacidosis, e.g. intercurrent infection or poor glucose control, should be further explored.

HYPOGLYCAEMIA

Hypoglycaemia is defined as a plasma glucose <2.5 mmol/L. The actual glucose level at which symptoms develop varies markedly.

CAUSES

DRUGS

- Insulin
- Sulfonylurea
- Alcohol
- Beta blockers
- Quinolones
- Pentamidine
- Quinine

ENDOCRINE

- Pituitary insufficiency
- Addison's disease

NEOPLASTIC

- Pancreatic islet cell tumours; insulinoma
- Non-pancreatic tumours; retroperitoneal fibrosarcoma, haemangiopericytoma

LIVER DISEASE

- Inherited glycogen storage disorders
- Cirrhosis
- Acute liver failure
- Alcohol

OTHER

- Post-prandial dumping syndrome (post-gastrectomy, post-vagotomy and drainage)
- Immune-mediated (e.g. anti-insulin receptor antibodies in Hodgkin's disease)

SYMPTOMS AND SIGNS

The most common symptoms include sweatiness, palpitations, weakness, hunger, drowsiness, restlessness, tremor, seizures and coma. Occasionally, personality changes may be a presenting symptom. By far the most common cause of hypoglycaemia is an excess of insulin or oral hypoglycaemic agents in a known diabetic. Enquire about a history of diabetes mellitus and medication. Occasionally, relatives of diabetics may be covertly ingesting hypoglycaemic agents. Insulin has been used by athletes to improve stamina. Alcohol excess without food may lead to hypoglycaemia. A full medication history is important.

There may be a history of pituitary dysfunction. Causes of pituitary failure include tumour, trauma, pituitary surgery and infection. The symptoms of Addison's disease include weakness, weight loss, dizziness and pigmentation of the buccal mucosa and palmar creases. Islet cell tumours may produce symptoms of hypoglycaemia intermittently and to varying degrees. Classically, the symptoms develop during fasting. Personality or neurocognitive changes may develop. Diagnosis of insulinoma depends on the classical diagnostic triad, i.e. Whipple's triad: (1) attacks precipitated by fasting; (2) blood sugar is low during the attack; and (3) symptoms are relieved by administration of glucose. Check for a history of liver failure. Dumping syndrome may occur following gastric surgery when a high osmotic load is delivered to the jejunum. A history of lymphoma may be present in immune-mediated hypoglycaemia.

Examination may reveal classic signs of hypoglycaemia. Look for complications of diabetes. Look for evidence of chronic liver disease in alcoholics. Pituitary insufficiency may lead to a variety of examination findings depending upon the deficiency and may include hypotension, loss or gain of weight, breast atrophy, hypogonadism, weakness, central obesity or dry skin. Retroperitoneal tumours may lead to renal impairment. Look for features of chronic liver disease. Lymphadenopathy and hepatosplenomegaly may be apparent in Hodgkin's disease.

GENERAL INVESTIGATIONS

- **Blood glucose test strips**
  ↓ glucose.
- **Serum blood glucose**
  Hypoglycaemia.
- **LFTs**
  ↑ bilirubin and transaminases with liver failure.
- **Toxicology screen**
  Alcohol.
- **U&Es**
  ↑ urea and creatinine with renal failure associated with retroperitoneal disease.
- **Insulin and C-peptide levels**
  Normal or ↑ insulin (insulinoma, sulfonylurea treatment). Absent C-peptide with exogenous insulin. ↓insulin (non-pancreatic neoplasm, insulin receptor antibodies), alcohol, pituitary or adrenal failure.
- **Pituitary hormone levels**
  Reduced in pituitary failure (e.g. GH (growth hormone), TSH, LH, FSH, prolactin).

- **Prolonged oral glucose tolerance test**
  To identify dumping syndrome.
- **i.v. insulin suppression test**
  Insulinoma.
- **Arterial stimulation with venous sampling**
  Insulinoma.
- **CT/MRI**
  Insulinoma.

- Profound hypoglycaemia is an emergency with potentially serious sequelae. It can be easily and rapidly identified by a blood glucose test strip estimation.

HYPERKALAEMIA

Hyperkalaemia is an elevated blood level of potassium (mild: 5.5–6.0 mmol/L, moderate: 6.0–6.4 mmol/L, severe: > 6.5 mmol/L). Hyperkalaemia is a medical emergency due to the risk of potentially fatal arrhythmias.

CAUSES (ALL CAUSES OF ACUTE HYPERKALAEMIA REQUIRE URGENT ASSESSMENT) ⚠

- Excess administration of potassium, especially rapidly
- Renal failure
- Haemolysis
- Massive blood transfusion
- Crush injuries (rhabdomyolysis)
- Tissue necrosis, e.g. burns, ischaemia
- Metabolic acidosis
- Adrenal insufficiency (Addison's disease)
- Drugs interfering with urinary excretion: ACE inhibitors and angiotensin receptor blockers, potassium-sparing diuretics (spironolactone and amiloride), NSAIDs (ibuprofen, naproxen), calcineurin inhibitors for immunosuppression (ciclosporin and tacrolimus), trimethoprim, pentamidine

SYMPTOMS AND SIGNS

Cardiac arrest. Mild breathlessness (hyperkalaemia associated with metabolic acidosis). Paraesthesiae, areflexia. Weakness. Palpitations. Abdominal pain. Hypoglycaemia. Hyperpigmentation associated with Addison's disease.

GENERAL INVESTIGATIONS

- **U&Es**
  K^+ > 5.4 mmol/L (patients with chronic renal failure will tolerate higher K^+ levels) – exclude haemolysis. Acute or chronic renal impairment.
- **FBC**
  Exclude haemolysis.
- **Blood gases**
  Metabolic acidosis.
- **Blood glucose**
  Diabetic ketoacidosis.
- **ECG**
  Tall T waves, flat P waves, prolonged PR interval, wide QRS, AV blocks and bradycardia.

- **Creatine kinase**
  ↑ in crush injuries.
- **Plasma cortisol**
  ↓ adrenal insufficiency (Addison's disease).

- **Hyperkalaemia is a medical emergency. The first sign of hyperkalaemia may be cardiac arrest due to an arrhythmia.**

HYPOKALAEMIA

Hypokalaemia is a reduced blood level of potassium <3.5 mmol/L.

CAUSES

INADEQUATE INTAKE

- Potassium-free i.v. fluids
- Reduced oral intake, e.g. coma, dysphagia

EXCESSIVE LOSS

- Renal
  - Thiazide or loop diuretics
  - Renal tubular disorders
- Gastrointestinal
  - Diarrhoea
  - Vomiting
  - Fistulas
  - Laxatives
  - Villous adenoma
- Endocrine
  - Cushing's syndrome
  - Steroid therapy
  - Hyperaldosteronism
  - Diabetic ketoacidosis (related to excessive diuresis and effects of insulin treatment)

SYMPTOMS AND SIGNS

Muscle weakness. Myalgia. Constipation. Paralytic ileus. Cardiac arrhythmia (ranging from ectopics to serious arrhythmias with sudden death at very low levels of potassium).

GENERAL INVESTIGATIONS

- **U&Es**
  Serum K^+ <3.5 mmol/L.
- **Blood bases**
  Metabolic alkalosis – pH↑HCO$_3^-$ ↑.
- **ECG**
  Flattened T waves. ST depression. U waves. Prolonged QT intervals.
- **Serum Mg**
  Mg↓ (magnesium is required for adequate processing of K^+).

- **Plasma aldosterone**
  Raised in Conn's syndrome (primary hyperaldosteronism).
- **Plasma renin**
  Low in Conn's syndrome.
- **Plasma cortisol**
  Diurnal variation lost in Cushing's syndrome.
- **Urinary free cortisol**
  Elevated in Cushing's syndrome.
- **ACTH levels**
  High in pituitary-dependent cases, low or undetectable with adrenal tumour; may be very high with ectopic ACTH secretion.

- In a patient with prolonged ileus postoperatively, always remember to check serum potassium.
- In a patient presenting with unexplained lethargy, fatigue and muscle weakness, check the serum potassium. Conn's syndrome is a possible diagnosis.

HYPERNATRAEMIA

The normal serum sodium level is 135–145 mmol/L. Hypernatraemia refers to a serum sodium level >145 mmol/L.

CAUSES

DECREASED WATER INTAKE

- Confusion

NON-RENAL WATER LOSSES

- Gastrointestinal losses (e.g. vomiting, diarrhoea)
- Pyrexia
- Burns

RENAL WATER LOSSES

- Osmotic diuresis (i.e. hyperglycaemia)
- Nephrogenic diabetes insipidus
  - Drugs (e.g. lithium)
  - Bence Jones proteins
  - Post-relief of obstructive uropathy
  - Recovering acute tubular necrosis
- Congenital diabetes insipidus

SODIUM EXCESS

- Excessive intravenous sodium therapy
- Chronic congestive cardiac failure
- Cirrhosis of the liver
- Steroid therapy
- Cushing's syndrome
- Primary hyperaldosteronism (Conn's syndrome)

SYMPTOMS AND SIGNS

Thirst usually occurs when the plasma sodium rises by 3–4 mmol/L above the upper limit of normal. Severe symptoms such as coma, seizures, muscular tremor and rigidity arise when the level is above 158 mmol/L. Lack of thirst is associated with central nervous system disease.

GENERAL INVESTIGATIONS

- U&Es
  Na^+ 150–170 mEq/L usually indicates dehydration.
  Na^+ >170 mEq/L usually indicates diabetes insipidus.
  Na^+ >190 mEq/L usually indicates long-term salt ingestion.

SPECIFIC INVESTIGATIONS

- Urine & plasma osmolality
  Central versus nephrogenic diabetes insipidus.
- CT head
  Central diabetes insipidus, e.g. cerebral tumour/trauma.

- Rapid correction of hypernatraemia can lead to cerebral oedema.

HYPONATRAEMIA

The normal serum sodium level is 135–145 mmol/L. Hyponatraemia refers to serum sodium levels of <135 mmol/L, and serum sodium of <120 mmol/L is considered severe.

CAUSES

HYPOVOLAEMIC

- Gastrointestinal losses
  - Diarrhoea
  - Vomiting
  - Enterocutaneous fistula
- Renal sodium losses
  - Diuretics
  - Osmotic diuresis (e.g. hyperglycaemia)
  - Renal failure
- Other sodium losses
  - Burns
  - Ascites
  - Crush injuries
  - Peritonitis

EUVOLAEMIC

- Endocrine
  - Severe hypothyroidism
  - Addison's disease
- Water load
  - Intravenous infusions
  - Water drinking (excessive)
  - TURP (transurethral resection of prostate) syndrome
- SIADH
  - Pulmonary disease (e.g. pneumonia, lung cancer)
  - Drugs (e.g. carbamazepine)
  - Intracranial disease (e.g. tumour, head injuries)

OEDEMATOUS

- Cardiac failure
- Nephrotic syndrome

SYMPTOMS AND SIGNS

Symptoms of hyponatraemia are related to how low the serum sodium is and how rapidly it has developed. They can range from asymptomatic to mild nausea, vomiting, headache, malaise to diminished reflexes, seizures, stupor or coma.

GENERAL INVESTIGATIONS

- U&Es
  $\downarrow$ Na$^+$. $\uparrow$ urea and creatinine (renal failure). $\uparrow$ K$^+$ (Addison's disease).

SPECIFIC INVESTIGATIONS

- Paired serum and urine osmolality
  SIADH is suggested by inappropriately concentrated urine (>100 mOsm/kg) with serum hypo-osmolality (<270 mOsm/kg).
- Paired serum and urinary sodium
  SIADH is suggested with inappropriately concentrated urinary sodium (>20 mmol/L).

- Falsely low sodium values can occur with high circulating levels of lipids, proteins and in severe hyperglycaemia.

- Most patients with hyponatraemia do not require treatment with intravenous sodium chloride, but, if this is required, the rate of correction of serum sodium levels must be carried out with great care to minimise the risk of central pontine demyelination.

HYPERCALCAEMIA

Hypercalcaemia is a serum calcium >2.62 mmol/L (normal range 2.1–2.6 mmol/L). It may be an asymptomatic laboratory finding. Symptoms usually become apparent with levels >3.50 mmol/L.

CAUSES

- Malignancy ⚠
  - Solid tumour with lytic bony metastases, e.g. Ca breast, bronchus
  - Solid tumours with humoral mediation, e.g. inappropriate PTH secretion with carcinoma of the bronchus, carcinoma of the kidney
  - Multiple myeloma
- Hyperparathyroidism (primary, secondary, tertiary)
- Hyperthyroidism
- Drugs, e.g. thiazide diuretics, lithium
- Addison's disease
- Paget's disease of bone
- Excess intake of vitamin A, vitamin D or calcium
- Sarcoidosis
- Familial hypocalciuric hypercalcaemia

SYMPTOMS AND SIGNS

These depend on the patient's age, duration and rate of increase of plasma calcium and the presence of concurrent medical conditions. Symptoms and signs are usually described using the well known adage 'bones' (i.e. abnormal curvature of spine, fractures), "stones" (i.e. renal stones), abdominal "groans" (i.e. abdominal pain – pancreatitis, constipation, peptic ulcer, vomiting) and "moans" (i.e. fatigue, depression, confusion, psychosis). Other signs and symptoms include polyuria/nocturia, haematuria, renal failure, hypertension and arrhythmias.

GENERAL INVESTIGATIONS

- Fasting calcium and phosphate
  Ca ↑ PO_4 ↓.
- U&Es
  ↑ creatinine ↑ urea. Renal failure.
- ECG
  Short QT interval. Widened T waves.
- Serum amylase
  ↑ in acute pancreatitis associated with hyperparathyroidism.

SPECIFIC INVESTIGATIONS

- **PTH levels**
  ↑ hyperparathyroidism.

- **Protein electrophoresis and Bence Jones protein**
  Multiple myeloma.

- **AXR**
  Stones. Nephrocalcinosis.

- **US**
  Renal stones. Carcinoma of the kidney (inappropriate PTH secretion). Parathyroid lesions.

- **Skull X-ray**
  Myeloma. Abnormal sella turcica in MEN associated pituitary tumour. Paget's disease of bone.

- **Sestamibi scan**
  Hyperparathyroidism.

- **24-Hour urinary calcium excretion**
  ↑ calcium excretion in hyperparathyroidism (calcium-restricted diets).

- In a patient with depression or psychosis, always check the serum calcium. Hyperparathyroidism may be a cause.

- In a patient presenting with polyuria, if diabetes has been excluded, check the serum calcium.

HYPOCALCAEMIA

Hypocalcaemia is a serum calcium of <2.1 mmol/L (normal range 2.1–2.6 mmol/L) with an ionised fraction <0.8 mmol/L.

CAUSES

ASSOCIATED WITH HIGH SERUM PHOSPHATE

- Chronic renal failure
- Hypoparathyroidism
- Rhabdomyolysis
- Phosphate therapy

ASSOCIATED WITH LOW OR NORMAL SERUM PHOSPHATE

- Hypomagnesaemia
- Acute pancreatitis ▲
- Critical illness (i.e. sepsis, burns) ▲
- Osteomalacia (inc. Vit D deficiency)

MASSIVE BLOOD TRANSFUSION DUE TO CITRATE-BINDING

HYPERVENTILATION WITH RESPIRATORY ALKALOSIS AND REDUCTION IN IONISED PLASMA CALCIUM

DRUGS

- Bisphosphonates
- Calcitonin

SYMPTOMS AND SIGNS

Mildly low levels may often result in no symptoms. Circumoral paraesthesia, peripheral tingling and paraesthesia, cramp, tetany (carpo-pedal spasm), hypotension, hyperactive tendon reflexes, Chvostek's sign (tapping over the facial nerve causes facial spasm), Trousseau's sign (inflating blood pressure cuff to above systolic pressure causes carpal spasm), laryngospasm (life-threatening), cardiac arrhythmias and rarely dystonia and psychosis.

GENERAL INVESTIGATIONS

- Serum calcium magnesium and phosphate
  Ca ↓ PO$_4$ may be low, normal or high. ↓ Mg – magnesium deficiency may lead to hypocalcaemia.

- U&Es
  ↑ creatinine ↑ urea. Renal failure.

- **Serum amylase**
  Ca ↓ associated with acute pancreatitis.
- **ECG**
  Prolonged QT interval.

SPECIFIC INVESTIGATIONS

- **ABGs**
  pH ↑ (hypocalcaemia associated with respiratory alkalosis).
- **PTH levels**
  Hypoparathyroidism.
- **Serum vitamin D**
  Vitamin D deficiency.

- The first symptom of hypocalcaemia is circumoral paraesthesia.
- If symptoms occur after thyroid or parathyroid surgery, the serum calcium should be checked and appropriate treatment initiated.

HYPOMAGNESAEMIA

The normal range of serum magnesium is 0.7–1.0 mmol/L.
Hypomagnesaemia refers to a serum level below 0.7 mmol/L.

CAUSES

EXCESSIVE LOSSES

- Diuretics
- Severe diarrhoea
- Prolonged vomiting
- Polyuria (poorly controlled diabetes)
- Prolonged and excessive nasogastric aspiration

INADEQUATE INTAKE

- Starvation
- Alcoholism
- Malabsorption syndrome
- Parenteral nutrition

SYMPTOMS AND SIGNS

Symptoms of low magnesium levels are very similar to those of low
calcium with muscle weakness, lethargy, irritability, confusion, seizures
and arrhythmias. In addition, there may be co-existing symptoms due
to hypocalcaemia or hypokalaemia. Severe symptoms do not usually
occur until serum levels drop below 0.5 mmol/L.

GENERAL INVESTIGATIONS

- Serum magnesium
  Serum magnesium level is diagnostic and can indicate level of
  severity.
- U&Es
  ↓ K^+ (Mg^+ and K^+ tend to move in and out of cells in the same
  direction).
- Serum Ca
  ↓ Ca (present in up to 60% of cases).

- If symptoms related to hypocalcaemia and hypokalaemia
  are resistant to calcium and potassium supplements,
  respectively, remember to check the serum magnesium
  level.

METABOLIC ACIDOSIS

Metabolic acidosis is caused by increased production of hydrogen ions from metabolic causes or from excessive bicarbonate loss (pH ↓, HCO_3^- ↓).
Compensatory mechanisms are:

- ↓ pCO_2 by hyperventilation
- ↓ H^+ by kidneys (unless in renal failure).

CAUSES (ALL CAUSES OF METABOLIC ACIDOSIS REQUIRE URGENT ASSESSMENT) ⚠

EXCESSIVE PRODUCTION OF H^+

- Diabetic ketoacidosis
- Lactic acidosis secondary to hypoxia, e.g. shock, ischaemic gut
- Septicaemia
- Starvation
- Drugs, e.g. ethanol, paracetamol, salicylates

DECREASED H^+ EXCRETION

- Renal failure

EXCESSIVE LOSS OF BASE

- Diarrhoea
- Fistula – pancreatic, intestinal or biliary

EXCESSIVE INTAKE OF ACID

- Parenteral nutrition

SYMPTOMS AND SIGNS

These may be non-specific. Specific symptoms include chest pain, palpitations, headache, nausea, vomiting, abdominal pain, weight loss. Deep rapid breathing (Kussmaul respirations) classically associated with diabetic ketoacidosis. Extreme acidosis may result in lethargy, stupor, coma, seizures, arrhythmias, ventricular tachycardia.

GENERAL INVESTIGATIONS

- Arterial blood gases
  pH usually <7.35. Bicarbonate usually <12 mmol/L. Elevated lactate in sepsis, ischaemia, diabetic ketoacidosis, overdose.
- FBC
  WCC ↑ in sepsis, infarction, septicaemia.
- U&Es
  ↑ K^+, acute kidney injury.

- **Blood glucose**
  ↑ in diabetic ketoacidosis.
- **Blood/urinary ketones**
  Raised in diabetic ketoacidosis.
- **Serum salicylate**
  Salicylate poisoning.

To distinguish between the main types of metabolic acidosis, it is necessary to measure the *anion gap*.

Anion gap = $([Na^+] + [K^+]) - ([Cl^-] + [HCO_3^-])$

This is normally about 8–16 mmol/L. An elevated anion gap, i.e. >16 mmol/L, may indicate a particular type of acidosis.

Increased anion gap

- Lactic acidosis.
- Ketoacidosis.
- Chronic renal failure.
- Intoxication, e.g. salicylate, ethanol, ethylene glycol, metformin.
- Massive rhabdomyolysis.

- Rapidly increasing metabolic acidosis over minutes or hours is not due to renal failure. Severe sepsis, tissue hypoperfusion or tissue necrosis should be suspected, especially when there is an associated clinical deterioration.

METABOLIC ALKALOSIS

Metabolic alkalosis is caused by an increase in HCO_3^- or decrease in H^+ ($\uparrow$ pH, $\uparrow HCO_3^-$). Compensatory mechanisms are:

- $\uparrow pCO_2$ by hypoventilation (limited by hypoxia)
- $\downarrow HCO_3^-$ by kidneys.

CAUSES

EXCESS LOSS OF H⁺

- Vomiting
- Nasogastric aspiration
- Gastric fistula
- Diuretic therapy (thiazide or loop)
- Cushing's syndrome (mineralocorticoid effect)
- Conn's syndrome (mineralocorticoid excess)

EXCESSIVE INTAKE OF BASE

- Ingestion of HCO_3^- (usually iatrogenic)
- Antacids, e.g. milk-alkali syndrome

SYMPTOMS AND SIGNS

The patient is usually asymptomatic in mild cases, although if breathing spontaneously will hypoventilate. In cases of moderate to severe alkalosis, there may be tetany, seizures, confusion or coma.

GENERAL INVESTIGATIONS

- Blood gases
  pH > 7.54 confirms diagnosis. HCO_3^- normally high >29 mmol/L.
- U&Es
  K^+, Na^+ and Cl^- usually fall below normal range.
- Plasma cortisol
  Diurnal variation lost in Cushing's syndrome.
- Plasma aldosterone
  Raised in Conn's syndrome.

- Metabolic alkalosis will cause a left shift of the oxyhaemoglobin curve, reducing oxygen availability to the tissues.

RESPIRATORY ACIDOSIS

Respiratory acidosis is caused by CO_2 retention due to inadequate pulmonary ventilation ($\downarrow$ pH, $\uparrow$ pCO_2). Compensatory mechanisms are:

- $\uparrow$ HCO_3^- by bicarbonate buffer system
- $\downarrow$ H^+ by kidneys (can take several days).

CAUSES (ANY CAUSE OF HYPOVENTILATION) (ALL CAUSES OF RESPIRATORY ACIDOSIS REQUIRE URGENT ASSESSMENT) ⚠

IMPAIRED GASEOUS EXCHANGE

- Chronic obstructive pulmonary disease
- Alveolar disease, e.g. pneumonia, ARDS (acute respiratory distress syndrome)
- Thoracic injury, e.g. pulmonary contusions

CNS DEPRESSION

- Head injury
- Drugs, e.g. opiates, anaesthetics
- Coma
- Stroke
- Encephalitis

NEUROMUSCULAR DISEASE

- Myasthenia gravis
- Guillain–Barré syndrome
- Muscular dystrophy
- Motor Neurone Disease

SKELETAL DISEASE

- Kyphoscoliosis
- Ankylosing spondylitis
- Flail chest

ARTIFICIAL VENTILATION (UNCONTROLLED AND UNMONITORED)

SYMPTOMS AND SIGNS

A history of the underlying disorder may be evident such as trauma, drug ingestion or an established medical history of chronic obstructive pulmonary disease. The symptoms of respiratory acidosis can range from anxiety, disorientation, confusion, or lethargy to somnolence. On examination, tachycardia and a bounding arterial pulse can occur with carbon dioxide retention. In severe disease, cyanosis and hypotension can result. Papilloedema may be a feature of underlying raised intracranial pressure. Features of a flail chest or any severe chest wall deformity may be evident.

GENERAL INVESTIGATIONS

- **ABGs**
  pH < 7.35.
  pCO_2 > 5.8 kPa.
  ↑ HCO_3^-.

- **CXR**
  Underlying pulmonary disease.

- **Pulmonary function tests**
  COPD, which usually manifests as an obstructive defect (FEV1 ↓, FVC normal, with no reversibility). Skeletal disease (reduced chest movement).

- **EMG and nerve conduction studies**
  Myasthenia gravis and Guillain–Barré syndrome.

- **CT/MRI head**
  Central (brain stem) lesion.

- Associated hypoxaemia secondary to hypoventilation is a major threat to life and must be reversed rapidly.

RESPIRATORY ALKALOSIS

Respiratory alkalosis is a common disorder in critically ill patients. It occurs when carbon dioxide is lost via excessive pulmonary ventilation ($\uparrow$ pH, $\downarrow$ $p$$CO_2$). Compensatory mechanisms are:

- $\downarrow$ HCO_3^- by bicarbonate buffer system
- $\uparrow$ H^+ by kidneys (slow process – may take several days).

CAUSES (ANY CAUSE OF HYPERVENTILATION)

CENTRAL NERVOUS SYSTEM

- Pyrexia
- Pain
- Anxiety
- Hysteria
- Head injury
- Stroke ▲
- Encephalitis ▲

RESPIRATORY DISORDERS

- Pneumonia
- Pulmonary oedema
- Pulmonary embolus ▲

PHYSIOLOGICAL

- Pregnancy
- High altitude
- Severe anaemia

DRUGS

- Salicylates ▲

OTHER CAUSES

- Sepsis ▲
- Mechanical ventilation
- Metabolic acidosis (overcompensation) ▲

SYMPTOMS AND SIGNS

Symptoms may include light-headedness, perioral paraesthesia, dizziness and numbness of the hands and feet. Acute development of low carbon dioxide levels can occasionally cause cerebral vasoconstriction, leading to confusion, syncope, and seizures.

SECTION B

GENERAL INVESTIGATIONS

- ABGs
  pH > 7.45.
  pCO_2 < 4.4 kPa.
  ↓ HCO_3^- (compensatory mechanism due to bicarbonate buffer system).

- Serum calcium
  ↓ Ca^{2+} (due to increased calcium binding to serum albumin).

- Serum salicylate level
  If overdose is suspected.

- CT/MRI head
  Intracranial lesion as a cause of hyperventilation.

- Prolonged artificial ventilation with inadequate monitoring should be remembered as a cause of respiratory alkalosis.

URAEMIA

Blood urea is a useful test of renal function. However, other factors such as liver failure, dehydration and protein breakdown may alter levels of blood urea. The normal level of blood urea is 2.5–7.8 mmol/L. However, values may be lower in pregnancy and the newborn, and in the elderly, values may be slightly increased due to lack of renal concentration.

CAUSES

INCREASED BLOOD UREA

- Renal failure (acute and chronic)
- Dehydration
- Shock ⚠
- Congestive cardiac failure
- Gastrointestinal haemorrhage (digested blood increases blood urea) ⚠
- Excessive protein intake
- Excessive protein catabolism

DECREASED BLOOD UREA

- Malnutrition
- Liver failure
- Overhydration, e.g. prolonged i.v. fluids
- Pregnancy (increased plasma volume)
- Impaired protein absorption
- SIADH
- Anabolic steroid use

SYMPTOMS AND SIGNS

- Signs of uraemia, e.g. oliguria, anuria, nausea, fatigue, confusion, thirst, oedema (peripheral and pulmonary), uraemic frost (rare)
- Signs of dehydration, e.g. dry skin, loss of skin turgor
- Signs of congestive cardiac failure, e.g. oedema, JVP ↑. GI haemorrhage, e.g. tachycardia, hypotension, haematemesis and melaena. Decreased intake, e.g. oedema, ascites
- Signs of liver failure. SIADH, e.g. head injury, small cell lung cancer.

GENERAL INVESTIGATIONS

- U&Es
  Urea ↑ Na ↓ in SIADH (<130 mEq/L).

- **Creatinine**
  Cr ↑. Disparity between creatinine and urea (urea↑creatinine normal) in gastrointestinal haemorrhage.
- **FBC**
  Anaemia. PCV ↑ in dehydration. PCV ↓ in overhydration.
- **LFTs**
  Liver failure. Hypoalbuminaemia.
- **MSU**
  Red cells, casts and protein in intrinsic renal disease.
- **CXR**
  Pulmonary oedema. Cardiomegaly.
- **Urine electrolytes**
  See Table on p. 340 in Oliguria.
- **Urine osmolality**
  Acute renal failure versus physiological oliguria. See Table on p. 340 in Oliguria.
- **Ultrasound**
  Urinary tract obstruction.
- **MAG 3 scan**
  Renal function. Renal infarction (absent outline of kidney).

> • A grossly raised blood urea in association with metabolic acidosis, hyperkalaemia, fluid overload and clinical symptoms, e.g. coma, pericarditis, is an indication for urgent haemodialysis.

SECTION C

HAEMATOLOGICAL PRESENTATIONS

ANAEMIA

Anaemia is defined as a haemoglobin concentration of <13.5 g/dL in men and <11.5 g/dL in women. Classification of anaemia according to red cell indices is useful because specific investigations can be tailored accordingly.

CAUSES

MICROCYTIC (MCV <80 fL)

- Iron deficiency
- Anaemia of chronic disease
- Thalassaemia (more common in certain groups)

NORMOCYTIC (MCV 80–95 fL)

- Acute blood loss
- Haemolytic anaemia
  - Hereditary spherocytosis
  - Sickle cell disease (most common in sub-Saharan Africa)
  - G6PD deficiency (varies with ethnicity)
  - Autoimmune haemolytic anaemia
  - Malaria (geographic variability)
  - Drugs (e.g. dapsone, quinine, sulphonamides)
  - Red cell trauma (burns, mechanical heart valves)
- Mixed deficiencies
- Secondary anaemia (liver and renal disease)
- Bone marrow failure
- Pregnancy

MACROCYTIC (MCV > 95 fL)

- Megaloblastic anaemia
  - Pernicious anaemia
  - Vitamin B_{12} deficiency
  - Folate deficiency
- Alcoholism
- Liver disease
- Hypothyroidism
- Hyperthyroidism (Graves' disease)
- Addison's disease
- Marrow infiltration
- Drugs, e.g. azathioprine, methotrexate.

SYMPTOMS AND SIGNS

Important aspects of the history are to enquire about symptoms suggestive of the diagnosis of anaemia and to establish any underlying cause.

Symptoms of anaemia

The symptoms of anaemia are dependent on the degree of anaemia, speed of onset, age and the presence of co-existing disease. Mild to moderate chronic anaemia may be asymptomatic in young, fit individuals. Symptoms of anaemia include tiredness, lethargy and dyspnoea. Anaemia can precipitate or worsen angina and lower limb claudication.

History of the underlying disorder

Blood loss is a common cause of iron deficiency anaemia and frank bleeding can easily be established from the history. Occult bleeding from the gastrointestinal tract is an important cause of chronic blood loss. Patients may have melaena and may also experience upper abdominal pains from peptic ulceration, gastritis, gastro-oesophageal reflux or gastric carcinoma (p. 2). The causes of lower gastrointestinal bleeding are detailed on p. 369. The amount and frequency of blood loss with menstruation should be documented and the presence of haemoptysis and haematuria should be ascertained. Malabsorption can cause a deficiency of substrate or coenzyme requirements for the synthesis of haemoglobin. Gastrectomy or atrophic gastritis with pernicious anaemia may impair both iron and vitamin B_{12} absorption due to alterations in pH and effects on intrinsic factor, respectively. Impairment of vitamin B_{12} absorption may also result from extensive disease or resection involving the terminal ileum and predisposes to megaloblastic anaemia. A history of travel to areas where malaria and hookworm infections are endemic should be sought.

Dietary history

It is important to take a dietary history, as folate deficiency results from poor dietary intake. This is in contrast to iron, as dietary deficiency of iron alone rarely results in anaemia unless accompanied by increased utilisation or blood loss. Owing to intrinsic stores of vitamin B_{12}, dietary deficiencies may take up to two years before becoming clinically apparent. The amount of alcohol intake should also be noted because alcohol excess may result in a macrocytic anaemia.

Past medical and drug history

A number of chronic diseases can result in anaemia, but it is important to exclude other concomitant causes before attributing anaemia to the effects of the primary illness. Diseases predisposing to macrocytic anaemia have been listed above. Aplasia of the marrow may occur as a complication of viral hepatitis or exposure to radiation and result in aplastic anaemia. Drugs such as chemotherapeutic agents, chloramphenicol and sulphonamides may also precipitate bone marrow failure. Respiratory tract infections with mycoplasma, infectious mononucleosis, lymphomas and connective tissue disease are associated with autoimmune haemolytic anaemia.

Family history

Haemoglobinopathies such as thalassaemia and sickle cell disease may be inherited. Alternatively, hereditary enzyme defects (G6PD) or red cell membrane defects (hereditary spherocytosis) may also result in intravascular haemolysis.

Examination

Classically, patients with anaemia have pallor of the palmar skin creases and conjunctivae; however, diagnosis based solely on these findings is unreliable. With iron deficiency, spoon-shaped nails (koilonychia) may be noted; these findings may be accompanied by angular cheilitis and glossitis. Jaundice can be a complication of haemolytic anaemia or can result from chronic liver disease.

Subacute combined degeneration of the cord is a complication of severe vitamin B_{12} deficiency. Neurological examination reveals symmetrical loss of light touch, vibration and proprioception of the feet due to dorsal column involvement. In addition, Romberg's sign may be elicited. Less common features are peripheral neuropathy, optic atrophy and dementia.

With anaemia, examination of the cardiovascular system may reveal evidence of a hyperdynamic circulation with tachycardia, bounding pulse and a systolic flow murmur.

Splenomegaly is associated with hereditary spherocytosis, thalassaemia and sickle cell disease.

SPECIFIC INVESTIGATIONS

Microcytic anaemia

- **FBC and blood film**
  Low haemoglobin concentration occurs with microcytosis (MCV < 80 fL) and hypochromia (MCH < 27 pg). The platelet count may be raised when anaemia is associated with acute bleeding. Microcytic, hypochromic red blood cells with accompanying pencil cells may also be seen on the blood film.

- **Serum iron and TIBC**
  Serum iron reduced and TIBC raised with iron deficiency. With chronic disease, both are reduced, and with thalassaemia, both are normal.

- **Serum ferritin**
  Concentration of serum ferritin, a protein-iron complex, will be reduced with iron deficiency. It is not affected by chronic disease or thalassaemia. Ferritin is also an acute-phase reactant and so may be raised even in confirmed iron deficiency anaemia.

- Faecal occult blood and faecal microscopy
  Detects blood loss from the gastrointestinal tract. Hookworm ova
  can be identified on microscopy.

- Hb electrophoresis
  Allows the specific diagnosis and classification of thalassaemia and
  sickle cell disease.

Normocytic anaemia

- FBC and film
  Low haemoglobin levels are accompanied by normal red cell
  indices (MCV 80–95 fL, MCH > 27 pg), which can also occur in
  the presence of co-existing microcytic and macrocytic anaemia
  (mixed deficiency), although this will usually be picked up on the
  blood film. Certain haematology laboratories report RDW, which
  is increased in the presence of differing red corpuscle sizes. The
  reticulocyte count will be increased with haemolytic anaemia and
  following acute blood loss. Red blood cell fragments (schistocytes),
  spherical red blood cells (spherocytes) or 'bite' cells present on
  blood film also indicate haemolytic anaemia.

- Tests for haemolysis
  Unconjugated bilirubin, urine urobilinogen and faecal stercobilinogen
  are raised with all causes of haemolysis. Serum haptoglobins are
  absent. Plasma haemoglobin is raised specifically with intravascular
  haemolysis. Reference to haematology textbooks will be required for
  confirmatory tests for individual haemolytic disorders.

- Urinalysis
  Haemosiderin and haemoglobin will be present in the urine,
  specifically with intravascular haemolysis.

- Bone marrow aspiration
  Aspiration of the bone marrow will reveal erythroid hyperplasia
  with haemolytic anaemia; with aplastic anaemia, bone marrow
  hypoplasia with fat replacement results.

Macrocytic anaemia

- FBC and film
  Low haemoglobin is accompanied by macrocytosis (MCV > 95 fL).
  The reticulocyte count is low and accompanying low platelet
  and white cell counts may indicate megaloblastic anaemia.
  Hypersegmented neutrophils may be seen on the blood film.

- Serum vitamin B_{12} assay
  Serum levels of vitamin B_{12} can be estimated and deficiency readily
  ascertained. If the aetiology of vitamin B_{12} deficiency is not apparent,
  a Schilling test can be performed to clarify if the problem lies within
  the stomach, terminal ileum or is due to intrinsic factor.

- Antiparietal cell antibodies and anti-intrinsic factor antibodies
  Pernicious anaemia results from lack of intrinsic factor production
  or blocking antibodies.

- **Serum and red cell folate**
  Both of these tests are low with folate deficiency; however, in the presence of vitamin B_{12} deficiency, the red cell folate may actually be increased.

- **Bone marrow aspiration**
  Megaloblasts are seen in marrow aspirates with vitamin B_{12} or folate deficiency.

- **Further tests**
  Further tests for individual diseases responsible for macrocytosis or secondary anaemia need to be tailored according to the clinical presentation.

- **Examination of the peripheral blood film is an important guide to the type of anaemia, the underlying cause and the response to treatment.**

- **Remember that shortness of breath may be an early presenting symptom of anaemia.**

CLOTTING DISORDERS

Disorders of clotting can present with an increased tendency to clotting (thrombophilia) or a decreased ability to form clots and therefore an increased risk of bleeding.

CAUSES

INCREASED CLOTTING

CONGENITAL
- Factor V Leiden deficiency
- Protein C deficiency
- Protein S deficiency
- Antithrombin III deficiency

ACQUIRED
- Malignancy
- Pregnancy
- Infection
- Prolonged immobility
- Autoimmune: anti-phospholipid syndrome (can be related to SLE)
- Drugs: oral oestrogen-containing contraception, heparin-induced thrombocytopenia

REDUCED CLOTTING

CONGENITAL
- Haemophilia A and B
- von Willebrand's disease

ACQUIRED
- Vitamin K deficiency
- Obstructive jaundice
- Fat malabsorption
- Liver disease
- Autoimmune diseases, e.g. systemic lupus erythematosus
- Drugs – heparin, warfarin, thrombolytic therapy
- Disseminated intravascular coagulation (DIC)
- Massive transfusion

SYMPTOMS AND SIGNS

Onset and duration

All thrombophilias present with an increased tendency for blood clots to form in the venous circulation, leading to conditions such as pulmonary embolisms (PE), deep vein thrombosis (DVT) or portal vein thrombosis. Of the inherited causes, Factor V Leiden is the most common and mildest. Acquired thrombophilias will have symptoms of the associated cause such as malignancy or infection.

Increased bleeding disorders will present at different ages, depending on the underlying cause. Patients with haemophilia A or B usually present at a young age with excessive blood loss following injuries or surgical procedures, such as circumcision. Muscle haematomas and painful haemarthroses may be accompanying features.

Medical history

Inherited thrombophilias may have no prior medical history. For acquired causes, prior history of malignancy, auto-immune disease or recent surgery or trauma leading to prolonged bed rest is important to consider. Recurrent miscarriages can be a feature of anti-phospholipid syndrome.

Concomitant disease constitutes most causes of acquired coagulation disturbances. As coagulation factors are synthesised in the liver, disease of the liver naturally predisposes to clotting abnormalities. Vitamin K is a fat-soluble vitamin essential for the production of clotting factors II, VII, IX and X. Conditions that impair the absorption of fat will therefore result in decreased production of these factors, such as obstructive jaundice, pancreatic or small bowel disease.

Severe infections, malignancy, obstetric complications and burns may give rise to DIC. This is characterised by widespread consumption of clotting factors and platelets, resulting in severe coagulation disturbances.

Drug history

Coagulation abnormalities may be iatrogenic. Oestrogen-containing contraceptives increase the risk of thrombus formation. Therapeutic anticoagulation is achieved with heparin, either unfractionated or low molecular weight, and warfarin. Unfractionated heparin can paradoxically cause clotting due to heparin-induced thrombocytopenia, a complication resulting from platelet activation. Thrombolytic agents may produce severe derangement of clotting and widespread bleeding. Coagulation disturbances can result from dilution from massive blood transfusions (when the patient's entire circulating volume has been replaced by transfusion within 24 hours).

Examination

Vein thrombosis of a limb will usually present with pain, erythema and swelling of the affected limb only. A patient presenting with dyspnoea due to PE may have bloody sputum, or there may be no overt examination findings, and diagnosis depends upon clinical presentation and investigation. Well's criteria should be used to clarify the likelihood of a PE or DVT as the cause for presentation.

A general examination is performed to identify any stigmata from haemophilia. Early-onset osteoarthritis and pseudotumours may result from episodes of repeated haemorrhage. Skin haematomas or, rarely, skin necrosis may be seen with excessive warfarin dosage. In acquired coagulation disorders, signs of liver disease may bring attention to the underlying disorder.

GENERAL INVESTIGATIONS

■ FBC
Low platelet count or abnormal platelet function results in prolonged bleeding time but not clotting results.

■ Clotting screen
PT, APTT and TT are measured. Thrombophilias will often not demonstrate any abnormalities. Bleeding disorder abnormalities are listed in the following table.

Disorder	PT	APTT	TT
Haemophilia	N	↑	N
von Willebrand's disease	N	↑	N
Liver disease	↑	↑	N
Warfarin/vitamin K deficiency	↑	↑	N
Heparin	N or ↑	↑	↑
DIC	↑	↑	↑

PT, Prothrombin time; *APTT,* activated partial thromboplastin time; *TT,* thrombin time; *N,* within normal range.

SPECIFIC INVESTIGATIONS

■ Thrombophilia screen
Can be used to identify protein C, S and Factor V Leiden deficiency and lupus anticoagulant/anti cardiolipin antibodies for antiphospholipid syndrome. The screen is of limited clinical value, however, as it is unlikely to change clinical management.

■ Clotting factor assays
Clotting factor assays are required to differentiate between haemophilia A, haemophilia B and von Willebrand's disease. Low levels of factor VIII are found in both haemophilia A and von Willebrand's disease. Low levels of factor IX indicate haemophilia B. As the name implies, von Willebrand's factor is low in von Willebrand's disease and the bleeding time is also prolonged.

■ Fibrinogen and fibrin degradation products
With DIC, the platelet count and serum fibrinogen levels are low, whereas the fibrin degradation products such as D-dimers are increased.

- Prolonged bleeding can result from abnormal platelet function, despite normal platelet counts.

LEUCOCYTOSIS

Leucocytosis is an increase in the absolute count of circulating white blood cells. The normal range is 4–11 × 10⁹/L. It may involve any of the types of white cells, but a polymorphonuclear leucocytosis, i.e. neutrophilia, is the most common.

CAUSES

NEUTROPHILIA

PHYSIOLOGICAL
- Neonates
- Exercise
- Pregnancy
- Childbirth
- Lactation
- Stress

BACTERIAL INFECTION, e.g. acute appendicitis, pyelonephritis

ACUTE NON-INFECTIVE INFLAMMATION
- Surgery
- Burns
- Infarction, e.g. myocardial infarction, mesenteric infarction ⚠
- Crush injuries ⚠
- Rheumatoid arthritis

ACUTE HAEMORRHAGE AND HAEMOLYSIS

METABOLIC
- Uraemia
- Diabetic ketoacidosis ⚠
- Gout

CHRONIC MYELOPROLIFERATIVE DISEASE
- CML (chronic myeloid leukaemia)
- Polycythaemia rubrum vera
- Myelofibrosis

NON-HAEMATOLOGICAL MALIGNANCY
- Carcinoma
- Lymphoma

DRUGS
- Corticosteroids

MISCELLANEOUS
- Convulsions
- Electric shock
- Post-neutropenia rebound
- Post-splenectomy (temporary)

LYMPHOCYTOSIS

VIRAL INFECTIONS
- EBV/CMV (infectious mononucleosis)
- Rubella
- Varicella zoster (chickenpox)
- Measles
- Mumps
- Influenza
- Viral hepatitis

BACTERIAL INFECTIONS
- Pertussis
- TB
- Brucellosis
- Syphilis

CHRONIC LYMPHOCYTIC LEUKAEMIA

POST-SPLENECTOMY (TEMPORARY)

MONOCYTOSIS

BACTERIAL (USUALLY CHRONIC INFECTIONS)
- TB
- Brucellosis
- Typhoid
- Subacute infective endocarditis

PROTOZOAL
- Malaria
- Trypanosomiasis
- Leishmaniasis

MALIGNANT
- Myelodysplasia
- Leukaemia – monocytic and myelomonocytic
- Hodgkin's
- Carcinoma

EOSINOPHILIA

- Allergy, e.g. asthma, drug reaction
- Allergic bronchopulmonary aspergillosis
- Hypersensitivity pneumonitis
- Parasitic infections, e.g. filariasis, schistosomiasis
- Malignancy, e.g. Hodgkin's disease
- Cholesterol emboli
- Pulmonary eosinophilia

BASOPHILIA

- Chronic myeloproliferative disease
- Hypersensitivity reactions
- Hypothyroidism

SYMPTOMS AND SIGNS

It is important to seek a history of symptoms of infection and to examine the patient for signs of infection or an underlying haematological malignancy. A full description of the signs and symptoms of haematological disease is beyond the scope of this book and the reader is referred to a textbook of haematology.

GENERAL INVESTIGATIONS

- **FBC**
  Hb ↓ malignancy. WCC ↑. Differential count for type of white cell.

- **Blood film**
  'Toxic' granulation – infection. Immature granulocytes, blast cells – white cell dyscrasias.

- **Blood culture**
  Sepsis.

- **Bone marrow**
  Indicated for leukaemoid reaction, leucoerythroblastic blood film, leucocytosis due to blasts. Diagnosis of various types of white cell dyscrasia.

- **Mantoux test**
  TB.

- **Antibody screen**
  SLE.

- **Rheumatoid factor**
  Rheumatoid arthritis.

- **U&Es**
  ARF. CRF.

- **Blood sugar**
  Diabetic ketoacidosis.

- **CXR**
  Malignancy. Allergic bronchopulmonary aspergillosis. Hypersensitivity pneumonitis. Pulmonary eosinophilia.
- **CT**
  Malignancy.
- **ECG**
  Myocardial infarction.
- **Monospot**
  Infectious mononucleosis.
- **VDRL**
  Syphilis.
- **Brucella agglutination test**
  Brucellosis.

- In patients with leucocytosis it is important to seek a history of symptoms of infection and to examine the patient not only for signs of infection, but also for the possibility of an underlying haematological disorder, i.e. exclude lymphadenopathy and hepatosplenomegaly.

LEUCOPENIA

Leucopenia is a reduction in circulating white blood cells. The normal range is $4-11 \times 10^9$/L. In practice, the commonest form is neutropenia – a deficiency of neutrophil granulocytes. Neutropenia may be selective or part of a pancytopenia.

CAUSES

NEUTROPENIA

PANCYTOPENIA
- Bone marrow depression, e.g. cytotoxic agents, malignant infiltration
- Severe B_{12} or folate deficiency
- Hypersplenism

SELECTIVE NEUTROPENIA
- Physiological
  - Benign ethnic neutropenia, e.g. Afro-Caribbeans
- Infection
  - Overwhelming sepsis, e.g. septicaemia ⚠
  - Brucellosis
  - TB
  - Typhoid
- Auto immune
  - Systemic lupus erythematosus (SLE)
  - Felty's syndrome (rheumatoid arthritis)
  - Autoimmune neutropenia
- Drug induced, e.g. chemotherapy agents, carbimazole, cotrimoxazole, penicillins, clozapine, NSAIDs

LYMPHOPENIA
- Acute infection
- Trauma
- Surgery
- Radiotherapy
- Chemotherapy
- Steroid therapy
- SLE
- Uraemia
- Cushing's syndrome
- Hodgkin's disease
- Immunodeficiency syndromes, e.g. HIV

SYMPTOMS AND SIGNS

The history and physical examination provide a guide to the subsequent management of a patient with neutropenia. Simple observation is appropriate initially for an asymptomatic patient with an isolated mild neutropenia who has an unremarkable history and examination. Take a full drug history. Check for any recent infections or surgery. Check particularly for recent viral illnesses. Severe leucopenia may result in opportunistic infections. Patients with neutropenia may present with recurrent stomatitis, gingivitis, oral ulceration, sinusitis and perianal infection.

GENERAL INVESTIGATIONS

- **FBC**
  Hb ↓ in malignancy, bone marrow depression. WCC ↓ – type of white cell involved.

- **U&Es**
  Uraemia. Renal involvement, e.g. SLE.

- **Mantoux test**
  TB.

- **Antibody screen**
  SLE.

- **Antineutrophil antibody screen**
  Autoimmune neutropenia.

- **Serum B$_{12}$ and folate**
  B$_{12}$ and folate deficiency.

- **Rheumatoid factor**
  Felty's disease.

- **Viral titres**
  HIV.

- **Bone marrow**
  Bone marrow depression.

- Neutropenia with counts of $<0.5 \times 10^9$/L may result in severe life-threatening sepsis, e.g. candidiasis, septicaemia, opportunistic infections. Patients in this group who have an identified source of infection or are pyrexial with suspected sepsis require immediate treatment with broad-spectrum i.v. antibiotics.

POLYCYTHAEMIA

Polycythaemia is an increase in red cell concentration above the normal limit, usually accompanied by a corresponding increase in haematocrit and haemoglobin concentration. Polycythaemia can be 'real' due to a true increase in red cell concentration or 'apparent' due to low plasma volume (e.g. dehydration). Primary polycythaemia (polycythaemia vera) is due to a neoplasm of the myeloid cells whilst secondary polycythaemia is due to raised erythropoietin levels. This may be caused by chronic low oxygenation or erythropoietin production from renal tumours.

CAUSES

TRUE POLYCYTHAEMIA (INCREASED RED CELL MASS)

- Primary polycythaemia
  - Polycythaemia vera
- Secondary polycythaemia
  - Appropriate erythropoietin production (hypoxia)
  - Smoking (due to carbon monoxide exposure)
  - Chronic obstructive pulmonary disease
  - Long-term exposure to high altitude
  - Cyanotic heart disease
  - High-affinity haemoglobinopathy
- Inappropriate erythropoietin production
  - Renal carcinoma or cysts
  - Renal artery stenosis
  - Renal amyloidosis
  - Hepatocellular carcinoma
  - Massive uterine fibroids
  - Cerebellar haemangioblastoma

APPARENT POLYCYTHAEMIA (REDUCED PLASMA VOLUME, NORMAL RED CELL MASS)

- Low plasma volume polycythaemia
  - Dehydration
  - Burns
  - Enteropathy
- Stress; Gaisböck's syndrome

SYMPTOMS AND SIGNS

The condition may be asymptomatic for months or years. Presenting features of polycythaemia vera are fatigue, aquagenic pruritus (skin itching after a hot bath), sweating and, occasionally, weight loss.

Patients may also present with complications such as stroke, deep vein thrombosis, leukaemia or hyperviscosity (headache, blurred vision and confusion). On examination, there is plethora and cyanosis. Scratch marks or spontaneous bruising may be visible on the skin. The conjunctival vessels are engorged and dilated retinal veins may be evident on funduscopy. Splenomegaly may be palpable on examination of the abdomen. Hypertension may be present in some patients.

GENERAL INVESTIGATIONS

- **FBC**
  Hb 17.5 g/dL in men and 15.5 g/dL in women with accompanying rise in red cell count. Haematocrit >52% in men and 48% in women (figures may vary globally). Thrombocytosis and neutrophil leucocytosis present in up to 50% of cases of polycythaemia vera.

- **Blood film**
  Occasional metamyelocytes and myelocytes on blood film. Polycythaemia vera will have increased haematocrit, neutrophils and platelets.

- **ABG**
  O_2 concentration in blood is normal in primary polycythaemia but reduced in secondary polycythaemia, due to respiratory failure or cardiac disease, with right to left shunt.

- **Total red cell volume**
  Red cells, in a sample of blood from the patient, are tagged with 51Cr, and the labelled red cells are re-injected. The dilution of the isotope in a subsequent venous blood sample is used to calculate the red cell mass. The normal range is 25–35 mL/kg in men and 22–32 mL/kg in women.

- **Plasma volume**
  125I-albumin is used to estimate total plasma volume, the normal range is 35–45 mL/kg. This is usually performed in conjunction with the estimation of total red cell volume to distinguish between real and apparent polycythaemia.

- **Bone marrow aspiration**
  In polycythaemia vera, there is a hypercellular bone marrow with erythroid hyperplasia. Megakaryocytes may be prominent and increased reticulin deposition is common.

- In polycythaemia vera, the higher the haematocrit, the greater the risk of thrombotic episodes. Regular phlebotomy is required to maintain the haematocrit below 45%.

- Consider urgent referral to a haematologist if there are symptoms of hyperviscosity (including bleeding, visual disturbances, chest pain and shortness of breath).

- Consider further investigations for persistant haematocrit >0.52 in males and >0.48 in females.

THROMBOCYTOPENIA

Thrombocytopenia is a low platelet count below 150×10^9/L. The causes of a low platelet count can be grouped according to reduced production, decreased survival or sequestration in the spleen.

CAUSES

REDUCED PRODUCTION

- Aplastic anaemia
- Drugs, e.g. tolbutamide, alcohol, cytotoxic agents
- Viral infections, e.g. EBV, CMV
- Myelodysplasia
- Bone marrow infiltration, e.g. carcinoma, leukaemia, myeloma, myelofibrosis
- Megaloblastic anaemia
- Hereditary thrombocytopenia

DECREASED PLATELET SURVIVAL

IMMUNE

- ITP
- Drugs, e.g. penicillins, heparins, quinine, sulphonamides, methotrexate, gold
- Infections
- Post-transfusion

NON-IMMUNE ⚠

- Disseminated intravascular coagulation (DIC)
- Thrombotic thrombocytopenic purpura
- Haemolytic uraemic syndrome

HYPERSPLENISM

- Sequestration of platelets

SYMPTOMS AND SIGNS

Drug history including over-the-counter drugs, e.g. quinine. Alcohol intake. Easy or spontaneous bruising, petechial rash, epistaxis, haematuria, mucosal bleeding. Cirrhosis/hypersplenism. History of malignancy with marrow infiltration. DIC.

Petechiae and bruising on examination. Signs of infection. Lymphadenopathy. Hepatosplenomegaly.

GENERAL INVESTIGATIONS

■ FBC
Isolated thrombocytopenia is likely to be due to increased destruction. Thrombocytopenia due to marrow failure is likely to be associated with anaemia, leucopenia.

■ Blood film
Red cell fragmentation (DIC). Platelet size (large in ITP and some hereditary conditions). WBC (atypical lymphocytes/lymphoblasts).

■ Bleeding time
Prolonged if platelet count $<80 \times 10^9$/L.

■ Coagulation screen
Clotting times normal in autoimmune thrombocytopenia but may be abnormal in other causes, e.g. DIC.

■ Platelet function test
Associated abnormal platelet function, e.g. uraemia.

■ Serology
Antinuclear antibodies (autoimmune disease). Monospot (glandular fever). Antiplatelet antibodies (unreliable). Paul–Bunnell test (glandular fever). CMV serology.

■ U&Es, creatinine
Haemolytic uraemic syndrome, thrombotic thrombocytopenic purpura.

■ LFTs
Hepatitis, e.g. due to EBV, CMV.

■ Bone marrow
Megakaryocytes increased in number and size in ITP. Absence or reduction in megakaryocytes rules out ITP. Aplastic anaemia. Leukaemia. Marrow infiltration (carcinoma, lymphoma, myeloma).

- Primary haemostasis is only impaired when platelet count falls to $<80 \times 10^9$/L.

- Spontaneous bruising, purpura and mucosal bleeding are rare until the platelets are $<20 \times 10^9$/L, unless there is also a defect in platelet function.

- Always take a careful and detailed drug history.

- In the pale patient with purpura, a serious underlying bone marrow disorder is likely.

THROMBOCYTOSIS

Thrombocytosis is a high platelet count >400/450 × 10⁹/L. It may be secondary to a myeloproliferative disorder or another pathological process.

CAUSES

ESSENTIAL (PRIMARY)

- Essential thrombocythaemia (myeloproliferative disorder)
- Alternative chronic myeloproliferative disorders, e.g. chronic myeloid leukaemia, myelofibrosis, polycythaemia rubrum vera.

REACTIVE (SECONDARY)

- Haemorrhage
- Haemolysis
- Trauma
- Surgery
- Postpartum
- Chronic inflammation, e.g. rheumatoid arthritis, inflammatory bowel disease
- Iron deficiency anaemia
- Infection
- Malignant disease
- Hyposplenism (splenectomy, splenic atrophy)

SYMPTOMS AND SIGNS

Ask about headaches, dizziness, chest pain and a burning sensation in the hands. History of trauma, blood loss, surgery, splenectomy, chronic inflammatory disease, infection and malignancy. Episodes of spontaneous arterial or venous thrombosis, e.g. stroke, DVT, venous thromboembolism. Hepatosplenomegaly on examination. Increased platelet count at routine blood test.

GENERAL INVESTIGATIONS

- **FBC**
  Platelets ↑. Hb ↓ (iron deficiency anaemia). Hb ↑ (polycythaemia rubrum vera). MCV ↓ (iron deficiency anaemia). PCV ↑ (polycythaemia rubrum vera). WBC ↑ (infection, chronic myeloid leukaemia).

- **Blood film**
  Microcytic hypochromic anaemia in iron deficiency.
  Thrombocytosis, giant platelets, platelet clumping, megakaryocyte fragments in essential thrombocythaemia.

- **ESR**
  Chronic inflammation. Malignancy including myeloma.
- **Serum iron and TIBC**
  Serum iron ↓ TIBC ↑ in iron deficiency.
- **Serum ferritin**
  Reduced in iron deficiency. Raised in acute inflammation/infection.
- **Bone marrow**
  Essential thrombocythaemia – hypercellularity, increased megakaryocytes, large megakaryocytes. Polycythaemia ruba vera – increased cellularity due to hyperplasia for erythropoietic cells, granulocytopoietic cells and megakaryocytes. Chronic myeloid leukaemia – marked hypercellularity due to myeloid hyperplasia. Myelofibrosis – 'dry tap' (aspiration unsuccessful).

- **Persistent platelet counts over 600×10^9/L warrant investigation and treatment for malignancy.**
- **In myeloproliferative disorders associated with thrombocytosis, there is not only an increased risk of thrombosis but also an increased risk of haemorrhage due to platelet dysfunction.**